PRIMARY AND SECONDARY LUNG DISEASE

Collected Reprints (1970-2015)

By

WILLIAM C. ROBERTS, MD

and

COLLEAGUES

ISBN: 979-8-88680-077-7
Printed in the United States of America on acid-free paper.

Preface

Various conditions primarily affecting the lungs have secondary effects on the heart, and various conditions primarily affecting the heart have secondary effects on the lungs. Most of the conditions listed here in the Table of Contents have primary effects on the lungs, and most were conceived by Dr. Ronald G. Crystal when he was the Chief of the Pulmonary Branch at the National Heart, Lung, and Blood Institute. One clearly cannot forget the lungs as a heart specialist or the heart as a lung specialist.

—William C. Roberts, MD

Table of Contents

*Articles are numbered based on WCR's CV.

Pulmonary Parenchymal Ossific Nodules in Idiopathic Hypertrophic Subaortic Stenosis

L. MAXIMILIAN BUJA, MD
and WILLIAM C. ROBERTS, MD, FACC
Bethesda, Maryland

Attention is called to the occurrence of pulmonary parenchymal ossific nodules in 2 siblings, both young adults, with idiopathic hypertrophic subaortic stenosis. This association has not been described previously.

Ossific nodules in the pulmonary parenchyma frequently are observed radiographically and morphologically in patients with rheumatic mitral valvular disease, especially stenosis.[1-3] Similar nodules have been observed rarely in patients with interstitial pulmonary fibrosis (Hamman-Rich syndrome)[4] and in at least 1 patient with each of the following conditions: left atrial myxoma, constrictive pericarditis, systemic hypertension, coronary arterial disease and aortic regurgitation.[5,6] This report describes pulmonary ossific nodules in 2 siblings with idiopathic hypertrophic subaortic stenosis. The association of such nodules with this entity has not been recorded previously, and we did not observe them at autopsy examination of the lungs of 7 other patients with idiopathic hypertrophic subaortic stenosis.

Case Reports

Case 1. At age 26, this man was asymptomatic when examined at the National Heart Institute, Bethesda, Md. A grade 2–3/6 systolic murmur was heard over the left sternal border and apex. Electrocardiogram showed sinus rhythm, biatrial enlargement and T wave abnormalities. Chest roentgenograms (Fig. 1) showed cardiomegaly and multiple densities throughout both lung fields. (These lesions were reported to have been observed on a chest roentgenogram taken 5 years earlier.) Repeated radiograms during the subsequent 7 years showed no increase in the number or size of the pulmonary parenchymal nodules. Results of the histoplasmin skin test were positive; those of skin tests for blastomycosis, coccidiomycosis and tuberculosis were negative. On cardiac catheterization the intravascular pressures (mm Hg) were right atrial mean 3; right ventricular 35/3; pulmonary arterial 35/24; left atrial mean 16, with *a* waves 26 and *v* waves 20; simultaneous left ventricular and brachial arterial 150/26 and 120/70, respectively, yielding a 30 mm Hg peak systolic gradient at rest which increased to 85 mm Hg with provocation (ouabain). The cardiac index was 2.1 liters/min per m^2.

At age 33 (6 months before death) exertional and nocturnal dyspnea and atrial fibrillation developed. Three weeks before death the patient was again hospitalized. The precordial systolic murmur was now only intermittently audible. Electrocardiogram showed atrial fibrillation and intraventricular conduction defect. The rhythm reverted to normal after transthoracic electrical countershock.

From the Section of Pathology, National Heart and Lung Institute, National Institutes of Health, Bethesda, Md. 20014.
Manuscript received December 30, 1968, accepted February 25, 1969.
Address for reprints: Dr. William C. Roberts, Section of Pathology, National Heart and Lung Institute, National Institutes of Health, Bethesda, Md. 20014.

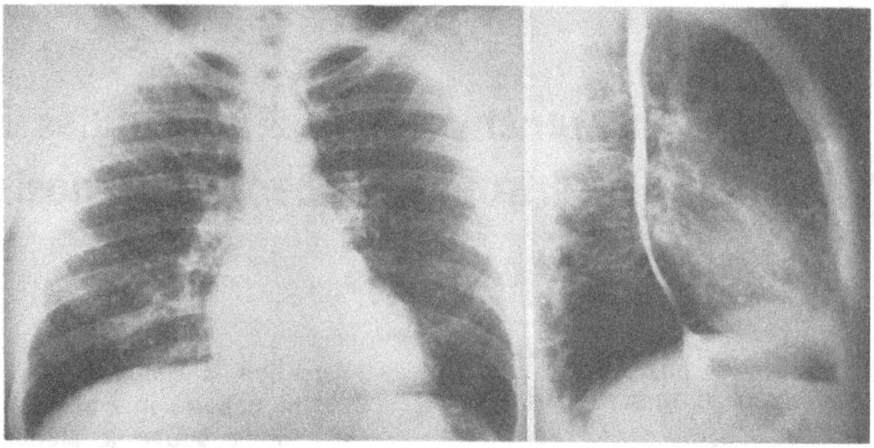

Figure 1. Case 1. Chest roentgenograms taken at age 26. Anteroposterior **(left)** and lateral **(right)** views.

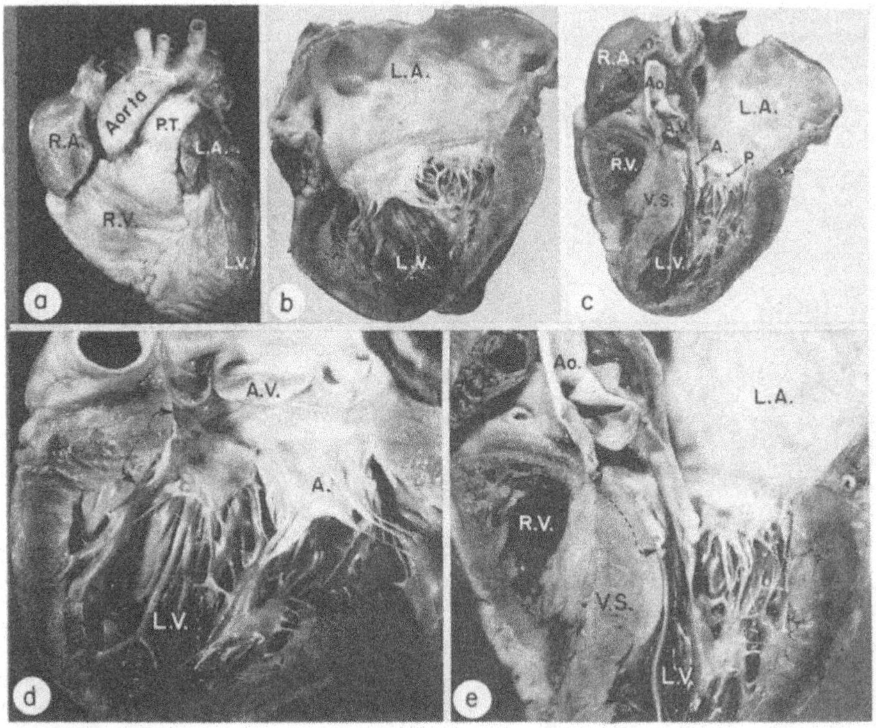

Figure 2. Case 1. Heart at autopsy. **a,** exterior view. All chambers are enlarged L.A. = left atrium; L.V. = left ventricle; P.T. = pulmonary trunk; R.A. = right atrium; R.V. = right ventricle. **b,** open left side showing dilated left atrium, focally thickened mitral leaflets and chordae and hypertrophied left ventricle. A thrombus is present at the apex of the left ventricle. **c,** coronal section. The ventricular septum (V.S.) is thicker than the free wall of the left ventricle. A close-up view of the outflow tract is shown in **e.** A. and P. = anterior and posterior mitral leaflets, respectively; Ao. = aorta. **d,** opened aorta, aortic valve (A.V.) and left ventricle. The endocardium in the outflow tract is thickened, and this thickening corresponds to similar thickening on the ventricular aspect of the anterior mitral leaflet (A.). The aortic valve is normal.

Repeat catheterization showed the pulmonary arterial pressure to be 52/25; mean pulmonary arterial wedge 22, with *a* waves 24 and *v* waves 26; and simultaneous left ventricular and brachial arterial pressures 120/26 and 120/80 mm Hg, respectively. A 33 mm Hg gradient was provoked by isoproterenol. The cardiac index was 2.0 liters/min per m^2. Six days after catheterization atrial fibrillation recurred, and 4 days later sudden unilateral hemiparesis appeared. The next day the left femoral arterial pulse was absent, and the patient died.

At necropsy the left external iliac, right internal iliac and left internal carotid arteries were completely occluded by thromboembolic material, as were several small mesenteric arteries. A thrombus (1.5 by 1.5 by 1.5 cm) was present in the apex of the left ventricle. Several renal and splenic infarcts were present.

The heart (Fig. 2) weighed 450 g. The ventricular septum was 2.7 cm thick, and the left ventricular free wall was 1.3 cm thick. An endocardial plaque was present in the left ventricular outflow tract. The mitral valve leaflets and several chordae tendineae were thickened. The left atrium was dilated, and the endocardium of its posterosuperior wall was thickened. There was narrowing of the lumens of the anterior descending (25 to 50 percent), left circumflex (50 to 75 percent) and left marginal (90 percent) coronary arteries.

The lungs together weighed 1,050 g. On postmortem radiograms and plastic (vinyl) cast preparations (Fig. 3) circumscribed nodules measuring between 0.1 to 0.6 cm were observed in all lobes. The ossific nodules (Fig. 3) consisted of mature lamellar bone with osteocytes and bone marrow but no iron or sim-

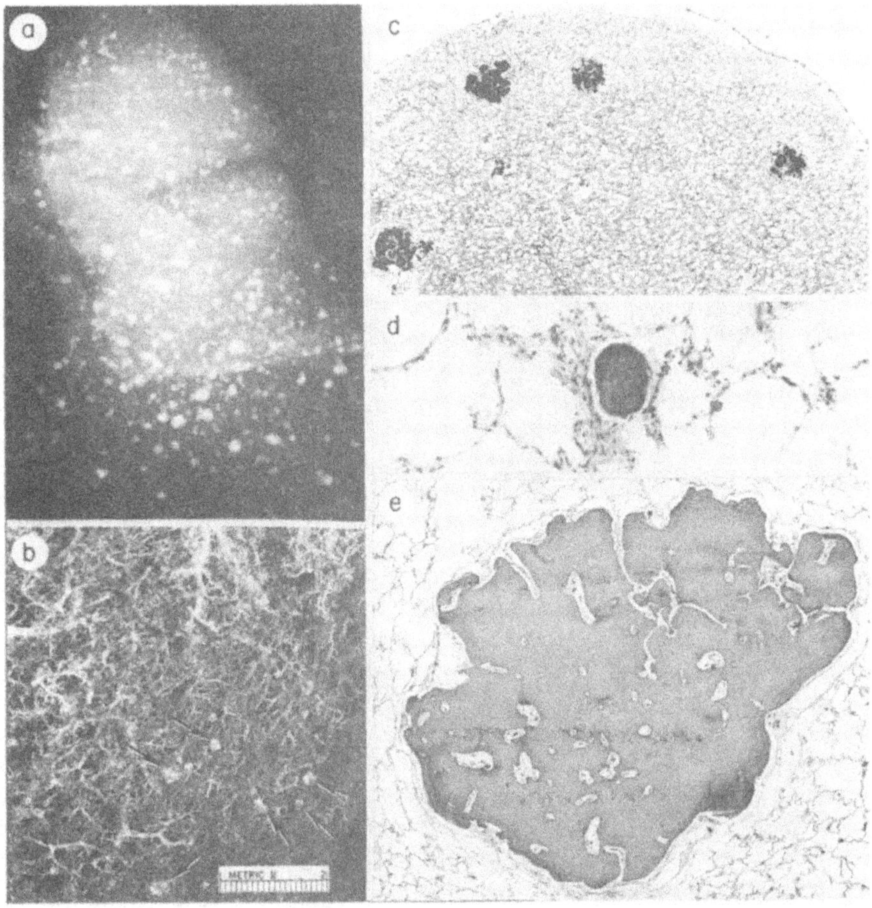

Figure 3. Case 1. Lung at autopsy. **a,** postmortem radiograph of left lung showing numerous pulmonary parenchymal ossific nodules. **b,** a plastic (vinyl) cast preparation of right lung demonstrating normal pulmonary arteries. Pulmonary ossific nodules are indicated by arrows. **c,** photomicrograph of lung showing four ossific nodules. Elastic van Gieson, × 6, reduced by 39 percent. **d,** minute ossific nodule located entirely within an alveolus. Hematoxylin and eosin stain, × 160, reduced by 39 percent. **e,** more usual-sized ossific nodule consisting of mature, lamellar bone with osteocytes in lacunae and spaces containing bone marrow. Hematoxylin and eosin, × 20, reduced by 39 percent.

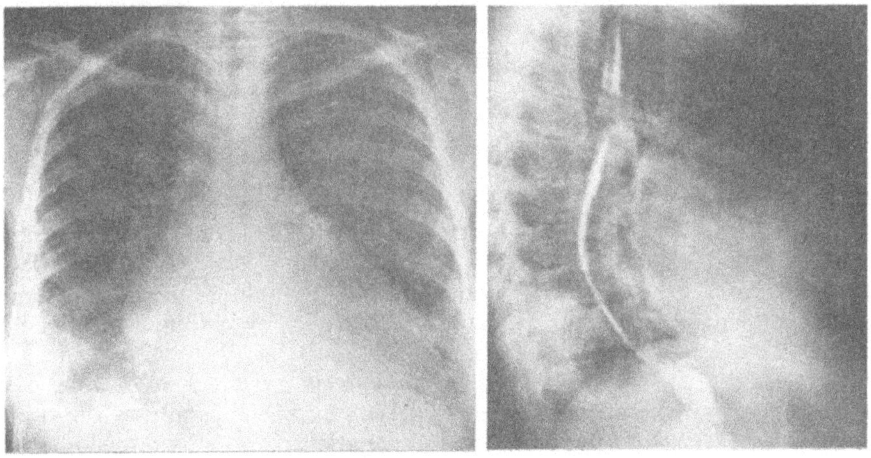

Figure 4. Case 2. Chest roentgenograms taken at age 25. Anteroposterior **(left)** and lateral **(right)** views.

ple calcium salts (Prussian blue and Von Kossa stains).* Hemosiderin-laden macrophages were present in a few alveoli. No microorganisms were seen. The capillaries were congested, and the interlobular septa were edematous. The pulmonary blood vessels were normal histologically.

Case 2. This 26 year old woman was the sister of the patient in Case 1. She had had exertional and nocturnal dyspnea and persistent dependent subcutaneous edema for 3 years before she was examined at the National Heart Institute at age 25. A grade 3/6 blowing systolic murmur was heard over the apex, left axilla and left sternal border. The feet were edematous. Electrocardiogram showed atrial fibrillation, left ventricular hypertrophy with strain, left ventricular conduction delay and an occasional premature contraction. Chest roentgenograms (Fig. **4**) showed left atrial enlargement and right pleural effusion. On cardiac catheterization the intravascular pressures (mm Hg) were right atrial mean 10; right ventricular

* The Von Kossa method stains the phosphate and carbonate ions of calcium phosphate and carbonate molecules that remain in tissue after the calcium has been removed to facilitate histologic sectioning. The method is positive only for simple molecules and is negative once the calcium phosphate and carbonate are formed into the complex crystals of mature bone. Thus, the stain is positive only in areas of recent calcific deposition or areas of bone destruction.

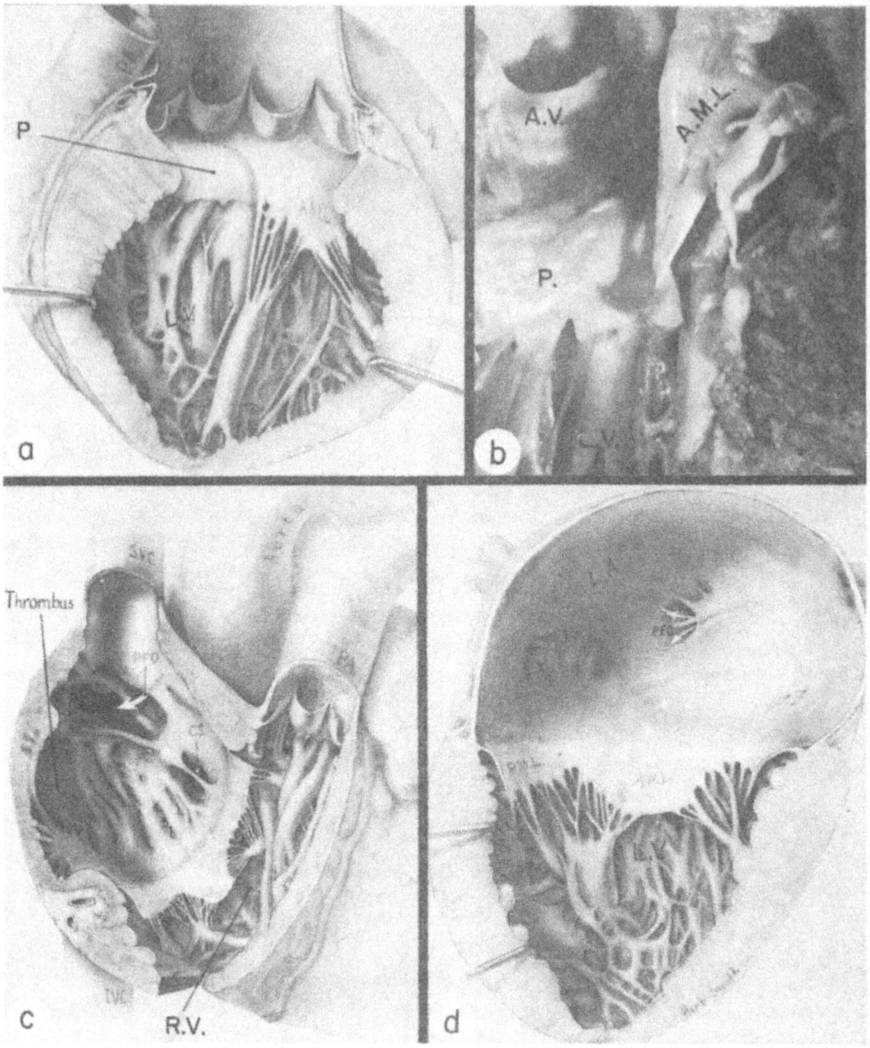

Figure 5. Case 2. Heart at autopsy. **a,** drawing of opened aorta and hypertrophied left ventricle (L.V.). A thick endocardial plaque (P) covers the left ventricular aspect of the cephalad portion of the ventricular septum which is severely hypertrophied. The anterior leaflet of the mitral valve (A.M.L.) and some of the chordae tendineae are thickened. P.A. = pulmonary trunk; L.A. = left atrium. **b,** a close-up of an actual photograph of the left ventricular outflow tract. A.V. = aortic valve. **c,** drawing of the opened right side of the heart. The right atrium is dilated and contains a thrombus. The fossa ovale region is probe-patent but valvular-competent (P.F.O.). The tricuspid valve is normal, and the right ventricular (R.V.) cavity is very small. S.V.C. = superior vena cava; C.S. = ostium of coronary sinus; I.V.C. = inferior vena cava. **d,** drawing of opened left atrium (L.A.), thickened mitral valve and left ventricle. The left atrium is dilated. P.M.L. = posterior mitral leaflet.

50/8; pulmonary arterial 40/25; left atrial mean 19—with v waves 23; left ventricular 103/2; and aortic 95/55. The cardiac index was 1.8 liters/min per m^2. Symptoms of cardiac dysfunction progressed, and she died with severe congestive heart failure 1 year later at another hospital.

At autopsy the heart weighed 350 g and was very similar to the heart of the patient's brother (Case 1). The cephalad portion of the ventricular septum was disproportionally thickened, and an endocardial plaque present in the left ventricular outflow tract corresponded to fibrous thickening of the ventricular aspect of the anterior mitral leaflet (Fig. 5). The left atrium was dilated, and the aortic valvular cusps were normal. An antemortem thrombus was present in the right atrium. The coronary arteries appeared normal.

The lungs showed changes of severe chronic pulmonary congestion and pulmonary hypertension. The alveolar septa were focally but extensively thickened; many alveoli contained hemosiderin-laden macrophages; parenchymal cholesterol granulomas were frequent;[7] acute pneumonia was present in the right lower lobe; large areas of atelectasis were present bilaterally; the visceral pleura over the lower lobes was thick; and many ossific nodules, similar to those seen in the lungs in Case 1, were found throughout the pulmonary parenchyma (Fig. 6).

The muscular pulmonary arteries and arterioles showed medial hypertrophy and intimal proliferation. A few smaller pulmonary arteries contained organized thromboemboli. The lumens of the pulmonary veins also were severely narrowed by fibrous intimal tissue.

Discussion

Differential diagnosis: The pulmonary parenchymal nodules observed in these 2 cases were similar radiographically and morphologically to those seen in patients with rheumatic mitral valvular disease.[1–3] Such nodules consist of mature lamellar bone. They measure 0.1 to 1.0 cm in diameter and are located within the pulmonary parenchyma, often purely intra-alveolar. They may be present in any lobe, most frequently the lower lobes, and they may contain

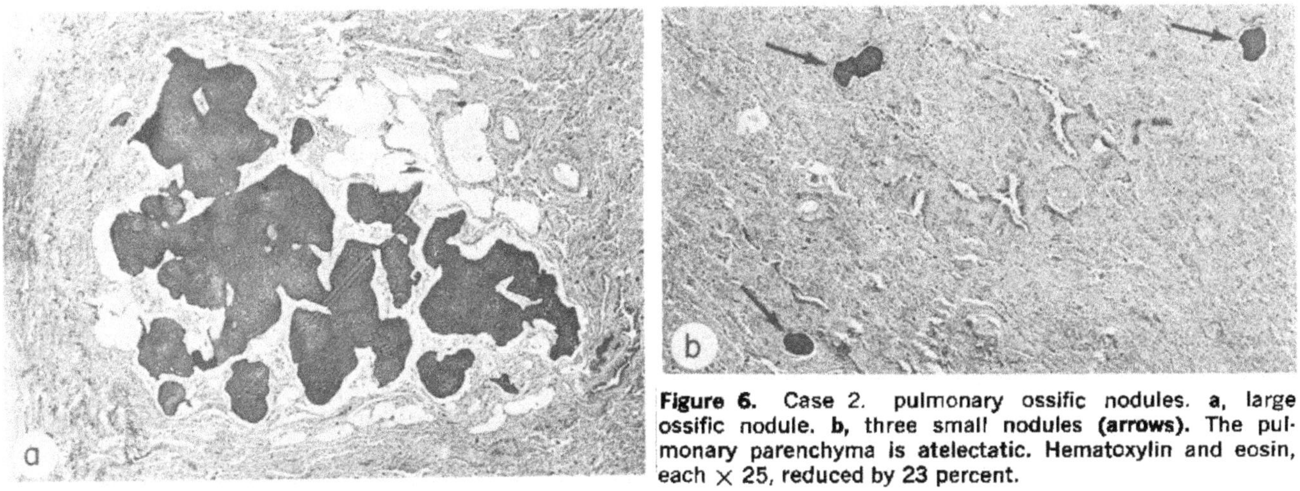

Figure 6. Case 2. pulmonary ossific nodules. **a**, large ossific nodule. **b**, three small nodules (arrows). The pulmonary parenchyma is atelectatic. Hematoxylin and eosin, each × 25, reduced by 23 percent.

bone marrow or iron or calcium salts. They are free of microorganisms. The ossific nodules are distinctly different morphologically from pulmonary alveolar microliths,[8] pulmonary corpora amylacea[9] and branching interstitial pulmonary bone occasionally observed in older patients.[1] Pulmonary ossific nodules, corpora amylacea and alveolar microliths have not been reported to occur together in the same patient. Pulmonary alveolar microlithiasis presents a distinctive roentgenographic appearance similar to that produced by acute pulmonary edema. However, the patients with pulmonary microliths are asymptomatic at least initially despite the striking radiographic appearance. Later in these subjects chronic cor pulmonale may develop. Interestingly, pulmonary alveolar microlithiasis is familial.[8] Pulmonary ossific nodules as occurred in each of our 2 cases have not been reported previously in more than 1 member of a single family. Pulmonary corpora amylacea are not visible radiographically, and there is no evidence that they produce pulmonary dysfunction.

The nodules observed on chest roentgenograms of patients with healed histoplasmosis, miliary tuberculosis, chickenpox or some pneumoconioses may simulate the radiographic appearance of pulmonary parenchymal ossific nodules. The nodules in the lungs of Patient 1 were diagnosed radiographically during life as healed histoplasmosis.

Mechanism of formation of pulmonary parenchymal ossific nodules: The mechanism of formation is speculative. The only finding that appears to be common to patients with these nodules is pulmonary venous hypertension, but the exact relation of the increased pressure to the ossific nodules is unknown.[2,3,5] Pulmonary nodules have been observed in patients with[3,5] and without[2] overt congestive cardiac failure. Organization of pulmonary edema fluid to form osteoid and finally bone has been suggested as a possible mechanism of formation of the pulmonary parenchymal ossific nodules.[2,3,5] Development of the ossific nodules by transformation of intraalveolar hemosiderin deposits also has been suggested[10] but seems unlikely. Ossific nodules may be observed in portions of lung entirely free from hemosiderin deposits, and ossific nodules have not been described in subjects with idiopathic pulmonary hemosiderosis, a condition that produces the largest deposition of iron in the alveolar spaces.[11] The ossific nodules were not observed at various stages of formation in either of our 2 patients. Indeed, whether the nodules were large or small, their morphologic features were similar. This fact suggests that all of the ossific nodules in an individual patient formed at the same time. Ossific nodules have been observed experimentally in rabbits given irradiation to the lungs 1 to 2 months before sacrifice.[12]

Relation of ossific nodules to degree of cardiac dysfunction: Although pulmonary venous hypertension occurred in our 2 cases, neither the number nor the size of the pulmonary ossific nodules was proportional to the degree of rise in pulmonary venous pressure. Patient 2 had severe cardiac failure for several years with extensive pulmonary parenchymal and vascular changes of chronic congestion. In contrast, Patient 1 was asymptomatic until 6 months before death, and his lungs were virtually normal except for the presence of numerous ossific nodules. Although Patient 2 had far more evidence of chronic pulmonary congestion than did Patient 1, she had far fewer ossific nodules. However, at autopsy the hearts of both patients were strikingly similar although the degree of cardiac dysfunction was quite different.

Acknowledgment

We thank Doctors Eugene Braunwald and Stephen E. Epstein for use of the clinical information in the 2 cases described.

References

1. **Wells HG, Dunlap CE:** Disseminated ossification of the lungs. Arch Path (Chicago) 35:420–426, 1943
2. **Fleming HA, Robinson CLN:** Pulmonary ossification with cardiac calcification in mitral valve disease. Brit Heart J 19:532–538, 1957
3. **Galloway RW, Epstein EJ, Coulshed N:** Pulmonary ossific nodules in mitral valve disease. Brit Heart J 23:297–307, 1961
4. **Ventura JC:** Disseminated nodular pulmonary ossification with Hamman-Rich syndrome. J Lancet 86:60–63, 1966
5. **Epstein EJ, Chapman R, Coulshed N, et al:** Pulmonary ossific nodule formation in the absence of mitral valve disease. A report of four cases. Amer Heart J 65:816–825, 1963
6. **Hudson REB:** Cardiovascular Pathology, Vol. I. Baltimore, Williams & Wilkins, 1961, p 1015
7. **Glancy DL, Frazier PD, Roberts WC:** Pulmonary parenchymal cholesterol-ester granulomas in patients with pulmonary hypertension. Amer J Med 45:198–210, 1968
8. **Sosman MC, Dodd GD, Jones WD, et al:** The familial occurrence of pulmonary alveolar microlithiasis. Amer J Roentgen 77:947–1012, 1957
9. **Michaels L, Levine C:** Pulmonary corpora amylacea. J Path Bact 74:49–56, 1957
10. **Ellman P, Gee A:** Pulmonary hemosiderosis. Brit Med J 2:384–390, 1951
11. **Soergel KH, Sommers SC:** Idiopathic pulmonary hemosiderosis and related syndromes Amer J Med 32:499–511, 1962
12. **Engelstad RB:** Über die Wirkungen der Röntgenstrahlen auf die Lungen. Acta Radiol (Stockholm) 15: Suppl 19:1–93, 1934

Pulmonary Alveolar Hemorrhage

A Common Finding in Patients with Severe Cardiac Disease

L. MAXIMILIAN BUJA, MD
THOMAS A. FREED, MD
MICHAEL A. BERMAN, MD
ANDREW G. MORROW, MD, FACC
WILLIAM C. ROBERTS, MD, FACC

Bethesda, Maryland

In 89 (63 percent) of 141 autopsy cases of congenital (shunts) or acquired (valvular) cardiac disease, the patients had alveolar hemorrhage; 19 (13 percent) had pneumonia, and 9 (6 percent) had pulmonary emboli or infarcts. Alveolar hemorrhage was visible both grossly and histologically in 66 patients and on histologic examination only in 23 patients. Of the 113 patients without pulmonary emboli, pulmonary infarcts or pneumonia, alveolar hemorrhage occurred in 70 of 81 patients (86 percent) who died within 45 days after cardiac operations, and in 19 of 32 patients (50 percent) who died after recovery from operation or who had never been operated upon. Radiographic evidence of alveolar hemorrhage was present in 36 of 55 patients (65 percent) examined.

A number of factors may be involved in the production of alveolar hemorrhage. The lesion may occur secondary to severe left-sided cardiac failure, but it may also be caused by shock, hypoxia and factors related to use of cardiopulmonary bypass or mechanical respirators.

Pulmonary parenchymal infiltrates are frequently observed in chest roentgenograms of patients with symptoms of severe cardiac dysfunction and in the early postoperative period after cardiac operations. Most often the radiodense lesions are attributed to acute pulmonary edema, acute pneumonia or pulmonary infarction. Another frequent but less commonly recognized pulmonary parenchymal infiltrate in severely ill cardiac patients and in patients who have undergone cardiac operations is extensive alveolar hemorrhage. To determine the incidence and significance of alveolar hemorrhage, the lungs of 141 patients who died with cardiac shunts or cardiac valvular lesions were examined. This report provides a summary of the anatomic and roentgenographic observations in these cases.

Patients Studied

An average of 6 histologic sections of lung were examined in each of 91 patients with congenital cardiac disease with shunts and in each of 50 patients with functionally severe (classes III and IV, New York Heart Association) valvular cardiac disease who underwent necropsy. Of the 91 patients with shunts, 21 had ventricular septal defect; 11, atrial septal defect; 3, patent ductus arteriosus; 9, a combination of these lesions; and 47, Fallot's tetrad. At cardiac catheterization, 34 of the 91 patients had left to right shunts with pulmonary arterial systolic pressures ranging from 15 to 130 mm Hg (average 60); 18 had mixed shunts with pulmonary arterial systolic pressures ranging from 18 to 138 mm Hg (average 81); and 39 patients had right to left shunts, with

From the Section of Pathology, Cardiology Branch and Clinic of Surgery, National Heart and Lung Institute, and the Department of Radiology, Clinical Center, National Institutes of Health, Bethesda, Md. 20014. Manuscript received December 29, 1969, accepted February 20, 1970.
Address for reprints: William C. Roberts, MD, Section of Pathology, National Heart and Lung Institute, National Institutes of Health, Bethesda, Md. 20014.

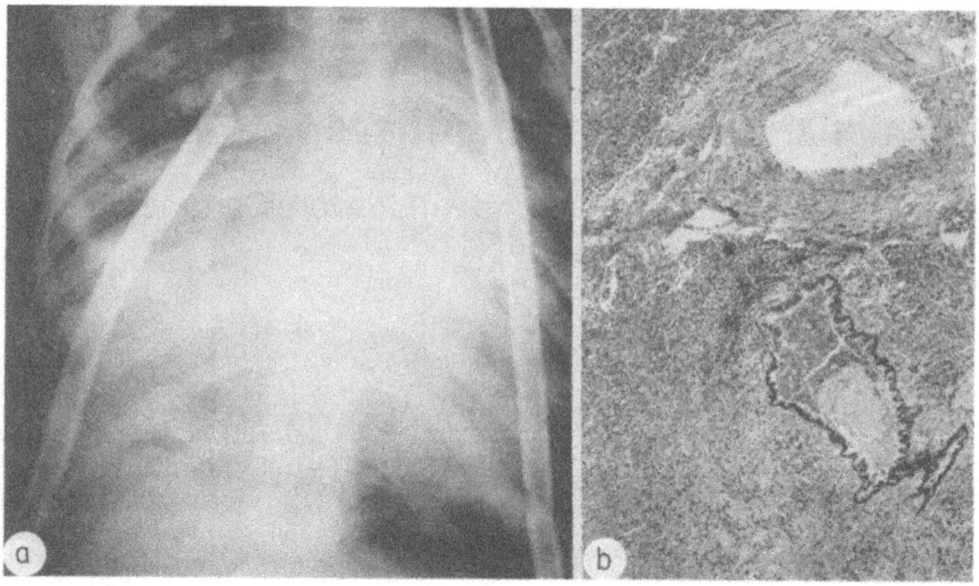

Figure 1. Chest roentgenogram **(a)** and photomicrograph of section of lung **(b)** of an 8 year old boy in whom a ventricular septal defect, complicated by pulmonary arterial hypertension, had been closed 36 hours before death. In the immediate postoperative period he had hypotension because of excessive bleeding, and extensive pulmonary infiltrates developed **(a)**. Dyspnea and tachycardia subsequently occurred and finally cardiac arrest. At autopsy, the alveoli and many bronchi were filled with blood **(b)**. Hematoxylin and eosin × 52, reduced by 31 percent.

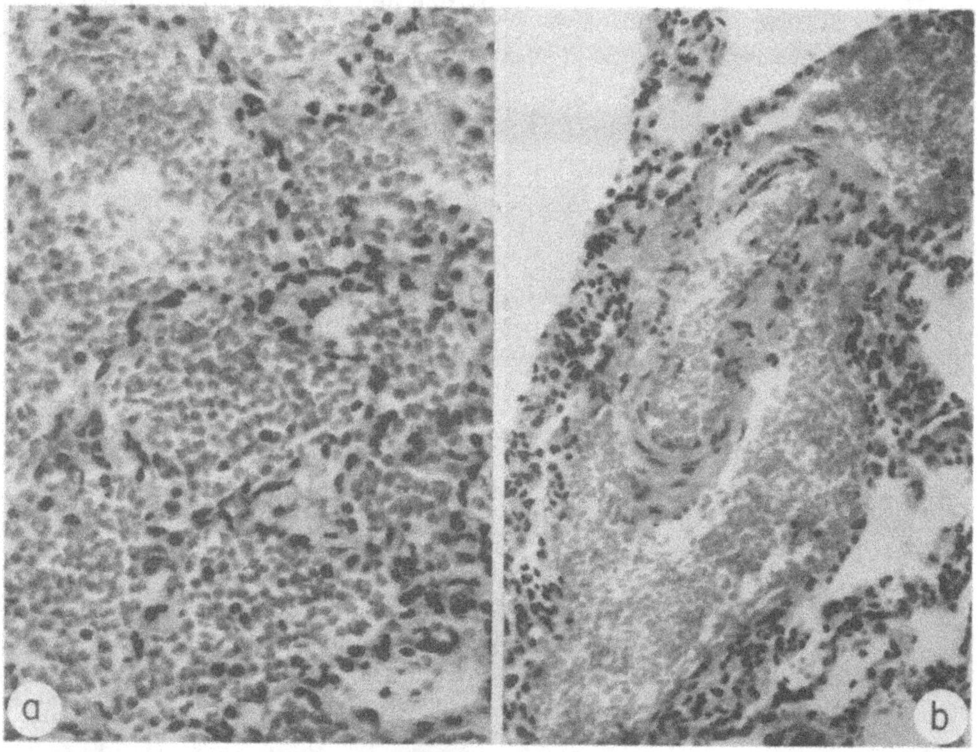

Figure 2. Photomicrographs of sections of lung of a 7 year old girl with a ventricular septal defect. Residual shunt, aortic regurgitation and congestive cardiac failure occurred after attempted closure of the ventricular septal defect 7 months before death. She had severely increased left atrial pressure after closure of the ventricular septal defect and died during attempted closure of the defect at a second operation. At autopsy, numerous alveoli were filled with blood **(a)** which also surrounded many muscular pulmonary arteries **(b)**. Hematoxylin and eosin × 400 **(a)** and × 250 **(b)**, reduced by 14 percent.

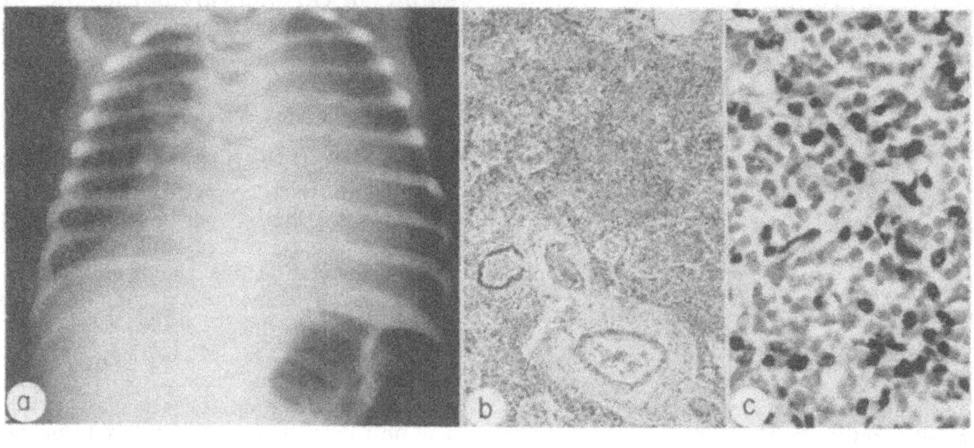

Figure 3. Chest roentgenogram and sections of lung of an 8 day old infant with complete isthmic aortic interruption, patent ductus arteriosus and ventricular septal defect. The child had never undergone operation. She had progressive congestive cardiac failure and extensive pulmonary infiltrates **(a)** due to alveolar hemorrhage **(b** and **c)**. Hematoxylin and eosin × 63 **(b)** and × 628 **(c)**, reduced by 36 percent.

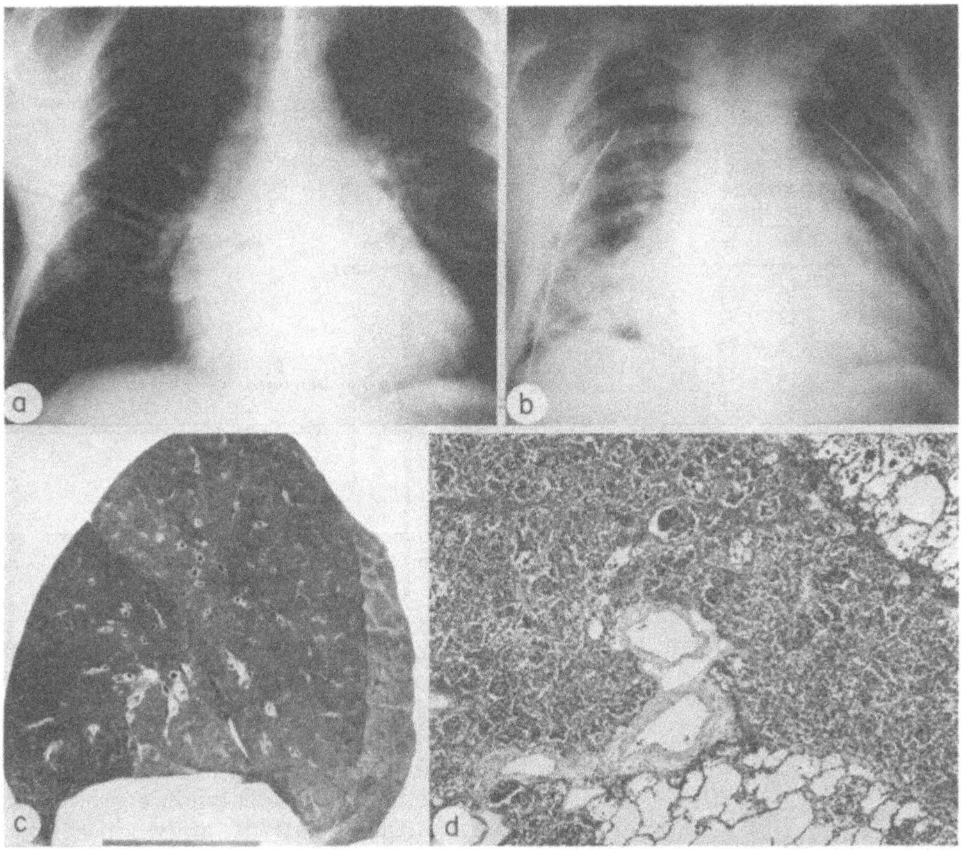

Figure 4. Pre- *(a)* and post-operative *(b)* roentgenograms, right lung **(c)**, and histologic section of a lung *(d)* of a 46 year old man whose mitral valve was replaced 6 days before death because of severe regurgitation. Postoperatively, he had increased left atrial pressure (*v* wave to 50 mm Hg), respiratory insufficiency, pulmonary infiltrates **(b)** and hemoptysis. He died in the operating room during attempted repair of a peribasilar leak. At autopsy, the right lower pulmonary lobe **(c)** was consolidated and similar foci were present in other lobes of both lungs, secondary to alveolar hemorrhage **(d)**. Hematoxylin and eosin × 40, reduced by 13 percent.

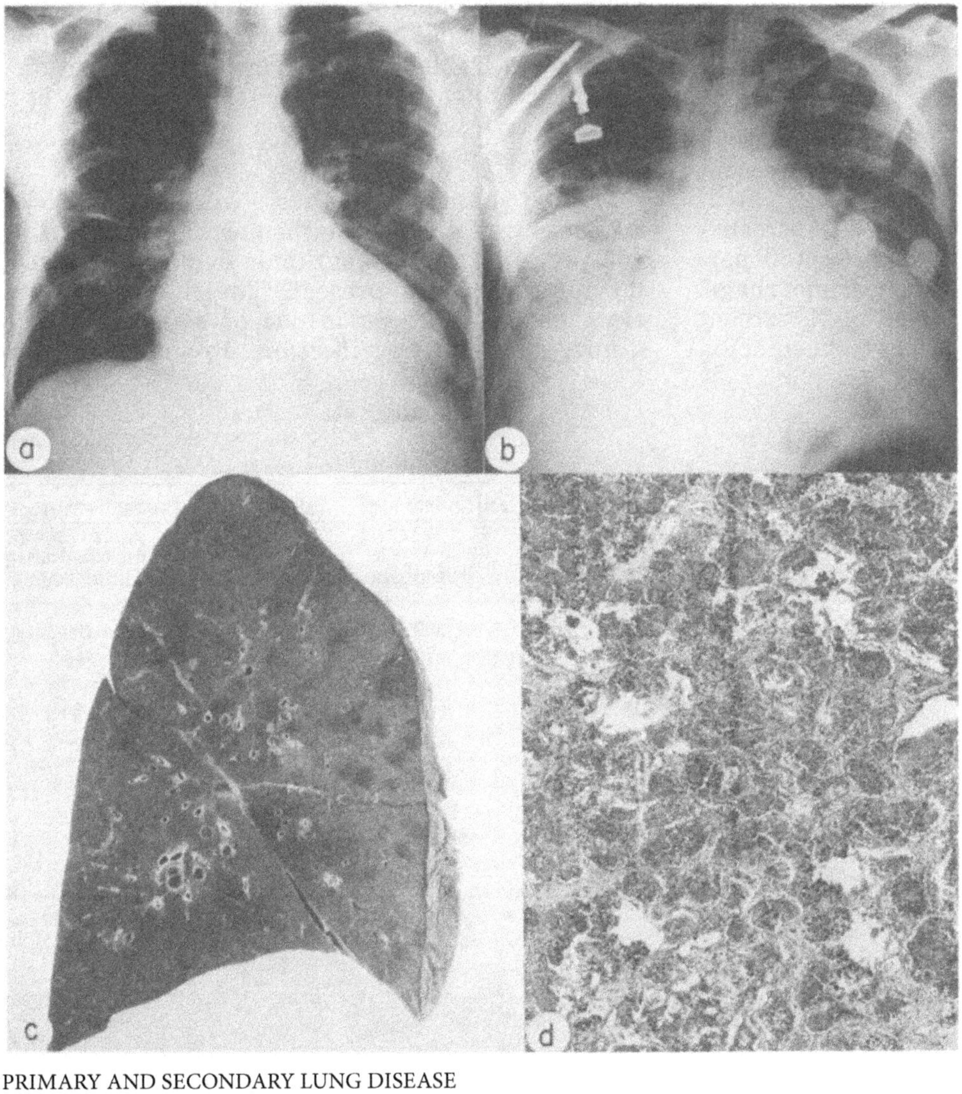

Figure 5. Chest roentgenograms **(a and b)**, cut section of right lung **(c)** and histologic section of lung **(d)** of 54 year old man with mitral and aortic stenosis and regurgitation in functional class IV. He never underwent operation. Roentgenogram **(a)** was taken 14 days before death. Dyspnea, hemoptysis and severe hypotension developed 3 days before death. Radiograph taken 2 days later showed bilateral pulmonary infiltrates **(b)**, the result of alveolar hemorrhage **(c and d)**. No pulmonary emboli were found, and the alveolar septa showed no evidence of ischemic damage. Several bronchi are plugged by hemorrhagic material. Hematoxylin and eosin × 40 **(d)**, reduced by 30 percent.

TABLE I
Associated Necropsy Pulmonary Findings in 113 Patients with Severe Cardiac Disease

	89 Patients With Alveolar Hemorrhage		24 Patients Without Alveolar Hemorrhage	
	no.	%	no.	%
Alveolar capillary congestion	89	100	14	58
Dilated pulmonary lymphatics	74	83	10	42
Interlobular septal edema	64	72	9	38
Alveolar edema fluid	54	61	4	17
Intrabronchial hemorrhage	52	59	0	0
Focal atelectasis and alveolar hemorrhage	44	49	0	0
Pulmonary arterial adventitial hemorrhage	31	35	0	0
Interlobular septal hemorrhage	26	29	0	0
Hyaline membranes	2	2	0	0

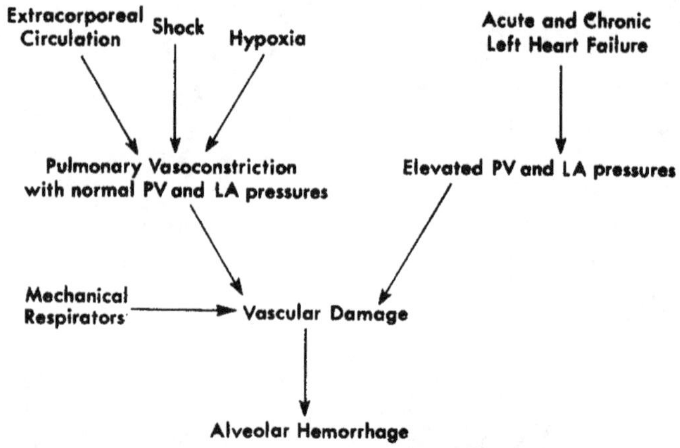

Figure 6. Etiologic factors and possible mechanisms responsible for alveolar hemorrhage. LA = left atrial; PV = pulmonary venous.

normal or low pulmonary arterial systolic pressures in 38 patients and severe pulmonary hypertension in 1 patient.

Of the 50 patients with valvular cardiac disease without shunts, 25 had mitral stenosis with or without regurgitation; 14, mitral and aortic stenosis with or without regurgitation; 1, pure mitral regurgitation; 2, mitral and aortic regurgitation; 7, aortic stenosis; and 1, pure aortic regurgitation. Pulmonary arterial systolic pressures ranged from 30 to 95 mm Hg (average 52).

Results

Necropsy Findings

Nine (6 percent) of the 141 patients had recent pulmonary emboli or infarcts, and each had valvular cardiac disease without shunts; 19 (13 percent) had extensive acute pneumonia, and 89 (63 percent) had focal pulmonary alveolar hemorrhage. Thus, alveolar hemorrhage occurred in 79 percent of the 113 patients without significant pneumonia or recent pulmonary emboli or infarcts. Microscopic-sized foci of acute pneumonia were present in 12 patients with alveolar hemorrhage, but in each the inflammatory infiltrate was small compared to the number of alveoli filled with erythrocytes. Alveolar hemorrhage was visible grossly in 66 (74 percent) of the 89 patients and on histologic sections only in 23 patients (26 percent). Other pulmonary lesions observed in the 113 patients with and without alveolar hemorrhage are summarized in Table I. Typical necropsy and radiographic findings are illustrated in Figures 1 to 5.

Roentgenographic Findings

Chest roentgenograms were examined in 55 of 89 patients with alveolar hemorrhage, and in 36 (65 percent) roentgenographic evidence of alveolar infiltrates was present. The findings varied from patchy mottling in one or several lobes to diffuse bilateral opacification. Progression from

TABLE II
Clinical Findings in the 113 Patients Studied

Finding	Total Group of Patients		Patients With Alveolar Hemorrhage			Patients Without Alveolar Hemorrhage		
	no.	%	no.	% of Total Group	% of 89 Patients With Alveolar Hemorrhage	no.	% of Total Group	% of 24 Patients Without Alveolar Hemorrhage
Presence or absence of operation	113	100	89	79	100	24	21	100
Death <45 days after operation	81	72	70	86*	79*	11	14	46
No operation, or death > 45 days after operation	32	28	19	59	21	13	41	54
Shock	62	55	56	90*	63*	6	10	25
Mechanical respirator	33	29	32	97*	36*	1	3	4
Acute left-sided cardiac failure	24	21	18	75*	20	6	25	25
Sudden death (arrhythmia)	24	21	12	50	13	12	50	50*
Generalized bleeding	10	9	6	60	7	4	40	17
Anticoagulant therapy	3	3	3	100	3	0	0	0

* $P < 0.05$.

scattered perivascular infiltrates to diffuse opacification of one or several lobes occurred in several patients. Air bronchograms frequently were identified. Diffuse pulmonary parenchymal changes often were present without enlargement of pulmonary veins, the "butterfly" distribution of acute pulmonary edema or other signs of left-sided congestive cardiac failure. Mediastinal shift and other signs of obstructive atelectasis were absent.

Clinical Findings

The clinical findings in the 113 patients without pulmonary emboli, pulmonary infarcts or significant pneumonia are summarized in Table II. Of the 81 patients who died within 45 days after operation, extracorporeal circulation was utilized in 66, and 58 (87 percent) had alveolar hemorrhage. Of the 15 in whom extracorporeal circulation was not utilized, 12 (80 percent) had alveolar hemorrhage. The difference was not significant. Likewise, no significant difference was found when the analysis was limited to the 57 patients who died within 2 days of operation. In addition, the presence or absence of alveolar hemorrhage did not correlate with the type of underlying cardiac disease, direction of shunt or severity of preoperative pulmonary hypertension.

Comments

This study has shown that pulmonary alveolar hemorrhage is a common lesion in patients with severe cardiac disease. It occurred in 89 (63 percent) of 141 patients with acquired or congenital cardiac disease. In the same group of patients acute pneumonia was found in only 19 (13 percent) and recent pulmonary emboli or infarcts in 9 (6 percent).

The cause of alveolar hemorrhage varies (Fig. 6). Shock, hypoxia and use of mechanical respirators and extracorporeal circulation have all been shown to be associated with alveolar hemorrhage.[1-8] These factors are believed to produce alveolar hemorrhage by direct effects on the lungs.[2,9-11] Left-sided congestive cardiac failure, either acute or chronic, also has been demonstrated to cause alveolar hemorrhage.[12,13] All of these factors, singly or in combination, occurred in the patients we studied, but delineation of a common clinical denominator was not possible. However, we suspect that alveolar hemorrhage, when unassociated with severely increased pulmonary venous pressure or with respirators, is simply the anatomic indicator of inadequate arterial perfusion of the lung (alveolar capillaries and septae).

References

1. **Moon VH:** Shock and Related Capillary Phenomena. London, Oxford University Press, 1938, p 209
2. **Hardaway RM, James PM, Anderson RW, et al:** Intensive study and treatment of shock in man. JAMA 199: 779–790, 1967
3. **Rigby RA, Christy JH:** Recovery following prolonged gram-negative shock and "shock lung" Amer J Med 45: 959–966, 1968
4. **Fishman AP, Fritts HW, Cournand A:** Effects of acute hypoxia and exercise on the pulmonary circulation. Circulation 22:204–215, 1960
5. **Penaloza D, Sime F:** Circulatory dynamics during high altitude pulmonary edema. Amer J Cardiol 23:369–378, 1969
6. **Nash G, Blennerhassett JB, Pontoppidan H:** Pulmonary lesions associated with oxygen therapy and artificial ventilation. New Eng J Med 276:368–374, 1967
7. **Kirklin JW:** Pulmonary dysfunction after open-heart surgery. Med Clin N Amer 48:1063–1068, 1964
8. **Tiley NL, Hester WJ:** Physiologic and histologic changes in the lungs of patients dying after prolonged cardiopulmonary bypass: an inquiry into the nature of post-perfusion lung. Ann Surg 166:759–765, 1967
9. **Lee WH Jr, Krumhaar D, Fonkalerud EW, et al:** Denaturation of plasma proteins as a cause of morbidity and death after intracardiac operations. Surgery 50:29–39, 1961
10. **Subhnandan R, Thal AP:** The effect of endotoxin and vasoactive agents on dibenzylene pretreated lungs. Surgery 58:185–195, 1965
11. **Veith FJ, Hagstrom JWC, Panossian A, et al:** Pulmonary microcirculatory response to shock, transfusion, and pump-oxygenator procedures: a unified mechanism underlying pulmonary damage. Surgery 64:95–109, 1968
12. **Oppenheimer BS, Schwartz SP:** Paroxysmal pulmonary hemorrhages. Amer Heart J 9:14–25, 1933
13. **Friedberg CK:** Diseases of the Heart. Philadelphia, W. B. Saunders, 1966, p 1042

Diffuse Fibrotic Lung Disease: A Correlative Study

Jack D. Fulmer, M.D.; William C. Roberts, M.D.;** and Ronald G. Crystal, M.D.**

Diffuse fibrotic lung disease is a complex, clinically protean disorder which we view through a number of separate monitors: morphologic, physiologic, and biochemical. Our laboratory has undertaken a large scale, multidisciplinary study of the etiology, pathogenesis, pathophysiology, and therapy of this disorder (Fig 1). This paper will present correlative clinical, physiologic, and pathologic data in a selected group of patients with diffuse fibrotic lung disease. Biochemical approaches to this disorder are described elsewhere in this volume.[1]

Material and Methods

Twenty patients (ten men, ten women, mean age 50 years) have been evaluated. Thirteen patients had open lung biopsy either prior to or during their evaluation at NIH. All patients presented initially with dyspnea, and all had a radiographic pattern of diffuse infiltrative process. Seventeen patients had idiopathic fibrotic lung disease; the remainder had fibrotic lung disease associated with collagen-vascular disease. Vital capacity (VC) and total lung capacity (TLC) are widely distributed with a range between 28 and 84 percent predicted for VC and 44 to 86 percent predicted for TLC (Fig 2). Most patients have reduced VC and TLC, but an occasional patient with histologic evidence of fibrotic disease will have a normal VC and/or TLC. The diffusing capacity ($D_{L_{CO}}$) was consistently reduced in all patients (range 14 to 70 percent predicted). The ratio of forced expiratory volume in one second (FEV_1) to forced vital capacity was normal in all but one patient in whom there was a borderline reduction. Residual volume to total lung capacity ratio ranged from 20 percent to 52 percent (Fig 2). Analysis of the static volume-pressure relationships demonstrates that compliance is reduced in the majority of the patients (Fig 3).

Maximum expiratory flow volume curves, dynamic compliance, maximum flow-static recoil curves, upstream resistance and single breath oxygen test (ΔN_2 750-1250) were performed in all patients as monitors of airway time constants and mechanics. Independently, and in a single blind fashion, one of us (WCR) reviewed the histopathology and graded the small airways as to whether they were normal or exhibited varying degrees of obstruction from either bronchioli-

Section on Pulmonary Biochemistry* and Section on Pathology,** National Heart and Lung Institute, National Institutes of Health, Bethesda.

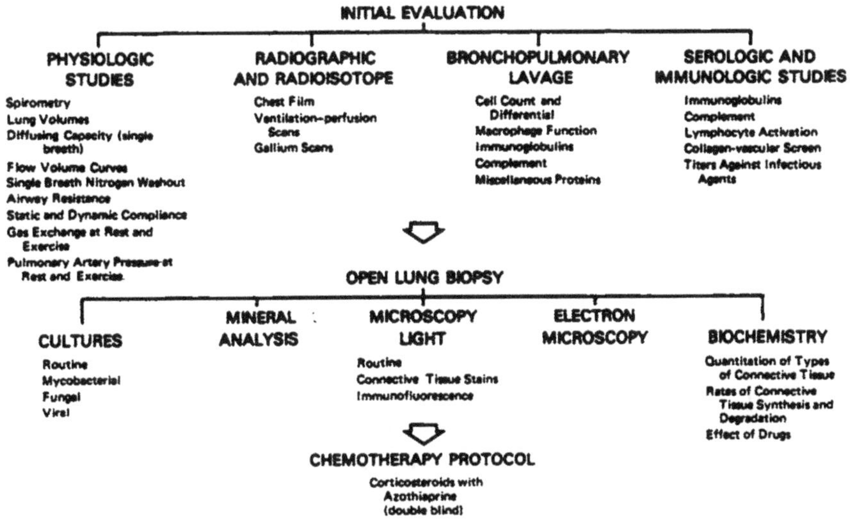

FIGURE 1. Protocol for the National Heart and Lung Institute, Intramural Division, Section on Pulmonary Biochemistry, Pulmonary Branch fibrotic disease study.

tis of peribronchial fibrosis and narrowing. A significant percentage of these physiologic and morphologic parameters were abnormal in these patients (Table 1). These data suggest agreement between the physiologic and morphologic data, and thus indicate that obstructive disease of airways is a feature of this disorder.

The volume-pressure data in these patients were analyzed using the peak transpulmonary pressure, slope of the volume-pressure curve and its position along the pressure axis. These parameters were compared to the severity of fibrosis (graded by WCR) on the open lung biopsy specimen. There was

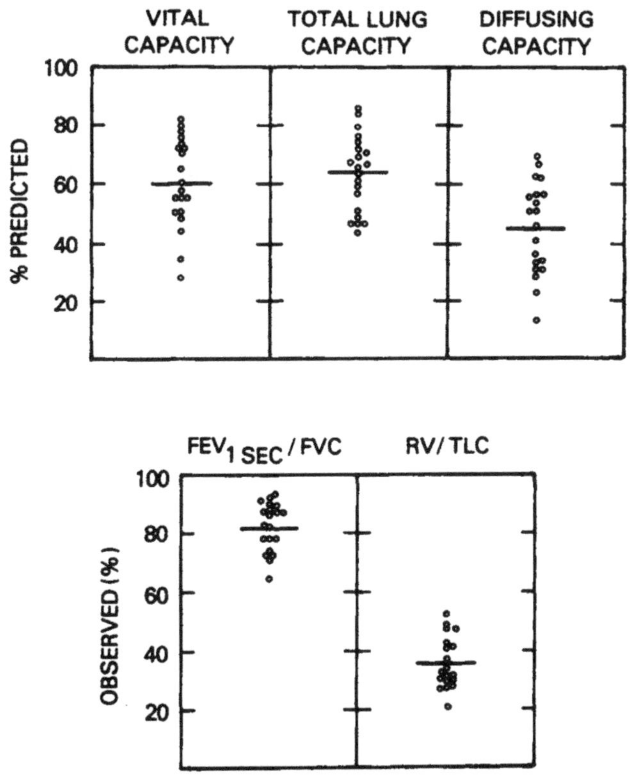

FIGURE 2. Lung volumes, simple mechanics and diffusing capacity in patients with pulmonary fibrosis of unknown etiology. Vital capacity, total lung capacity and diffusing capacity are expressed as percent predicted. Forced expiratory volume (1 sec)/forced vital capacity (FEV_1/FVC) and residual volume/total lung capacity (RV/TLC) are expressed as percentage of observed. Patients are represented by open circles.

correlation between peak transpulmonary pressure and severity of fibrosis, but there was no correlation between slope or position of the pressure-volume curve with severity of fibrosis nor was there correlation between maximum transpulmonary pressure, slope or position of the pressure-volume curve with degree of interstitial cellularity, alveolar cellularity or obstruction of airways. These data suggest that the relationship between factors associated with lung distensibility and factors which govern pressure-volume characteristics in patients are complex and likely interdependently related to chest wall strength, airways disease, location and amount of fibrosis, and amount of lung destruction.

Complete gas exchange studies were performed in 17 patients. All exhibited progressive arterial hypoxemia (PaO_2, range 38-60 mm Hg) and widening of the alveolar-arterial oxygen gradient (range 40-100 mm Hg) with graded exercise. There was no apparent correlation with severity of disease on biopsy with response to exercise. Five patients have been followed for up to nine months with serial lung volumes, diffusing capacity, and gas exchange studies. All five patients have subjectively worsened with no change in lung volumes, diffusing capacity or resting PaO_2. Preliminary longitudinal data suggest that quantitation of the rate of change of PaO_2 with oxygen consumption is a sensitive correlate with severity of breathlessness even in situations where TLC, $D_{L_{CO}}$ and resting PaO_2 remain stable.

RESULTS

The diagnostic usefulness of the change in dead-space to tidal volume ratio (V_D/V_T) with exercise has been debated.[2,3] Eighty percent of patients studied exhibited an abnormal response in V_D/V_T with exercise. Correla-

Table 1—*Comparison between Physiologic Monitors of Airway Mechanics and Histopathologic Evidence of Airway Obstruction*

Physiologic Parameter	% Abnormal	Comparison with Pathology
Maximum expiratory flow volume curve	45	good
Dynamic compliance	59	good
Upstream resistance	32	poor
Single breath oxygen test	80	good

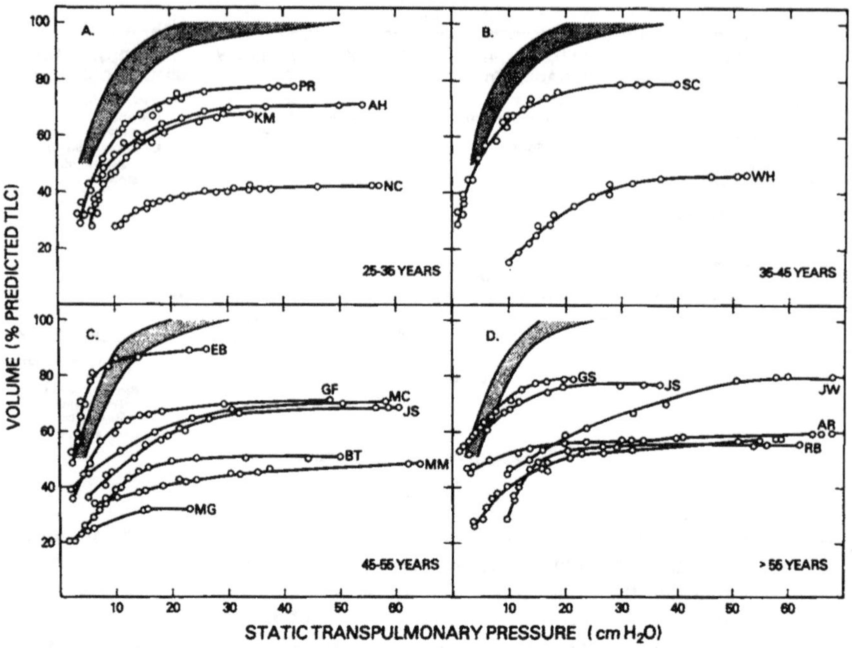

FIGURE 3. Static volume-pressure curves in patients with pulmonary fibrosis of unknown etiology. (A) Patients 25-35 years old; (B) 35-45 years old; (C) 45-55 years old; and (D) >55 years old. Lung volumes are presented as percent predicted total lung capacity (TLC). The shaded areas are normals matched for age.

tion of these data with evidence of pulmonary vascular disease on open lung biopsy was poor while correlation with evidence of obstruction of airways was good. These data suggest that distribution of ventilation is an important determinant in the V_D/V_T and emphasize the possible error in this test in diagnosis of pulmonary vascular disease.

In summary, correlative physiologic, pathogenic and clinical data are presented which suggest the following: 1) obstructive disease of airways with increased resistance to air flow is present in a significant percentage of patients with diffuse fibrotic lung disease; 2) although the peak transpulmonary pressure correlated with the degree of fibrosis, the lack of correlation of other parameters of the volume-pressure curve with the histopathology casts doubt on the usefulness of the volume-pressure relationships as a long-term monitor of diffuse fibrotic disease; 3) exercise physiologic testing with quantitation of the rate of change in PaO_2 with oxygen consumption appears to be the most sensitive correlate to clinical severity of disease; 4) the dead space-to-tidal volume ratio during exercise correlates poorly with evidence of pulmonary vascular disease, but appears to correlate well with evidence of obstruction of airways. The value of this test in the diagnosis of pulmonary vascular disease must be interpreted in light of co-existing abnormalities of distribution of ventilation.

REFERENCES

1 Hance AJ, Horwitz AL, Cowan MJ, et al: Biochemical approaches to the investigation of fibrotic lung disease. Chest 69:257-261, 1976

2 Nadel JA, Gold WM, Burgess JH: Early diagnosis of chronic pulmonary vascular obstruction. Am J Med 44:16-25, 1968

3 Williams HM, Adler JJ, Colp C: Pulmonary function studies as an aid in the differential diagnosis of pulmonary hypertension. Am J Med 47:378-383, 1969

Idiopathic Pulmonary Fibrosis

Clinical, Histologic, Radiographic, Physiologic, Scintigraphic, Cytologic, and Biochemical Aspects

Moderator: RONALD G. CRYSTAL, M.D. *Discussants:* JACK D. FULMER, M.D.; WILLIAM C. ROBERTS, M.D.; MORTON L. MOSS, M.D.; BRUCE R. LINE, M.D.; and HERBERT Y. REYNOLDS, M.D., F.A.C.P.; Bethesda, Maryland

Idiopathic pulmonary fibrosis is a fatal disorder that starts as an alveolitis and progresses to interstitial fibrosis. Correlative morphologic, physiologic, and biochemical studies in 29 patients have shown that the inflammatory process is best followed by serial bronchoalveolar lavage and ^{67}Ga citrate scanning, and the fibrotic process is best followed by quantitation of the exercise-induced drop in arterial oxygen tension per unit of oxygen consumed. Although biopsies in idiopathic pulmonary fibrosis seem to show increased amounts of fibrotic tissue, biochemical studies suggest that the disease is probably one of collagen rearrangement rather than collagen increase. Perhaps because of this, peripheral lymphocytes of these patients recognize collagen as "non-self" and, when exposed to it in vitro, produce lymphokines and cell lysis. The fibrotic process is probably irreversible, but the inflammatory and immune processes that cause it may be amenable to therapy if diagnosed early.

DR. RONALD G. CRYSTAL*: Forty one years ago, Hamman and Rich (1) described the clinical and morphologic features of four patients with progressive, rapidly fatal, diffuse pulmonary fibrosis. Clinicians soon began to diagnose this illness antemortem, and by 1957 more than 50 cases had appeared in the literature under the heading "Hamman-Rich syndrome" (2, 3). However, as more cases were described, it became apparent that the fulminating course of the original patients of Hamman and Rich manifested only part of the spectrum of the disorder now known as idiopathic pulmonary fibrosis (4-35).

More commonly, patients with idiopathic pulmonary fibrosis present with the insidious onset of breathlessness, sometimes after a flulike illness. It affects slightly more men than women; most patients are between the ages of 40 and 70 years, although the disease is sometimes found in children and young adults (36, 37). Almost all patients develop late inspiratory rales in the lower lung fields, clubbing of the fingers and occasionally the toes, and evidence of pulmonary hypertension. Although the inevitably fatal course of the disease can progress as rapidly as that described by Hamman and Rich, some patients can have the disorder for 15 to 20 years. However, this slower course is unusual; the average life span of a patient with idiopathic pulmonary fibrosis is only 47 months from the onset of symptoms (26).

In the early 1950s, as investigators developed the sophisticated tools to evaluate pulmonary disorders, Austrian and associates (38) described the "classic" physiologic concept of idiopathic pulmonary fibrosis. In general, patients have reduced lung volumes, reduced diffusing capacity, a normal forced expiratory volume in 1 sec/forced vital capacity ($FEV_1\%$), and arterial hypoxemia that worsens with exercise. These investigators coined the term "alveolar-capillary block," suggesting that the hypoxemia of idiopathic pulmonary fibrosis was secondary to an anatomic barrier to oxygen due to a thickened alveolar interstitium (38). This term was popular in the literature until 1962, when Finley, Swenson, and Comroe (39) presented data suggesting that the major cause of hypoxemia in these patients was not a diffusion barrier to oxygen, but rather was secondary to ventilation-perfusion mismatching. Clinicians had only recently adjusted to this new concept when it was challenged. Using sophisticated methods, Wagner and associates (40) showed that most of the hypoxemia in idiopathic pulmonary fibrosis is indeed secondary to ventilation-perfusion imbalance. With exercise, however, approximately 20% is due to a diffusion barrier to oxygen. Thus, our understanding of this phenomenon has come full circle. We will see later that, although ventilation-perfusion mismatching is

* Chief, Pulmonary Branch, National Heart, Lung, and Blood Institute.

► An edited transcription of a Combined Clinical Staff Conference at the Clinical Center, Bethesda, Maryland, 13 November 1975, by the National Heart, Lung, and Blood Institute, National Institutes of Health, U.S. Department of Health, Education, and Welfare.

Table 1. Classification of the Fibrotic Lung Disorders

Known Cause	Unknown Cause
Occupational and environmental* inhalants	Idiopathic pulmonary fibrosis
Drug reactions	Associated with a collagen-vascular disease†
Physical agents	Not associated with any known disorder
Infectious disorders	Associated with pulmonary arteritis‡
Cardiac disease	Sarcoidosis
Pulmonary vascular disease	Ankylosing spondylitis
Neoplastic disease	Congenital; familial
	Eosinophilic granuloma
	Idiopathic pulmonary hemosiderosis
	Alveolar microlithiasis
	Goodpasture's syndrome
	Alveolar proteinosis

* Including the group of disorders termed extrinsic allergic alveolitis; the fibrotic form is called chronic hypersensitivity pneumonitis.

† Including rheumatoid arthritis, progressive systemic sclerosis, systemic lupus erythematosus, dermatomyositis-polymyositis, Sjögren's syndrome, and the mixed connective tissue syndrome, but excluding patients with necrobiotic nodules or vasculitis.

‡ Including periarteritis nodosa; Wegener's granulomatosis; rheumatoid arthritis with necrobiotic nodules; and rheumatoid arthritis, progressive systemic sclerosis, and polymyositis-dermatomyositis with arteritis.

critically important in idiopathic pulmonary fibrosis, we are just beginning to understand what causes it.

For years, the morphologic features of idiopathic pulmonary fibrosis described by Hamman and Rich were accepted as definitive: a diffuse interstitial fibrosis with mononuclear cell infiltration (1, 2). It took the pioneering efforts of Scadding and Hinson (6, 18) and Liebow and co-workers (15, 21, 22) to point out that the spectrum of idiopathic pulmonary fibrosis was much broader and included marked intraalveolar cellularity as part of the histologic spectrum of the disease. Although most investigators have abandoned the designations "desquamative interstitial pneumonitis" (many intraalveolar cells with little interstitial disease) and "usual interstitial pneumonitis" (interstitial cellularity and fibrosis with little intraalveolar cellularity), these concepts remain important as probably representing the stages in the development of idiopathic pulmonary fibrosis (18, 29, 30, 33, 35).

As more clinicians recognized the importance of idiopathic pulmonary fibrosis, it became clear that many of these patients have serologic abnormalities that are associated with the collagen-vascular disorders. The physiologic and histologic features of idiopathic pulmonary fibrosis were noted in patients with rheumatoid arthritis (4, 25, 28, 33, 41-56), progressive systemic sclerosis (38, 52-66), polymyositis-dermatomyositis (65-80), and systemic lupus erythematosus (52-56, 81-85). As the association of these disorders became more evident, patients with idiopathic pulmonary fibrosis were screened with this in mind, and three groups emerged: those with a defined collagen-vascular disorder (41-85); those with serologic abnormalities that are seen in collagen-vascular disorders but that did not meet the criteria for a defined collagen-vascular disorder (33, 86-99); and those with no serologic abnormalities associated with the collagen-vascular disorders. Thus, for convenience, idiopathic pulmonary fibrosis is now categorized as "associated with a collagen-vascular disorder" (group 1) or "not associated with any known disorder" (groups 2 and 3) (Table 1). It is important to note, however, that with few exceptions, the two categories are identical. The major exceptions are that a small percentage of patients with rheumatoid arthritis have pulmonary necrobiotic nodules (46-48), and some patients with systemic lupus erythematosus, rheumatoid arthritis, progressive systemic sclerosis, or dermatomyositis-polymyositis have pulmonary arteritis (46, 48, 72, 84, 100). Even if these patients have pulmonary fibrosis, their disease is not considered to be idiopathic pulmonary fibrosis, and they will be excluded from our discussion. Likewise, patients with the lymphoproliferative form of Sjögrens syndrome (101), polyarteritis nodosa (102), Wegener's granulomatosis (103), and ankylosing spondylitis (104) clearly have a disorder different from idiopathic pulmonary fibrosis, and they will not be discussed.

Because idiopathic pulmonary fibrosis falls into the group of fibrotic lung disorders of unknown cause (Table 1), clinicians have tended to consider it a diagnosis of exclusion. However, as we will point out, this disorder has clearly defined clinical, histologic, radiographic, physiologic, scintigraphic, cytologic, and biochemical features that, taken as a whole, describe a characteristic and specific clinical entity. To give an overview of the current concepts of idiopathic pulmonary fibrosis, we will first present the general clinical, pathologic, and radiographic findings in 29 patients with this disorder. This will serve to place in context the newer physiologic, diagnostic, investigative, and therapeutic concepts that will follow.

Clinical Aspects of Idiopathic Pulmonary Fibrosis

Dr. Jack D. Fulmer*: A brief description of the clinical findings in this group of 29 patients will help to define idiopathic pulmonary fibrosis and its manifestations. Although these findings are not limited to this disorder, when considered in the setting of the whole clinical entity, they help to establish idiopathic pulmonary fibrosis as a specific and characteristic disease.

Eighty percent of the patients under discussion had idiopathic pulmonary fibrosis without any other associated disorder; the rest had a defined collagen-vascular disorder. Nationwide statistics are not available, but we think these relative percentages probably reflect only the pattern of our referrals. At least some manifestations of idiopathic pulmonary fibrosis are relatively common in rheumatoid arthritis (25, 33, 45-51) and progressive systemic sclerosis (33, 58, 61-63), so there are probably more patients with idiopathic pulmonary fibrosis associated with a collagen-vascular disorder than our patient population reflects.

The average age of all patients was 51.8 years. However, the group with associated collagen-vascular disorders were generally younger. There was a slightly higher percentage of men than women (1.1:1) in our idiopathic pulmonary fibrosis population, but in the group with collagen-vascular disorders women predominated. These age and sex distributions reflect the typical findings for idiopathic pulmonary fibrosis found in the literature (12, 13, 17). With the

* Chief, Clinical Service, Pulmonary Branch, National Heart, Lung, and Blood Institute.

Table 2. Clinical, Laboratory, and Physiologic Findings in Patients with Idiopathic Pulmonary Fibrosis

Presenting Symptoms	Percent of Patients	Laboratory	Percent of Patients	Physiologic Studies	Mean Values*
Breathlessness	100	↑ Sedimentation rate	94†	Vital capacity	61.7 ± 2.9‡
Cough	86	+ Antinuclear antibodies	7†		
Systemic§	48†	+ Rheumatoid factor	14†	Total lung capacity	62.9 ± 2.9‡
		+ Cryoimmunoglobulins	41†		
		+ Lupus erythematosus preparations	3†	Residual volume/ total lung capacity	34.4 ± 1.6‖
Physical		Abnormal serum protein			
Tachypnea	46	electrophoresis		$FEV_1\%$**	97.6 ± 2.3‡
Clubbing	72	↑ α2 macroglobulins	22		
Chest findings		↑ γ globulins	17	Diffusing capacity††	46.8 ± 3.5‡
Normal	14	Serum immunoglobulins			
Rales	65	↑ IgG	4		
Ronchi or bronchovesicular		↑ IgA	39		
sounds	21	↑ IgM	9		
Cardiac findings		Serum complement (C50) ↓	6†		
Normal	30	Polycythemia	3		
Augmented P_2	70				

* Mean ± SEM.
† These data refer only to patients with idiopathic pulmonary fibrosis with no associated collagen-vascular disorder; of the 29 patients with idiopathic pulmonary fibrosis, three had rheumatoid arthritis, one had systemic lupus erythematosus, one had a mixed collagen-vascular disease, and one had progressive systemic sclerosis.
‡ Percent predicted.
§ Systemic symptoms included flulike illness, fatigue, joint symptoms, fever, or weight loss.
‖ Percent observed.
** Forced expiratory volume in 1 sec/forced vital capacity.
†† Single breath, carbon monoxide.

exception of age and sex and the specific systemic abnormalities of each collagen-vascular syndrome in the group with associated collagen-vascular disorders, the manifestations of idiopathic pulmonary fibrosis in both groups were identical (49, 85) (Table 2).

The duration of symptoms from onset to evaluation at the NIH ranged from 0.5 to 10 years, but averaged 2.9 years. In the most extensive study of the natural history of idiopathic pulmonary fibrosis (26), the mean survival of patients was 4 years, with a range of 0.4 to 20 years. Although most of our patients are still alive, the relative number that have died would suggest that they are following a similar natural history.

The onset of idiopathic pulmonary fibrosis is usually associated with breathlessness, characteristically first noted during exercise (6, 17, 30). Most patients also noted a nonproductive cough early in the course of the disease, and about half noted constitutional symptoms such as a flulike illness, fatigability, weight loss, or arthralgias (Table 2).

In contrast to other pulmonary disorders associated with clubbing (105, 106), patients with idiopathic pulmonary fibrosis with clubbing rarely have hypertrophic osteoarthropathy. Excluding clubbing and varied constitutional symptoms, all of the clinical manifestations of idiopathic pulmonary fibrosis were limited to the chest. Early in the course of the disease, the chest examination may be normal. Later, in midcourse, the typical patient with idiopathic pulmonary fibrosis will have tachypnea (46%), harsh, dry rales at both bases (65%), and findings consistent with pulmonary hypertension (70%). Occasionally, patients will have only diffuse bronchovesicular breath sounds or rhonchi, or both. Although cardiac examination findings can be normal for years, the usual progression includes the development of a right ventricular heave and eventual right-sided failure (13). About 20% of the patients with idiopathic pulmonary fibrosis eventually die from a cardiovascular disorder, but most succumb to primary respiratory failure, often precipitated by infection (26).

Most patients with idiopathic pulmonary fibrosis have resting arterial hypoxemia that worsens with exercise. Polycythemia, however, is almost never seen (13), in marked contrast to other hypoxic states such as chronic obstructive lung disease or congenital heart disease (107). Almost all patients with idiopathic pulmonary fibrosis have an elevated sedimentation rate (94%). As pointed out by Dr. Crystal, idiopathic pulmonary fibrosis is definitely associated with abnormalities of the immune system (33, 86-98). However, of the routine studies available, none are specific for this disorder. Excluding patients with definable collagen-vascular disorders, abnormalities in antinuclear antibodies, rheumatoid factor, and γ-globulins are not as prominent in our group of patients as one would expect from reviewing the literature (compare Table 2 with References 88, 89). In addition, although an association had made between chronic hepatitis and idiopathic pulmonary fibrosis (108), none of our patients had liver function abnormalities. It is not generally recognized that many have circulating cryoimmunoglobulins (Table 2, Reference 33). The specific immunoglobulins involved have not been characterized as yet. There are other, probably much more important abnormalities of the immune system that are almost universal in idiopathic pulmonary fibrosis, and these will be discussed later.

The average patient with idiopathic pulmonary fibrosis had a total lung capacity of 62.9% predicted and a diffusing capacity of 46.8% predicted. However, two patients had normal lung volumes and one patient a normal diffusing capacity, even though they had morphologic evidence of mild to moderate fibrosis. Thus, although a

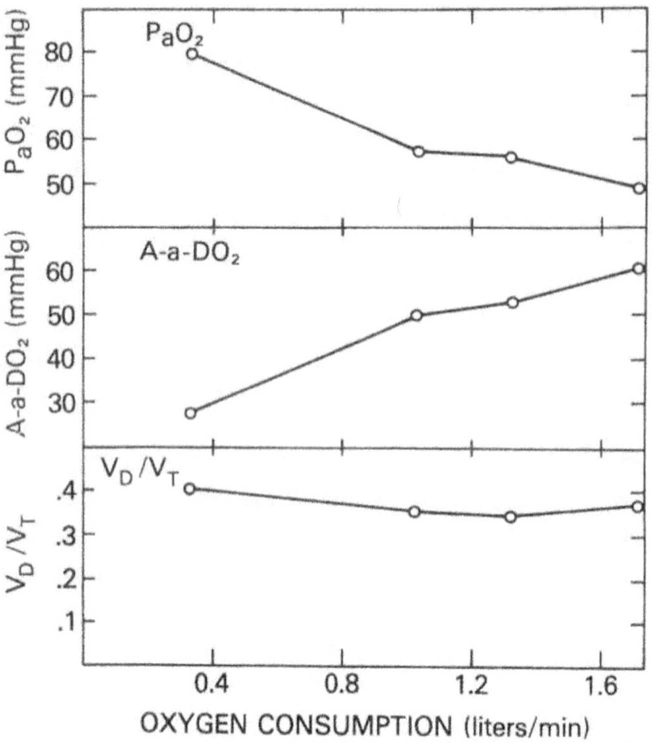

Figure 1. Gas exchange data from a 42-year-old man with idiopathic pulmonary fibrosis taken at rest and during treadmill exercise (see also Figures 2, 5c and d). **Top.** Progressive decrease in arterial oxygen tension (Pa_{O_2}) with exercise. **Middle.** Progressive increase in alveolar-arterial oxygen difference ($D[A\text{-}a]_{O_2}$) with exercise. **Bottom.** Dead space to tidal volume ratio (VD/VT) is abnormally high and does not decrease with progressive exercise. Oxygen consumption is proportional to power output.

reduced total lung capacity and diffusing capacity are the physiologic hallmarks of the disease, it is not mandatory that both be abnormal. Likewise, the average patient with idiopathic pulmonary fibrosis has resting arterial hypoxemia (69.3 mm Hg), but four of our patients have normal resting arterial oxygen tension (Pa_{O_2}). It is important to point out that a decreased diffusing capacity does not implicate a defect in oxygen diffusion but rather signifies a reduction of available alveolar-capillary bed (109).

Interestingly, 21% of our patients had decreased Pa_{O_2} values when they rose from the supine to the upright position, in direct opposition to what occurs in normal individuals. In idiopathic pulmonary fibrosis, the reversal of position-dependent changes in Pa_{O_2} is probably associated with alterations in pulmonary hemodynamics, causing greater ventilation-perfusion imbalance in the upright position (110).

It is generally thought that the hypoxemia of idiopathic pulmonary fibrosis is related to ventilation-perfusion mismatching, although limitation to oxygen diffusion may be present, especially during exercise (40). As we will discuss later, much of the ventilation-perfusion mismatching may be related to abnormalities in ventilation. However, the latter is not due to abnormalities in the large airways because almost all patients with idiopathic pulmonary fibrosis have normal values for FEV_1% (Table 2) and airway resistance by body plethysmography (111).

Even though the resting Pa_{O_2} can be normal in idiopathic pulmonary fibrosis, the resting alveolar-arterial oxygen gradient ($D[A\text{-}a]_{O_2}$) is almost invariably abnormal (97% of the patients). Even more sensitive physiologic monitors of idiopathic pulmonary fibrosis are the fall in Pa_{O_2} and the widening of $D(A\text{-}a)_{O_2}$ with exercise, findings that are universal in these patients (Figure 1, *Top and Middle*) (12, 30, 38).

Physiologic shunt at rest (as measured by 100% O_2) can be significant in idiopathic pulmonary fibrosis but usually develops late in the course of the disease (38, 39). Of our population, the four patients with the mildest disease had a physiologic shunt of less than 6%, whereas the four patients with the most advanced disease had a shunt of 15% to 30%. Thus, although physiologic shunt is generally not a significant cause of hypoxemia early in the disease, it becomes a major problem in the care of patients very late in their course, because even with very high inspired oxygen concentrations, they do not achieve adequate oxygenation.

Another characteristic of idiopathic pulmonary fibrosis is the increased physiologic dead space found in 60% of the patients even at rest (7, 12, 112). Whereas normal persons waste (that is, ventilate nonfunctional regions of lung) less than one third of their total ventilation, patients with idiopathic pulmonary fibrosis will often have dead space to tidal volume ratios (V_D/V_T) of greater than 0.4. In normal individuals the efficiency of ventilation improves with exercise (that is, the V_D/V_T falls) (113, 114); in more than 90% of patients with idiopathic pulmonary fibrosis it stays constant or may increase (Figure 1, *bottom*).

Also characteristic of idiopathic pulmonary fibrosis is the volume-pressure curve (Figure 2) that expresses the mechanical properties of lung and is usually discussed in terms of its position, shape, and slope (115). Typically,

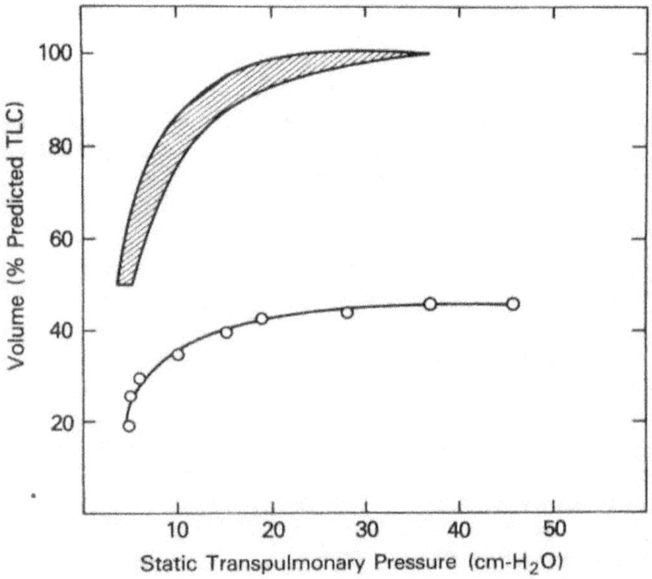

Figure 2. Volume-pressure relations of a 42-year-old man with idiopathic pulmonary fibrosis (see also Figures 1, 5c and d) showing a curve (○—○) that is shifted down and to the right of normal (*shaded area*). The volume data is presented as percentage of predicted total lung capacity (*TLC*).

patients with idiopathic pulmonary fibrosis have a volume-pressure curve shifted downward and to the right, whereas patients with emphysema have a curve shifted upward and to the left (112, 116). The reasons for these findings are controversial, but the curve graphically illustrates that after a certain point patients with idiopathic pulmonary fibrosis take in little volume of air, and to do so requires a large negative transpulmonary pressure. Although such a volume-pressure curve is not specific for idiopathic pulmonary fibrosis (it is seen in any infiltrative disease of lung) (115), taken in context, it helps to characterize the disorder.

Histologic Observations in Idiopathic Pulmonary Fibrosis

Dr. William C. Roberts*: This section will summarize our histologic observations from open lung biopsies in 29 patients with idiopathic pulmonary fibrosis and discuss the significance of some of these changes. There were no histologic differences between the groups with idiopathic pulmonary fibrosis and idiopathic pulmonary fibrosis associated with collagen-vascular disorders (12, 48).

The anatomic distribution of idiopathic pulmonary fibrosis is heterogeneous, a finding easily visualized with low power views of the biopsies (Figures 3*A*, 4*A*). Yet this same local heterogeneity is usually seen in multiple samples throughout the lung at postmortem evaluation of idiopathic pulmonary fibrosis, suggesting open lung biopsy specimens are, in general, representative of the disease process.

The major histologic abnormalities of idiopathic pulmonary fibrosis are listed in Table 3 and illustrated in Figures 3 and 4. A characteristic histologic feature of all biopsies was the apparent increased amounts of fibrous tissue in the alveolar septae. The distribution of this fibrous tissue, however, varied: in 23% of the patients it was focal, and most of the alveolar septae appeared normal; in another 23% there were more areas of the lung biopsy with apparently increased fibrous tissue than areas of normal-appearing lung; and in the remaining 54% most or all alveolar septae appeared thickened by fibrous tissue, the pulmonary architecture was considerably distorted, and the amount of area occupied by air appeared less than that occupied by tissue. Many patients had considerable peribronchiolar fibrosis and fibrous thickening of the interlobular septae and visceral pleura.

Inflammatory cells, mainly lymphocytes, macrophages, and plasma cells, were always seen in areas of increased fibrous tissue. A feature of idiopathic pulmonary fibrosis that is not often recognized is that eosinophils and neutrophils are present as well (2, 18, 29, 35). The number of mononuclear cells in the interstitium was quite variable: 13% of patients had considerable numbers, 54% had moderate numbers, and 33% were judged to have scattered cells. The normal lung has almost no inflammatory cells in the interstitium or alveolus, so the observation of even scattered interstitial inflammatory cells is important.

In many areas where the alveolar septae were thickened, the air side was lined by large cuboidal-shaped cells, often associated with collections of cells free in the alveolar sacs. The former has been referred to as "cuboidalization of alveolar lining cells" (19, 24, 117) and the latter as "desquamation" (15). Some degree of cuboidalization and desquamation was observed in all biopsies.

Normally, the epithelial surfaces of alveoli are covered by two types of cells: the alveolar type I cell (also called the type I pneumocyte, type A epithelial cell, small alveolar cell, or membranous pneumocyte) and the alveolar type II cell (also called the type II pneumocyte, large alveolar cell, granular pneumocyte, or vacuolated alveolar cell) (118). The type II cell is particularly important for its production of the material that lowers alveolar surface tension (119). The type I cell covers more than 90% of the alveolar surface area and is not visible by light microscopy; the type II cell covers the remaining surface area and is visible by light microscopy. Even though the vast majority of the epithelial surface is composed of type I cells, there are ordinarily 1.5 to 2 type II cells for every type I cell (118). In idiopathic pulmonary fibrosis, however, this ratio increases since the cuboidalization of the alveolar epithelial surface is most likely due to loss of type I cells and proliferation of type II cells. This change in alveolar epithelial cells is not specific for idiopathic pulmonary fibrosis because it occurs in most conditions associated with alveolar injury, including causes of pulmonary venous hypertension such as mitral stenosis (19, 117, 120, 121).

The term "desquamated" cells was originally used to describe free-floating cells within alveolar spaces, as these cells were thought to be alveolar type II cells that had been sloughed from the epithelial surface (15). As more patients with idiopathic pulmonary fibrosis were studied using electron microscopy, it became apparent that the term "desquamated" is probably improper because many of these cells are macrophages (29, 120, 122, 123). All of our patients with idiopathic pulmonary fibrosis have desquamated cells in alveoli. The relative numbers of these cells, however, varied (large in 7%, moderate in 43%, and only a few in 50%). The amount of "desquamation" varies not only from patient to patient, but also within the limited area of the same open lung biopsy specimen (Figure 3). This finding strengthens the concept that "desquamative interstitial pneumonitis" and "usual interstitial pneumonitis" are simply parts of the same disease rather than specific disease entities. Desquamative interstitial pneumonitis most likely represents early idiopathic pulmonary fibrosis, whereas usual interstitial pneumonitis represents the later stages of the disease (6, 18, 24, 29, 30, 33, 35). Since the morphology of both can appear in the same patient at the same time (Figure 3), it is probable that part of the heterogeneity of idiopathic pulmonary fibrosis within the same biopsy represents the same disease process at different stages.

Although idiopathic pulmonary fibrosis is classically considered a disorder of alveoli, 80% of the biopsies showed peribronchiolar fibrous tissue or peribronchial mononuclear inflammatory cells, or both. Many of the airway lumina contained cellular debris or mucus, or both (Figures 3*E*, 4*C*). In open lung biopsy specimens of normal lung, the

* Chief, Pathology Branch, National Heart, Lung, and Blood Institute.

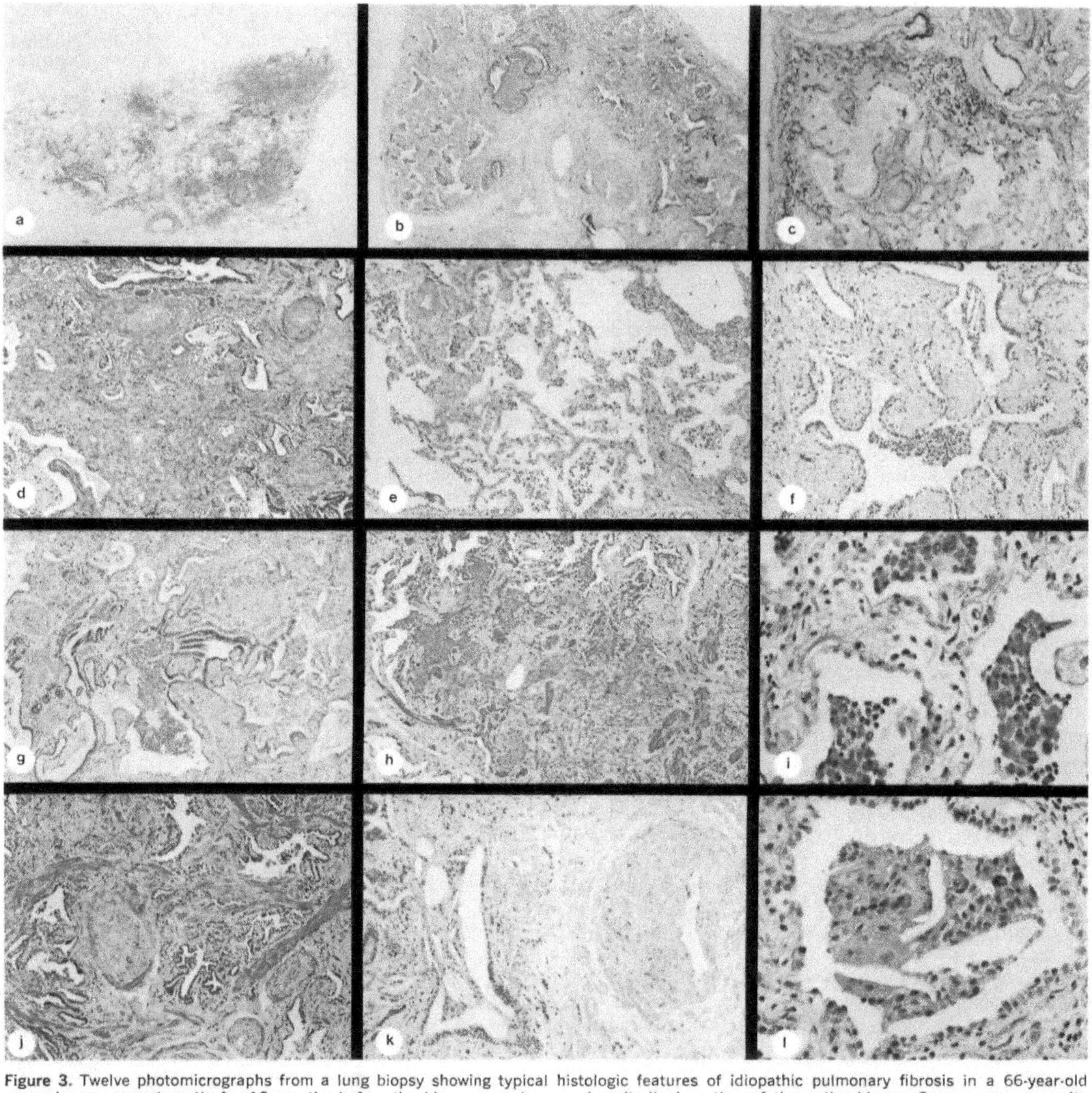

Figure 3. Twelve photomicrographs from a lung biopsy showing typical histologic features of idiopathic pulmonary fibrosis in a 66-year-old man who was symptomatic for 12 months before the biopsy was done. **a.** Longitudinal section of the entire biopsy. Some areas are quite scarred, others relatively normal. (Hematoxylin and eosin; original magnification, × 9.) **b.** Portion of thickened area showing marked distortion of pulmonary parenchyma, loss of alveolar space, marked increase in fibrous tissue, and "desquamation" in some air spaces. (Movat; original magnification, × 40.) **c.** Area encompassing a portion of that shown in *b*. There is both medial hypertrophy and intimal fibrous proliferation of the arteries. The latter produced luminal narrowing. The interlobular septae show increased fibrous tissue in some sites and edema fluid in others. The black represents elastic fibers. (Elastic van Gieson; original magnification, × 40.) **d.** Masson trichome stain showing huge amounts of fibrous tissue (*stained blue*). The arteries have narrowed lumina. Debris is present in some air spaces (original magnification, × 54). **e.** Area of lung with only mild increase in fibrous tissue but "desquamation" in alveolar sacs. (Hematoxylin and eosin; original magnification, × 80.) **f.** Close-up showing marked thickening of alveolar septae by fibrous tissue. Three cholesterol clefts are present in one alveolar space. (Movat; original magnification, × 130.) **g.** The alveolar spaces and airways here are filled with desquamated cells and mucinous material. There is smooth muscle proliferation in the alveolar septae, and the lumina of the arteries are narrowed. (Hematoxylin and eosin; original magnification, × 155.) **h.** Area showing alveoli packed with desquamated cells. The smooth muscle is prominent. (Movat; original magnification, × 80.) **i.** Periodic acid-Schiff (PAS) stain showing that the cytoplasm of the desquamated cells in the alveolar spaces is PAS-positive. The alveolar septae in this area appear edematous and also contain increased fibrous tissue. There is proliferation of the alveolar lining cells ("cuboidalization") (original magnification, × 360). **j.** Close-up showing proliferation of smooth muscle in the alveolar septae. The arteries have thick walls and narrowed lumina. (Movat; original magnification, × 80.) **k.** Close-up showing multiple cholesterol clefts in an alveolar space and an adjacent pulmonary artery with a narrowed lumen. (Movat; original magnification, × 140.) **l.** Close-up of cholesterol granuloma in an alveolus. The cholesterol clefts are indicative of pulmonary hypertension (124). (Hematoxylin and eosin; original magnification, × 380.)

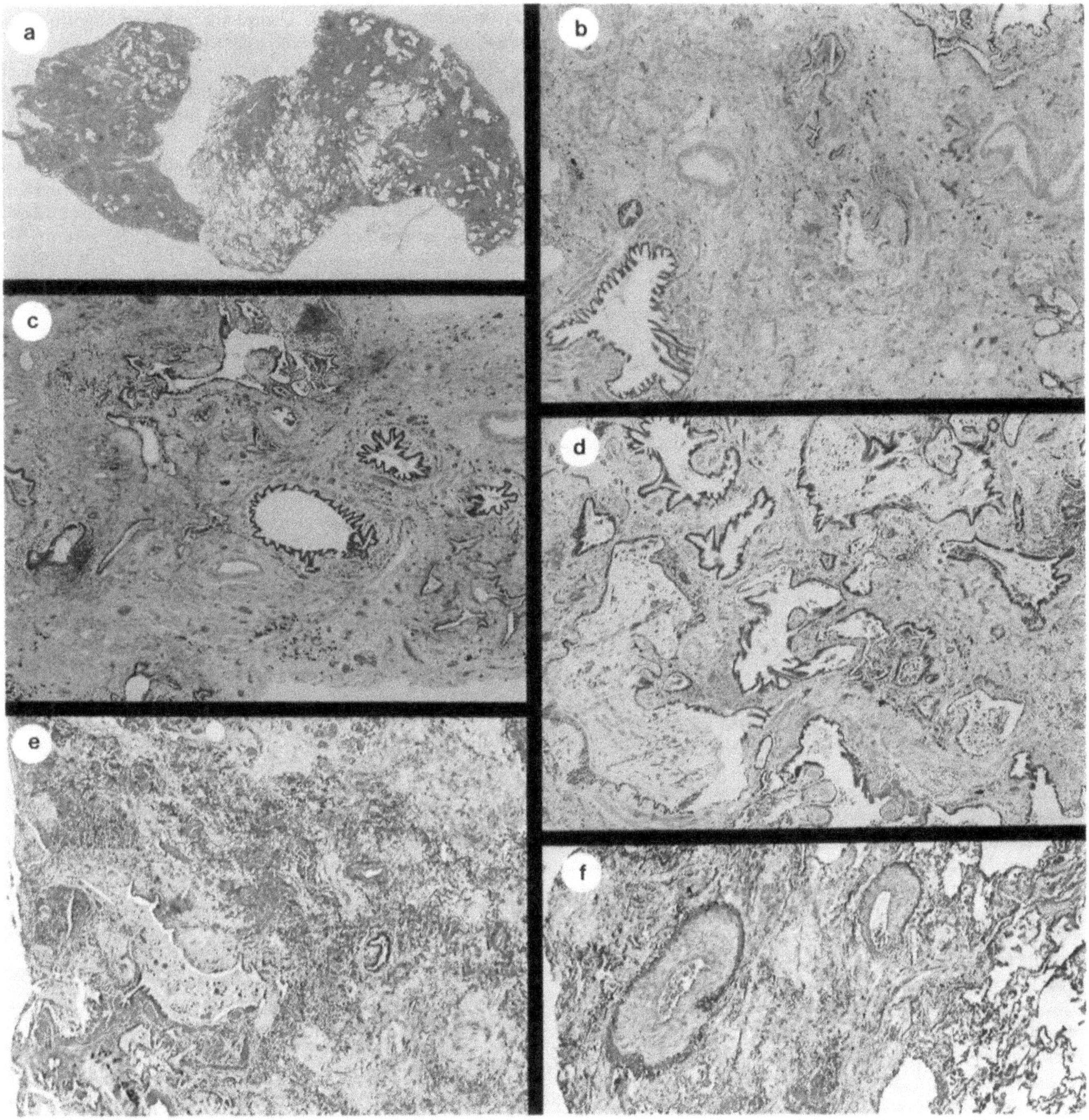

Figure 4. Lung biopsy in a 67-year-old man who had symptoms of respiratory insufficiency for only 6 months before this biopsy was obtained. **a.** Low-power view of the entire biopsy, which was in two pieces. Most of the pulmonary parenchyma is markedly thickened by fibrous tissue. Only a small area of near-normal lung remains. (Hematoxylin and eosin; original magnification, × 4.) **b.** Section showing loss of air space and replacement by fibrous tissue. A cholesterol granuloma is present in the air space near the center of the field. (Hematoxylin and eosin; original magnification, × 35.) **c.** Another area showing several airways, some of which are narrowed and others dilated. (Hematoxylin and eosin; original magnification, × 35.) **d.** Close-up of many dilated airways, some of which are filled with mucinous material. (Hematoxylin and eosin; original magnification, × 54.) **e.** Marked "condensation" of elastic fibers (*stained black*) in a subpleural location. (Movat; original magnification, × 54.) **f.** Another subpleural scar showing two pulmonary veins with narrowed lumina due to severe fibromuscular intimal proliferation. The lung parenchyma at the right is relatively intact. (Movat; original magnification, × 54.)

diameter of the small airways is always larger than the adjacent pulmonary artery. Using this as a criterion, 70% of the patients had narrowed airways and 30%, normal or dilated airways. All of those with dilated airways had narrowed airways in other areas of the biopsy.

Cholesterol-ester clefts were found in air spaces in 43% of our patients (Figure 3*G*). In a previous study (124), we suggested that these lesions indicate pulmonary hypertension. As a correlate of this finding, 70% of our biopsies showed thickening of the walls of the muscular pulmonary arteries by both medial hypertrophy and fibrous intimal proliferation. All patients with cholesterol clefts had these

Table 3. Histologic Observations from Open Lung Biopsies in 29 Patients with Idiopathic Pulmonary Fibrosis

Finding	Percent of Patients	Mild	Moderate	Severe
		←	%	→
Alveolar septal fibrosis	100	23	23	54
Interstitial inflammation	97	33	54	13
Alveolar "desquamation"	100	50	43	7
Cuboidalization of alveolar lining cells	100	33	27	40
Narrowed airways	70			
Normal or dilated airways	30			
Cholesterol-ester clefts	43			
Thickened pulmonary arteries	70			
Smooth-muscle proliferation	83			
Cystic changes	53			
Lymphoid nodules	50			
Granulomas	0			
Arteritis	0			

pulmonary arterial changes consistent with pulmonary hypertension. It also was noted that all of the patients with the more severe degree of interstitial fibrosis had concomitant pulmonary arterial changes.

Increased amounts of smooth muscle were seen in the interstitium in 83% of the patients. Smooth muscle proliferation is a recognized phenomenon in patients with idiopathic pulmonary fibrosis (125), but it is not clear whether this represents smooth muscle cells or rather increased numbers of interstitial mesenchymal cells with actin filaments, such as those described by Kapanci and associates (126).

Collections of lymphocytes in the lung parenchyma, some with centrally located histiocytes, were observed in half of the biopsies. This apparent increase in the number of parenchymal cells with the potential for immune competence may have significance in relation to the immune system abnormalities in idiopathic pulmonary fibrosis that will be discussed later.

Patients with idiopathic pulmonary fibrosis do not have arteritis, granulomas, or evidence of minerals in the lung (24, 102, 127-129). This important distinguishing feature of idiopathic pulmonary fibrosis is one of the major justifications for lung biopsy in these patients, because the presence of any of these abnormalities rules out idiopathic pulmonary fibrosis and indicates other possible disorders such as polyarteritis, extrinsic allergic alveolitis, or silicosis, all of which call for different therapeutic approaches.

The Chest X ray in Idiopathic Pulmonary Fibrosis

Dr. Morton L. Moss*: A detailed review of the chest X rays of this group of patients with idiopathic pulmonary fibrosis showed six radiographic patterns. The dominant patterns were reticular, reticulonodular, and ground glass (Figure 5). Seen less often were localized linear densities, nodular densities, and so-called "ill-defined" densities. In general, the radiographic findings of idiopathic pulmonary fibrosis involved both lungs equally but were predominant in the lower lung zones. Occasionally, these abnormalities were lobar or confined to the upper lung zones.

Reticular pattern refers to the netlike appearance of linear or curvilinear densities, or both, that are probably derived from the interstitial septal fibrosis and inflammation (130). The random orientation of the reticular net differentiates it from pulmonary vascular markings that are radially distributed from the hila. The reticular pattern can vary because of the thickness of the linear or curvilinear densities themselves, or because of the size of the translucent air spaces. These variables yield overall reticular patterns that can be defined as having fine, medium, or coarse textures. In general, the texture was fine early in the disease, with densities of less than 1 mm in width. As the disease progressed the texture coarsened, and the densities often were several millimeters in diameter. "Honeycombing," seen late in the disease, refers to a coarse reticular pattern with the translucencies measuring 0.5 cm to 1.0 cm in diameter (131, 132) (Figure 5*a*).

A reticulonodular pattern results from the superimposition of nodular densities (representing alveolitis, superimposition of thickened interstitium, or interstitium on end) on a reticular pattern (Figure 5*b*) (131). A ground glass pattern typically has a homogeneous, hazy appearance, probably resulting from an alveolitis (Figure 5*c*) (130). When this pattern surrounds airways, air bronchograms can be found, even though the lung is functional and not consolidated (Figure 5*d*) (130).

Less often, patients with idiopathic pulmonary fibrosis had localized areas of linear, nodular, or "ill-defined" densities either alone, in combination with each other, or in combination with the three more widespread patterns of reticular, reticulonodular, or ground glass densities. The isolated linear densities were often in the form of Kerley-B lines. Localized linear densities are probably an early form of the reticular pattern, while nodular and ill-defined densities are localized areas of alveolitis. The nodular densities are usually discrete 0.2- cm to 1.0-cm shadows, while ill-defined densities are poorly marginated and range from 1 cm to large amorphous densities of 4 cm to 5 cm.

Evaluation of the X rays of patients who have been followed from the onset of symptoms suggested that the radiographic evolution of idiopathic pulmonary fibrosis in our series was in general agreement with the data of Livingstone and co-workers (13). X rays of patients in the early course of disease showed localized linear, nodular, or "ill-defined" densities or a ground glass pattern, probably representing the alveolitis of idiopathic pulmonary fibrosis. With progression of the disease, reticular and reticulonodular patterns began to appear. In later stages the diaphragms were elevated, the pulmonary arteries were dilated, and a coarse reticular pattern developed. Terminal stages usually showed coarse reticulation often associated with cystic lesions and bullae. The cystic lesions were usually seen in the upper zones (132), although the bullae were randomly distributed. No matter how extensive their disease, patients with idiopathic pulmonary fibrosis seldom had fissure displacement or mediastinal shift. Occasionally, there was pleural thickening but never pleural effusion.

To evaluate the chest X ray as a tool in the diagnosis and

* Staff Radiologist, Diagnostic Radiology, Clinical Center.

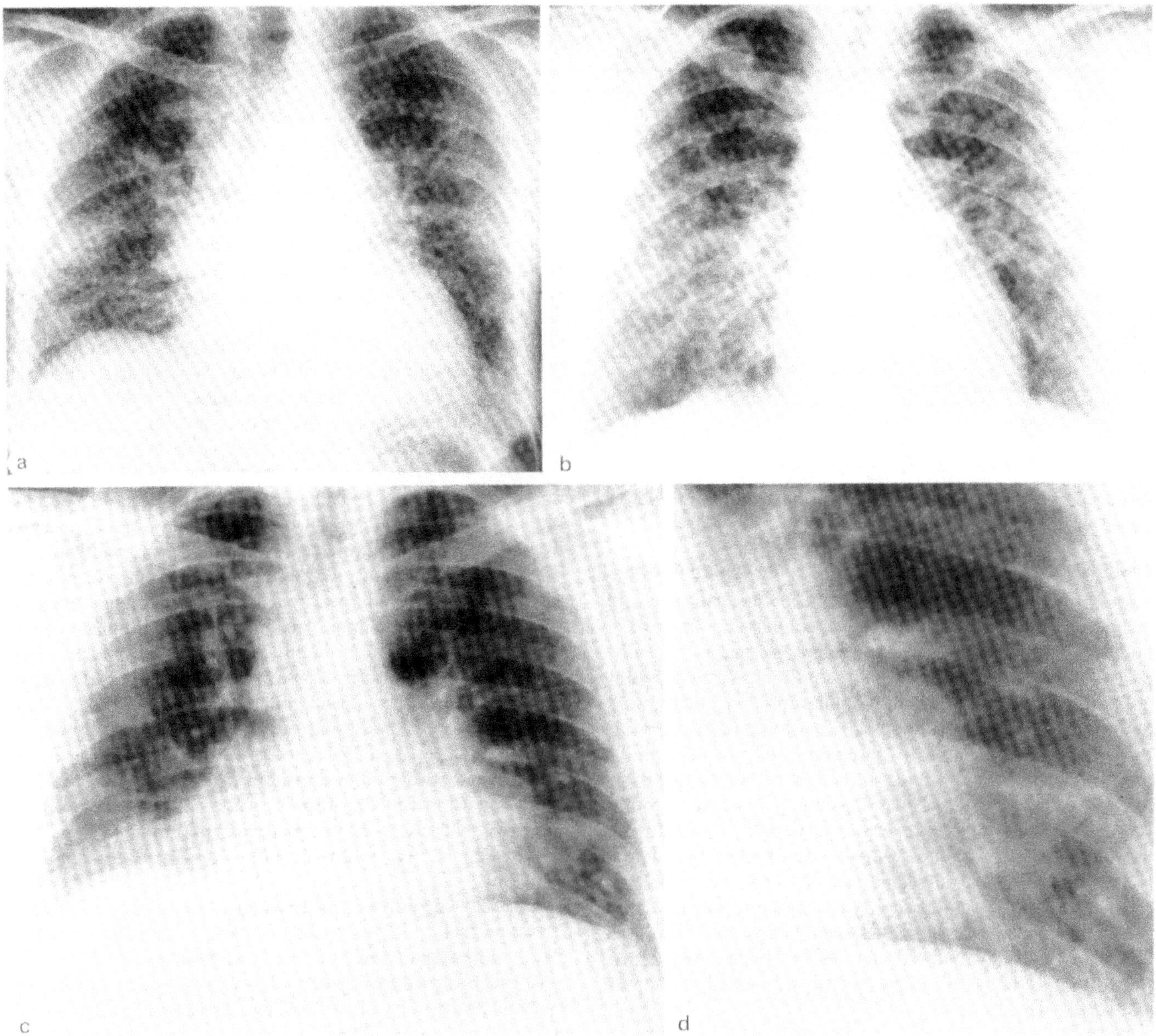

Figure 5. Three dominant radiographic patterns seen in patients with idiopathic pulmonary fibrosis. **a.** Coarse reticular pattern in a 56-year-old woman with symptoms for 4 years. Typical "honeycombing" is seen in the left lower lung field. **b.** Reticulonodular pattern in a 31-year-old woman with a 6-month history of progressive breathlessness after a flulike illness. **c.** Ground glass pattern in a 42-year-old man with symptoms for 2 years. **d.** A close-up of the left lower lung field of the X ray in panel C showing the homogeneous hazy appearance with air bronchograms.

staging of idiopathic pulmonary fibrosis, we graded the films of these patients as to the type and extensiveness of roentgenographic pattern and compared these data with the morphologic and physiologic findings. These comparisons showed a positive correlation between roentgenographic patterns indicating alveolitis and morphologic findings of marked cellularity. Furthermore, the honeycombing seen on chest X ray correlated well with the morphologic finding of cystic lesions accompanying severe fibrosis. Interestingly, there was a poor correlation between the degree of fibrosis seen on lung biopsy and the severity of disease estimated by chest film. However, this was not too surprising because the radiographic correlate of the fibrotic process can be masked by concomitant alveolitis. Furthermore, the chest X ray can, on rare occasion, be normal with morphologic evidence of fibrotic disease. In general, there was good agreement between the radiographic estimate of lung volume and the physiologic determination of lung volume by inert gas or body plethysmography. There was, however, no correlation between the degree of reduction in other physiologic variables and the radiologic estimate of severity of disease.

These comparisons would suggest that the chest X ray is useful in early idiopathic pulmonary fibrosis for a rough estimation of disease activity (for example, alveolitis). In midcourse idiopathic pulmonary fibrosis, X rays are not as reliable as physiologic and morphologic evaluations to gauge severity of disease and degree of fibrosis. They are

Table 4. Comparison of the Laboratory Evaluation of Idiopathic Pulmonary Fibrosis and the Degree of Fibrosis Found on Open Lung Biopsy Specimens

Physiologic Study	Correlation with Histopathology*
Chest X ray	Poor
Vital capacity	Poor
Total lung capacity	Poor
Diffusing capacity	Poor
Coefficient of retraction	Good
Resting arterial oxygen tension (Po_2)	Poor
Resting alveolar-arterial oxygen gradient ($D[A\text{-}a]O_2$)	Poor
Change in arterial Pao_2 and $D(A\text{-}a)O_2$ with exercise	Good

* The degree of fibrosis on the open lung biopsy specimens of 18 patients with idiopathic pulmonary fibrosis were graded as noted in Table 3. These rankings were compared with the physiologic values using a Spearmen rank correlation: poor = $P > 0.05$; good = $P < 0.05$.

of value again in later stages of disease for detecting cystic lesions and severe fibrosis (for example, coarse reticular pattern).

New Physiologic Concepts of Idiopathic Pulmonary Fibrosis

Dr. Fulmer: From the discussions of the histologic and radiographic features of idiopathic pulmonary fibrosis, a general pattern of the disease process emerges. It most likely begins as an alveolitis (ground glass or nodular appearance radiographically; inflammatory cells and "desquamation" seen histologically) and gradually develops into alveolar septal fibrosis (reticular or reticulonodular appearance radiographically; increasing numbers of alveolar septae appear fibrotic histologically). In all probability, idiopathic pulmonary fibrosis is a reversible process in the alveolitis stage, but once fibrosis occurs the anatomical derangements of the alveolar-capillary bed are such that affected portions of parenchyma are damaged permanently.

Therefore, assessment of the overall progression of disease must include methods that monitor the fibrotic process. This is important not only for prognosis but also for evaluating new therapies.

In common practice, patients with idiopathic pulmonary fibrosis are followed by four variables: the chest X ray, lung volumes (vital capacity or total lung capacity, or both), diffusion capacity, and resting arterial oxygen tension (12, 17, 133, 134). However, in our group of patients, none of these variables correlate with the degree of fibrosis determined histologically (Table 4). This, however, is not as surprising as it appears. As described earlier, the chest X ray, lung volumes, diffusing capacity, or resting Po_2 can be normal in patients with moderate degrees of fibrosis. In addition, there is often no overall correlation between the clinical severity of the disease (for example, what the patient feels) and any of these variables. Even the resting alveolar-arterial oxygen gradient, which was abnormal in 97% of our patients, does not correlate with the degree of fibrosis on the biopsy specimens (Table 4).

If the chest X ray, lung volumes, diffusing capacity, and resting arterial oxygen tension do not correlate with the degree of fibrosis in idiopathic pulmonary fibrosis, what physiologic tools can be used to stage and follow the fibrotic process? The two most useful variables are the volume-pressure curve for staging fibrosis (mild, moderate, or severe; *see* Table 3), and the exercise study to both stage and follow the fibrotic process.

To establish the usefulness of the static deflation volume-pressure curve in idiopathic pulmonary fibrosis (Figure 2), we correlated the degree of fibrosis on open lung biopsy with the slope ($\Delta V/\Delta P$) (115) and position (defined as the static transpulmonary pressure at 70% total lung capacity) of the curve; the maximum static transpulmonary pressure (Pst max) (116); and Pst max/observed total lung capacity (the coefficient of retraction) (135).

Comparison of $\Delta V/\Delta P$ and position of the curve with the morphologic grading of fibrosis showed that although a decreased slope is usually associated with the degree of fibrosis, the position of the volume-pressure curve (shift to right or left) does not correlate with the morphologic assessment of the degree of fibrosis. In contrast, Pst max did correlate with the degree of fibrosis; that is, as the degree of fibrosis increased, more transpulmonary pressure was required to achieve full inspiration. However, Pst max is not the perfect variable for staging the fibrosis of idiopathic pulmonary fibrosis because normal young persons can often develop large negative transpulmonary pressures (135, 136). The coefficient of retraction also correlates with the degree of fibrosis but more clearly separates patients with idiopathic pulmonary fibrosis from normal persons (135). Our current data suggest, however, that although the coefficient of retraction is useful for staging idiopathic pulmonary fibrosis, it may not be as useful in following the disease process because if patients improve without a major increase in lung volumes, the coefficient of retraction usually does not change significantly.

The lack of correlation between static monitors of lung function (chest X ray, lung volumes, diffusing capacity, Pao_2, volume-pressure curves) and progression of the disease explains what is obvious to the patient: as the disease evolves from early to midcourse, the patient feels fine at rest but invariably gives a history of breathlessness and fatigue with exercise. The physiologic correlate of this may be the decrease in Pao_2 with exercise that is always found (Figure 2). It is difficult, however, to quantitate exercise studies in these patients because the maximum amount of work they can do depends not only on their pulmonary status but also on their cardiovascular system, muscle

Table 5. Physiologic Evaluation of Airways in Patients with Idiopathic Pulmonary Fibrosis

Study	Patients with Abnormal Results
	%
$FEV_1\%$*	0
Airway resistance by body plethysmography	0
Dynamic compliance	70
Maximum expiratory flow-volume curves	45
Maximum flow-static recoil curve	31

* Forced expiratory volume in 1 sec/forced vital capacity.

strength, efficiency of muscle use, and willingness to achieve maximum effort (114). To obviate these problems, we have "normalized" the change in Pa_{O_2} and $D(A\text{-}a)\ O_2$ during exercise (Figure 2) to the relative amount of work done. The latter is directly proportional to oxygen consumption ($\dot{V}O_2$), so we have used $\Delta PO_2/\Delta \dot{V}O_2$ and $\Delta(D[A\text{-}a]O_2)/\Delta \dot{V}O_2$ to correlate with the degree of fibrosis in open lung biopsy specimens. There is a significant correlation between both exercise variables and degree of fibrosis (Table 4), and thus these measurements are extremely useful in staging the degree of fibrosis in idiopathic pulmonary fibrosis. We have also used the $\Delta PO_2/\Delta \dot{V}O_2$ and $\Delta(D[A\text{-}a]O_2)/\Delta \dot{V}O_2$ obtained in serial exercise studies to follow several patients for more than 1.5 years; so far the data show that this quantitative approach to exercise physiology is a sensitive and objective method of following the temporal changes in the fibrotic process (Figure 6).

As we discussed earlier, the major cause of hypoxemia in idiopathic pulmonary fibrosis has been attributed to ventilation-perfusion imbalance (40). Because air flow mechanics ($FEV_1\%$, airway resistance by body plethysmography) are usually normal in these patients (38, 39, 111), the abnormalities in distribution of ventilation have been ascribed to regional alterations in compliance (39). However, in other diseases such as asthma, recent data suggest that small airways disease, undetectable by $FEV_1\%$ and plethysmography methods, can result in significant ventilation-perfusion mismatching that causes hypoxemia (137-139). Nevertheless, when tests of small airways function such as dynamic compliance (140), maximum expiratory flow-volume curves (141), and maximum flow-static recoil curves (115, 142) are used to evaluate patients with idiopathic pulmonary fibrosis, a significant number show abnormal results (143, 144) (Table 5). This physiologic evidence of small airway disease correlates well with the morphologic observations that the small airways in idiopathic pulmonary fibrosis have peribronchiolar fibrosis and inflammation and that 70% of the patients with this disease show narrowed airways (Table 3). The clear association of abnormal physiologic function of small airways with the morphologic evidence of disease of these airways suggests that at least part of the ventilation abnormalities, and hence hypoxemia, of idiopathic pulmonary fibrosis may be due to small airways disease.

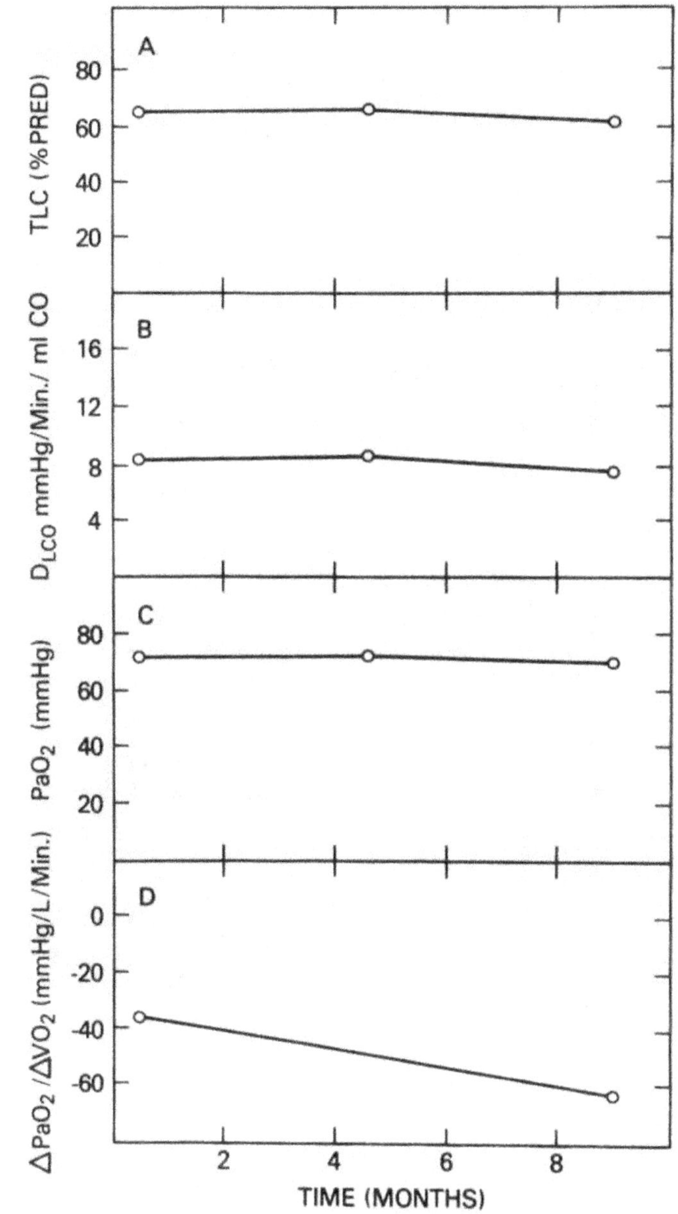

Figure 6. Temporal changes. **A.** In total lung capacity (*TLC*). **B.** In diffusing capacity (DLco). **C.** In resting oxygen tension (Po_2). **D.** Change in Pao_2 with exercise ($\Delta Pao_2/\Delta \dot{V}o_2$) in a 65-year-old woman with idiopathic pulmonary fibrosis. Over a 9-month period the patient developed progressive exertional breathlessness. The only objective finding was a further decrease in the $\Delta Pao_2/\Delta \dot{V}o_2$ on serial exercise testing.

Nuclear Scanning in Idiopathic Pulmonary Fibrosis

Dr. Bruce R. Line*: Nuclear scanning methods are useful in evaluating a chronic lung disorder such as idiopathic pulmonary fibrosis. Isotopic methods provide information about regional pulmonary function in terms of temporal and spatial tracer distribution images, in contrast to the static structural data provided by the standard chest X ray.

Three nuclear scanning methods are being used to study idiopathic pulmonary fibrosis: macroaggregated albumin labeled with technetium-99m (Tc-99m MAA) to evaluate lung perfusion; xenon-133 (^{133}Xe) or xenon-127 (^{127}Xe)† gas to evaluate ventilatory function; and gallium-67 citrate (^{67}Ga) to quantitate lung inflammation and hence the "alveolitis" of the disease.

The pulmonary capillary bed effectively filters particulate matter greater than 10 μm in diameter. After intravenous injection, particles of Tc-99m MAA (10 to 50 μm) mix with the right ventricular blood pool and are trapped in the pulmonary microcirculation. This microembolization produces little hemodynamic stress because fewer than one in 2000 capillaries are occluded (145, 146). The albumin particles are broken down and later consumed by the pulmonary reticuloendothelial system. The scintigraphic image obtained just after injection reflects the distribution of the

* Research Analyst, Division of Computer Research and Technology, and Clinical Associate, Department of Nuclear Medicine, Clinical Center.

† The recent availability of ^{127}Xe has resulted in a significant improvement in the quality of ventilation scans.

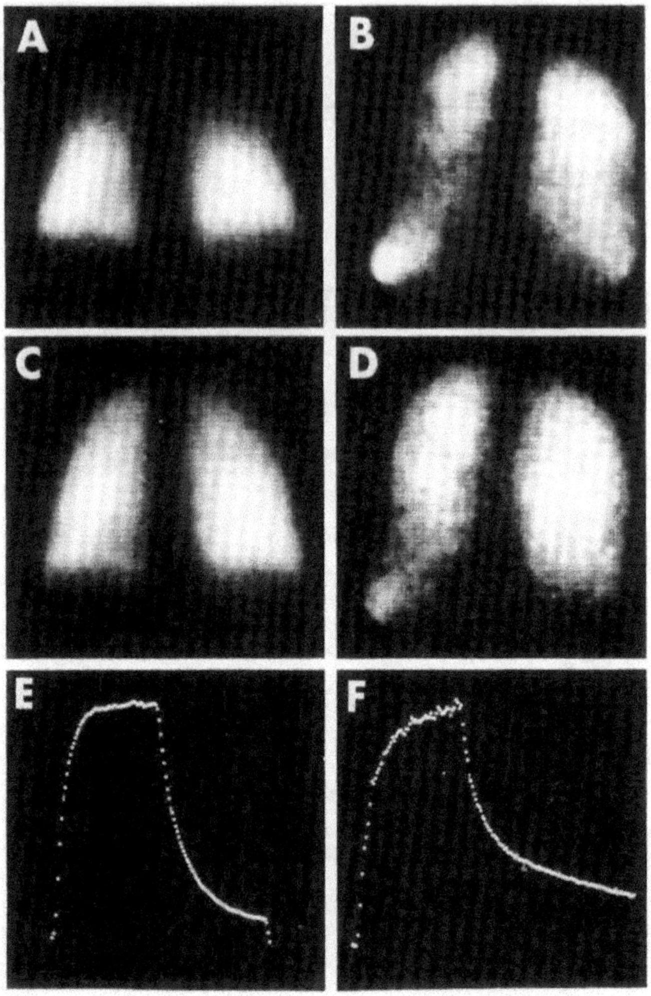

Figure 7. Perfusion and ventilation scans in a normal 57-year-old man (*A, C, E*) and a 48-year-old man with idiopathic pulmonary fibrosis (*B, D, F*). **A.** Normal perfusion scan with basal tracer prominence. **B.** Idiopathic pulmonary fibrosis perfusion scan; inhomogeneous pattern with marked upward shift. **C.** Normal equilibrium phase ventilation scan. **D.** Idiopathic pulmonary fibrosis equilibrium phase ventilation scan showing decreased tracer in the lower lung zones. **E.** Full thorax count profile of ventilation study showing normal wash-in, equilibrium, and wash-out phases. **F.** Rounded profile in idiopathic pulmonary fibrosis suggesting prolonged airspace time constants. The scans in A-D are all posterior views; the count profiles in E-F are also derived from posterior views.

right ventricular output. Because pulmonary blood flow is influenced by gravitational forces (147), a patient studied in the upright position normally shows little tracer in the upper lung zones with an increasing gradient of tracer intensity toward the lung base (Figure 7*A*). Excluding cardiac and diaphragmatic impressions, normal lung images show convex margins and have bilateral symmetry (148). Defects in tracer homogeneity may be related to a loss of capillary perfusion such as may accompany vasoconstriction in response to alveolar hypoxia (149) (pneumonia, asthma), parenchymal destruction (150) (idiopathic pulmonary fibrosis, emphysema), or pulmonary vascular occlusion (148) (embolic or thrombotic disease). Regional decreases in tracer localization may also be secondary to displacement of normal parenchyma by pleural fluid masses and bullae. In idiopathic pulmonary fibrosis, two basic findings appear in the perfusion scan: nonsegmental inhomogeneities and increased perfusion to the upper lung zones (Figure 7*B*).

These nonsegmental inhomogeneities are probably due to the localized loss of capillary bed and are usually seen in the lower lobes. Comparison of the chest X ray and the Tc-99m MAA scan shows correlation between areas of compromised perfusion and areas of reticular, reticulonodular, or ground glass densities, or a combination of these. Patients with idiopathic pulmonary fibrosis can also have nonsegmental inhomogeneities of the perfusion scan in radiographically normal areas, suggesting that a local deficit in capillary perfusion may be present before abnormalities are seen on the chest film.

Pulmonary hypertension has been associated with an upward shift in the gradient of capillary perfusion and a corresponding increase in apical tracer in upright perfusion images (110, 151). This has proven valuable in substantiating the diagnosis of pulmonary hypertension in patients with idiopathic pulmonary fibrosis.

The patency of airways and the functional integrity of alveoli can be assessed using the ventilation scan (152, 153). In comparison to the perfusion scan, which reflects the static distribution of macromolecules trapped in the pulmonary capillary bed, the ventilation scan is more complex, as it measures the dynamic bronchoalveolar distribution of a tracer gas. In the ventilation study, the patient rebreathes a mixture of tracer and air ("wash-in" phase) until the radioactivity measured over the chest stays constant ("equilibrium" phase). The patient then breathes room air until all of the radioactive gas leaves the lungs ("wash-out" phase).

The equilibrium picture of ^{127}Xe distribution reflects the relative proportion of lung that is being ventilated. For example, little radioactivity would be detected over areas of pneumonia or noncommunicating bullae. Patients with idiopathic pulmonary fibrosis have patchy, nonsegmental areas of decreased ventilation, reflecting regions of airway obstruction or alveolar destruction (Figures 7*C, D*). The equilibrium scintigraphs have been useful for detecting marginally functional parenchyma and indicating the presence of noncommunicating cysts or bullae in patients with idiopathic pulmonary fibrosis.

If the count rates over the lung fields are summed and plotted versus time, a curve is generated describing the rate of tracer accumulation or release from the lung. Patients with normal airways and alveoli will have a curve that is nearly "square," indicating rapid wash-in, flat equilibrium, and rapid wash-out phases (Figure 7*E*). With dysfunction of airways or alveoli, or both, the wash-in and wash-out phases are prolonged, so that the curve is rounded. About 70% of our patients showed a spectrum of abnormal curves, reflecting a slowness to come to equilibrium (Figure 7*F*). Regions of decreased compliance (for example, interstitial fibrosis) produce fast wash-in and wash-out phases. Therefore studies yielding prolonged phases indicate areas of increased compliance (such as the cystic areas of idiopathic pulmonary fibrosis) or airway dysfunction (such as the small airway disease of idiopathic pulmonary fibrosis).

The equilibrium phase (representing the total ventilated volume in each lung region) and the wash-out phase (representing the change in count rate per unit time in each region) may be combined to indicate the relative volume exchanged in each lung area per unit time (154, 155). This is computed in approximately one thousand small areas of the lung to generate a picture of dynamic regional ventilation. Whereas normal patients have homogeneous patterns of dynamic volume exchange, patients with idiopathic pulmonary fibrosis show disparity between lung zones, reflecting cystic areas or small airway disease (Figures 8*A* and *B*).

The data from the ventilation and perfusion scans can be combined to produce an image of the relative ventilation-perfusion ratio of each small region of the lung fields. In idiopathic pulmonary fibrosis, there is a general patchiness to the ventilation-perfusion matching throughout the lung. In addition, there is often a shift in perfusion to the upper lobes (reflecting pulmonary hypertension) so that areas of relatively low ventilation-perfusion ratios are seen in the upper zones (Figures 8*C* and *D*). This image has been used to estimate the proportion of regions with low ventilation-perfusion ratios such as functional shunt, as well as the proportion of areas of high ventilation-perfusion ratios such as areas of wasted ventilation. These findings support the concept that a significant portion of hypoxemia in patients with idiopathic pulmonary fibrosis is due to ventilation-perfusion mismatching (39, 40) and also confirm that the high dead space to tidal volume ratio found at rest in many of these patients (7, 12, 112) is well founded on anatomic grounds.

As discussed in the sections on the histology and radiology of idiopathic pulmonary fibrosis, alveolar inflammation is probably an early manifestation of the disease process. Whereas physiologic methods can detect the fibrotic process (coefficient of retraction, exercise $\Delta Po_2/\Delta \dot{V}o_2$), it has been extremely difficult to evaluate alveolar inflammation in this disease without resorting to repeated lung biopsies. Gallium-67 scanning has been investigated as a means to follow the alveolitis of idiopathic pulmonary fibrosis because studies have shown that this isotope localizes in regions of inflammation (156, 157). For example, ^{67}Ga will localize in the chest in disorders as diverse as pulmonary abscess, active tuberculosis, active sarcoidosis, silicosis, pleurisy, and bacterial pneumonia (158, 159). Although each condition varies in cause and histology, all are inflammatory disorders, and scan visualization gradually diminishes in intensity after appropriate therapy (156). Gallium-67 is used to detect and characterize the inflammation of idiopathic pulmonary fibrosis because it binds to neutrophils (probably in lysosomes) (157, 160), cells that are clearly found in the parenchyma in idiopathic pulmonary fibrosis.

Patients are scanned 48 to 72 h after the intravenous administration of 50 μCi of ^{67}Ga citrate/kg body weight. At the time of study, the tracer distributes primarily to liver, spleen, and skeletal tissues, with very little to normal lung (161,162). Sixty-seven percent of ^{67}Ga scans in patients with idiopathic pulmonary fibrosis showed increased pulmonary localization, whereas only 5% of control subjects showed an increase (163) (Figures 8*E* and *F*).

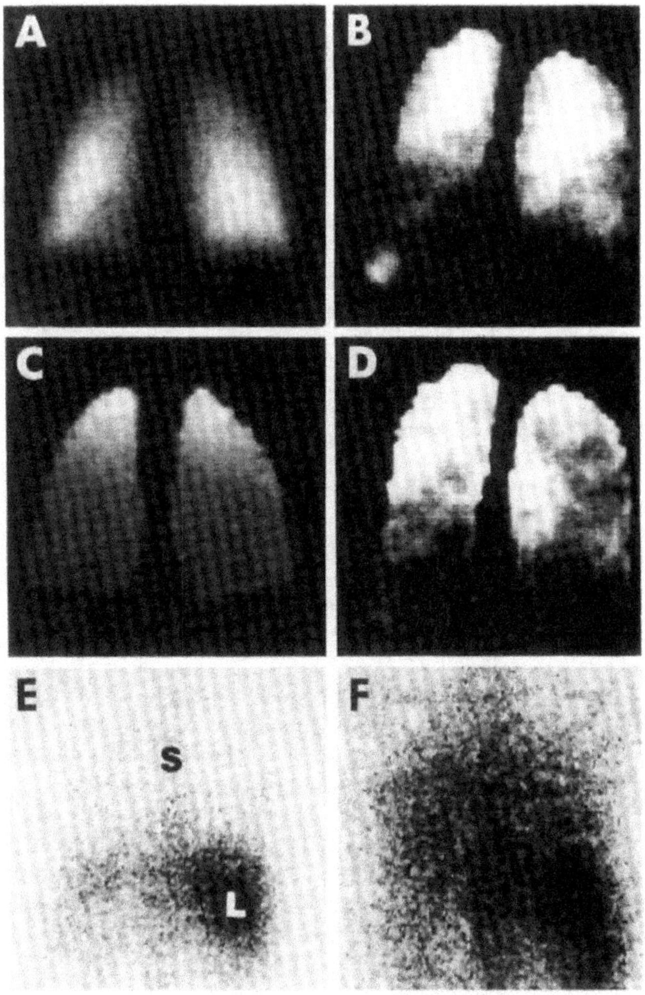

Figure 8. Dynamic ventilation, ventilation-perfusion, and gallium scans in a normal 57-year-old man (*A, C, E*) and a 48-year-old man with idiopathic pulmonary fibrosis (*B, D, F*). **A.** Normal dynamic ventilation; brighter regions indicate higher regional volume exchange per unit time. **B.** Idiopathic pulmonary fibrosis dynamic ventilation; patent but poorly ventilated basilar airspaces. **C.** Normal ventilation-perfusion ratio (V/Q) map; bright regions = high V/Q (relative dead space): gray = "good" V/Q match; dark = low V/Q (relative shunt). **D.** Same study as C but in idiopathic pulmonary fibrosis; there are patchy areas of high and low V/Q with fewer areas of "good" V/Q match compared with normal. **E.** Normal gallium scan; L= liver; S = spine; almost no gallium is taken up by normal parenchyma. **F.** Gallium scan in idiopathic pulmonary fibrosis showing prominent basilar tracer uptake, suggesting areas of active inflammation.

As a rule, interpretations of gallium scans are qualitative and include statements related to the presence and distribution of abnormal ^{67}Ga localization. It is difficult to quantitatively assess the degree of abnormality because of the wide spectrum of physiologic and technical influences on the ^{67}Ga image. However, by characterizing the percentage of lung involvement, the intensity of uptake, and the distribution of abnormalities, it is possible to rank the relative abnormality of gallium scans in idiopathic pulmonary fibrosis. Preliminary studies have shown that this quantitative assessment correlates well with the grading of alveolar and interstitial cellularity on open lung biopsy specimens of these patients. Thus the ^{67}Ga scan is a noninvasive, safe*, semiquantitative method of assessing the status of inflammation in idiopathic pulmonary fibrosis that may prove useful both in staging disease process and in evaluating the efficacy of treatment.

Bronchoalveolar Lavage in Idiopathic Pulmonary Fibrosis

Dr. Herbert Y. Reynolds†: One of the major limitations to understanding the pathogenesis of idiopathic pulmonary fibrosis is the inability to obtain samples of the same lung at different stages of the disease. However, the advent of the flexible fiberoptic bronchoscope and its adaptation to bronchoalveolar lavage has made it possible to evaluate repeatedly a representative sample of the fluid bathing the bronchoalveolar epithelial surface (165-167). We have adapted this method to study patients with idiopathic pulmonary fibrosis in order to [1] describe the cellular and protein components of their lower respiratory tract; [2] evaluate possible immune mechanisms that may contribute to the pathogenesis and continued activity of the disease; [3] determine if the therapy of idiopathic pulmonary fibrosis alters these components; and [4] correlate the cellular analysis of bronchoalveolar lavage fluid with the histologic findings.

We studied the bronchoalveolar lavage fluid in 19 of our 29 patients. To put these findings in perspective, we compared them to findings in seven patients with chronic hypersensitivity pneumonitis and 32 control subjects.

In all of these studies, the amount of lavage fluid retrieved varied from 31% to 48%. From the patients with idiopathic pulmonary fibrosis, an average of 18 million cells were recovered, with almost two times more cells found in fluid from untreated patients than treated patients. Interestingly, patients with idiopathic pulmonary fibrosis who did not smoke had more cells than those who did smoke; this is opposite to that found in control subjects (smokers normally have more than two times the cells of nonsmokers) (165). In general, patients with idiopathic pulmonary fibrosis had more cells recovered than those with chronic hypersensitivity pneumonitis, who in turn had more cells recovered than controls.

The variety in the types of cells recovered in lavage clearly distinguished the different local cellular responses of idiopathic pulmonary fibrosis and chronic hypersensitivity pneumonitis from each other and from controls (Table 6) (168). In general, patients with idiopathic pulmonary fibrosis had significant evidence of inflammation of the lower respiratory tract (an average of 33% neutrophils). The finding of these numbers of neutrophils in the lower respiratory tract was striking, since neutrophils in control lavage always represent less than 3% of the total cells. With treatment, perhaps secondary to corticosteroids, bronchoalveolar inflammation in idiopathic pulmonary fibrosis diminished (average neutrophils reduced to 14%, $P < 0.05$). Also striking was the invariable presence of eosinophils, a cell type almost never found in controls (165). In contrast to the reduction of lavage neutrophils with therapy, corticosteroids did not seem to influence the eosinophilic response in patients with idiopathic pulmonary fibrosis. Because these patients do not have a peripheral leukocytosis or eosinophilia, the findings suggest a local cellular response in the fluid bathing the bronchoalveolar epithelial surface. This is further strengthened by a comparison of the cells of patients with idiopathic pulmonary fibrosis to those of patients with chronic hypersensitivity pneumonitis. Lavage fluid of the latter group has an average of five times more lymphocytes than found in idiopathic pulmonary fibrosis, and an average of three times more lymphocytes than in controls.

The cell differential on bronchoalveolar lavage fluid in both groups of patients seems to correlate well with the histologic findings on open lung biopsy. Our findings corroborate those of Davis and co-workers (169), who have found cell analysis to be an accurate indicator of the alveolar cellular content in idiopathic pulmonary fibrosis. In addition, the lavage differential in idiopathic pulmonary fibrosis can predict which patients will show positive ^{67}Ga scans; those with more neutrophils tend to have more positive ^{67}Ga scans (163), as would be predicted from the evidence that ^{67}Ga is localized to areas of inflammation.

Quantitative determination of immunoglobulins (165-167) can also distinguish patients with idiopathic pulmonary fibrosis from control subjects and from patients with chronic hypersensitivity pneumonitis (Table 6). Compared with controls, both groups of patients have elevated IgG. Decreased IgE is seen only in patients with idiopathic pulmonary fibrosis, and IgM is found only in patients with chronic hypersensitivity pneumonitis. Therapy of idiopathic pulmonary fibrosis seems to reduce the bronchoalveolar fluid IgG levels, just as it reduces the neutrophil levels.

Not only are the IgG levels in lavage fluid from patients with idiopathic pulmonary fibrosis greater than those of controls, they are also more than two times higher than one would expect from transudation of serum alone*. Thus, the disease is probably associated with the local production of IgG or abnormalities in the mechanisms of lung IgG catabolism, or both. Part of the pathogenesis of idiopathic pulmonary fibrosis may be secondary to lung injury from locally produced IgG antibody in response to one or more as yet unidentified antigens. There is no evidence, however, of local complement use, since lavage fluid C4 and C6 levels were normal in idiopathic pulmonary fibrosis (Table 6).

These findings, together with the lack of elevated IgE or decreased complement, suggest that in this disorder the lung may act as a relatively independent immune organ; the immune reactions in this disease probably are not mediated by complement; and idiopathic pulmonary fibrosis is probably not an allergic disorder mediated by IgE (171, 172).

We have shown that limited bronchoalveolar lavage is an important tool for characterizing and understanding pulmonary disorders such as idiopathic pulmonary fibrosis.

* The total body dose of ^{67}Ga ordinarily amounts to less than 300 mrad/mCi of administered material (164).

† Chief, Pulmonary Section, Department of Medicine, Yale University School of Medicine, New Haven, Connecticut; formerly, Head, Section of Bacterial Diseases, Laboratory of Clinical Investigation, National Institute of Allergy and Infectious Diseases.

* The most rational basis for comparison of lavage proteins is to albumin, a protein synthesized external to lung that leaks across the alveolus and thus is representative of serum transudation (165-167, 170).

We have done this procedure in more than 150 patients with all forms of pulmonary disease. It is a simple extension of routine fiberoptic bronchoscopy and is well tolerated by patients. Analysis of the cell and protein content of the recovered lavage fluid is a direct attempt to evaluate those mechanisms that may contribute to the continued activity of the chronic lung disorders. These methods may also prove useful in following the response to specific therapy.

Biochemical Concepts and Overall Perspective of Idiopathic Pulmonary Fibrosis

Dr. Crystal: To begin to understand the biochemical basis of idiopathic pulmonary fibrosis, we must try to define the biochemical components of the deranged alveolar interstitium. Fibrosis is a histologic term that refers to the light microscopic assessment of an apparent excess of collagen, the macromolecule that is the major component of scar tissue. From studies of normal lung, we know that the alveolar interstitium contains at least two (and probably more) forms of collagen, distinguished from each other by their different amino acid sequences. The two major forms of collagen in the alveolar interstitium are termed collagen type I and collagen type III (173-179). Type I is the characteristic fibrillar collagen found in skin, bone, tendon, blood vessels, and lung. Type III is probably reticulin and is found in skin, blood vessels, intestine, and lung but not in bone or tendon*. In the normal human lung parenchyma, the ratio of type I to type III collagen is approximately 2:1 (178).

With light microscopy, the concentration of collagen in lung tissue from patients with idiopathic pulmonary fibrosis appears to be significantly greater than normal. This, however, is not the case, and studies of open lung biopsy specimens clearly show that collagen per unit dry weight is normal (143, 182, 183). There are several possible explanations for this: [1] the common light microscopy stains for collagen probably identify only fibrillar collagen. It is possible that the sum of fibrillar plus nonfibrillar interstitial collagen in idiopathic pulmonary fibrosis is normal, but there is a shift toward fibrillar collagen, thus giving the appearance of a relative increase in interstitial collagen; [2] collagen may be increased, but other lung components also increase in proportion, so that collagen per unit weight is constant; and [3] idiopathic pulmonary fibrosis is a disease of collagen rearrangement (more in some areas than others) rather than a total increase in fibrotic tissue. As we will see, all three still remain viable alternatives.

In other fibrotic disorders such as atherosclerosis, the ratio of type I to type III collagen increases (184). A recent study (178) of postmortem lung suggested that this is also true in idiopathic pulmonary fibrosis. Although type III collagen can form cross-banded fibers, it also exists in a loose fibril form. Thus, a change in the I/III ratio toward type I (but with the sum of I + III constant) might give the appearance of an increase in interstitial collagen when evaluated by light microscopy. Analagous to this hypothesis is the finding that tissues that are relatively compliant (fetal skin, lung, intestine, blood vessels) have a low type I/type III ratio (185); tissues with less compliance (adult skin, atherosclerotic blood vessel) have a higher ratio of type I to type III (184-186); and tissues that are very rigid (bone, tendon) have only type I and no type III (185). The lung in idiopathic pulmonary fibrosis is less compliant (*see* Figure 2), so a shift toward type I in this disease is certainly in concert with the concept that "stiffness" in lung is associated with more type I collagen.

Biochemical studies have not yet been done to verify that interstitial components other than collagen increase in idiopathic pulmonary fibrosis; however, one has only to look at the biopsy of a patient to appreciate the vast cellularity of the disease (Figures 3*B* and *D*). This is important because it suggests that this is a disease not only of collagen, but of many other components as well (143).

The most difficult hypothesis to approach biochemically is the possibility that the major collagen-related problem in idiopathic pulmonary fibrosis is a derangement of the connective tissue components of the normal alveolar

Table 6. Cells and Relative Concentrations of Proteins in Bronchoalveolar Lavage Fluid of Patients with Idiopathic Pulmonary Fibrosis and Chronic Hypersensitivity Pneumonitis Compared to Controls*†

	Controls§	Idiopathic Pulmonary Fibrosis‡		Chronic Hypersensitivity Pneumonitis‖
		Without Therapy	With Therapy	
Cells**				
Neutrophils	0-3	I (3+)††	I (2+)	I (1+)
Lymphocytes	8-18	N	N	I (4+)
Eosinophils	0	I (1+)	I (1+)	I (1+)
Alveolar macrophages	80-89	D (3+)	D (1+)	D (4+)
Proteins‡‡				
IgG, *mg/mg*	0.1-0.6	I (2+)	I (1+)	I (3+)
IgE, *ng/mg*	10-65	D (1+)	D (1+)	N
IgA, *mg/mg*	0.2-1.9	N	N	N
IgM, *mg/mg*	0	A	A	I (2+)
C4, $\times 10^{-3}$ *titer/mg*	0.5-3.0	N	N	N
C6, *titer/mg*	1-9	N	N	N

*Lavage was always carried out by positioning the bronchoscope in the lingula (B4 or B5) and infusing 100 ml of sterile saline (30- to 40-ml aliquots, immediately aspirated by suction).

† The quantitative data in this table were derived from Reynolds et al, *J Clin Invest*, in press.

‡ Nineteen patients with idiopathic pulmonary fibrosis (12 nonsmokers, seven smokers; seven receiving no therapy, 12 receiving a mean dose of 24.4 ± 4.0 mg daily of prednisone).

§ Controls consisted of 32 patients (age and sex matched to the patients with idiopathic pulmonary fibrosis; 11 nonsmokers, 21 smokers) with undiagnosed lesions limited to the right upper lobe; none had evidence of disease in the left lung.

‖ Seven patients with chronic hypersensitivity pneumonitis had a history of chronic intermittent respiratory and systemic symptoms related to their home or work environment; five had antibodies to thermophylic actinomycetes; granulomas in lung histopathology and reexposure to probable antigens helped confirm the diagnoses.

** Data presented as percentage of total cells.

†† I = increased compared with controls; N = normal and equal to controls; D = decreased compared with controls; A = absent; relative changes are indicated as 1 + to 4 +.

‡‡ Data presented relative to the lavage fluid albumin concentration (*See* text and references 165-168, 170).

* Type I collagen is the cross-banded material typically seen on electron micrographs; it is most of the material in the normal alveolar interstitium that stains blue with Masson trichrome. Most of the fine loosely bound fibrils on electron micrographs are type III collagen; this material is the silver staining "reticulin" seen by light microscopy (180, 181).

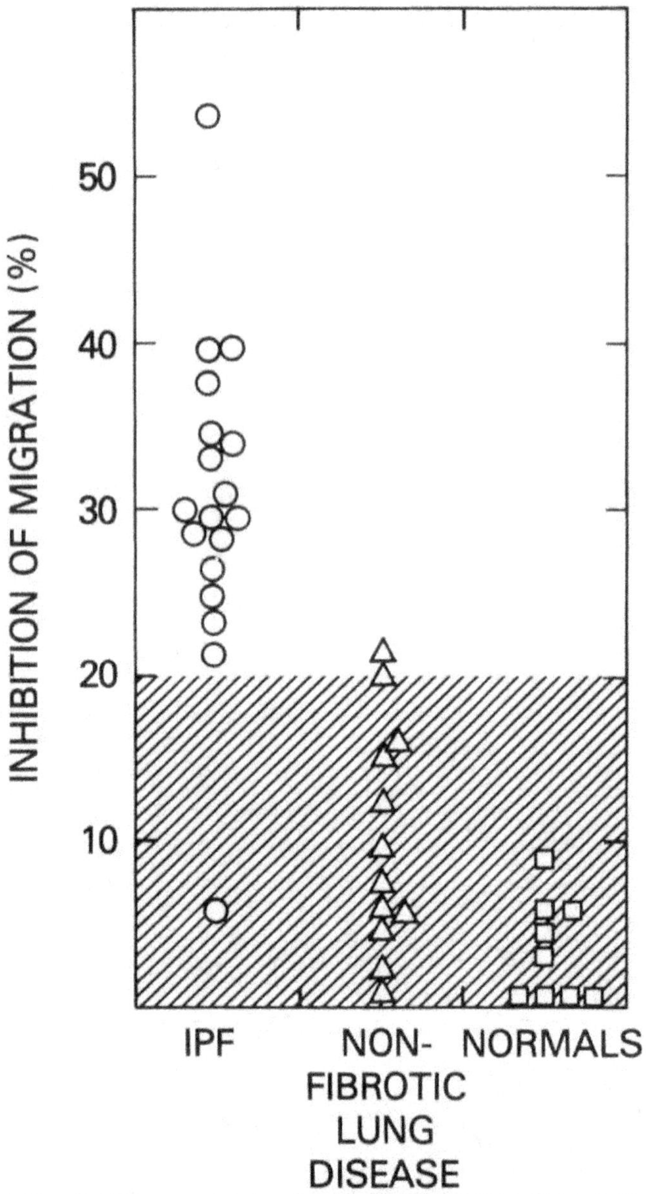

Figure 9. Collagen-induced production of migration inhibition factor by peripheral lymphocytes of patients with idiopathic pulmonary fibrosis. Lymphocytes were isolated from peripheral blood and exposed to 25 μg/ml of type I human lung collagen; production of migration inhibition factor was assayed using guinea pig peritoneal macrophages. Greater than 20% inhibition of migration was considered positive. Production of migration inhibition factor by lymphocytes of patients with idiopathic pulmonary fibrosis was completely obviated by exposing these lymphocytes to antihuman T-cell antiserum before incubation with the collagen antigen (187). Lymphocytes of patients with nonfibrotic lung disease seldom produce migration inhibition factor in response to collagen; lymphocytes of normal persons never do.

interstitium. We began by postulating that if collagen per unit weight was normal, perhaps it was turning over so rapidly that it would, by necessity, become deranged. To evaluate this, we quantitated the rate of collagen synthesis per cell in open lung biopsy specimens from our patients. However, in the eight biopsies evaluated thus far, the rate of collagen synthesis per cell (13.4 ± 2.6 μg of collagen/cell · h) is not significantly different from normal (15.9 ± 4.9 μg of collagen/cell · h) (143, 183). Thus, we have no evidence that collagen turns over more rapidly in idiopathic pulmonary fibrosis than normal.

As another, but much more indirect, approach to the question of derangement of the connective tissue in the idiopathic pulmonary fibrosis alveolar interstitium, we hypothesized that a derangement of collagen in the alveolar interstitium might result in the recognition of collagen as antigenic by the immune system. In studies in collaboration with Kravis and associates of the Navy Medical Research Institute (187), we showed that more than 95% of patients with idiopathic pulmonary fibrosis have circulating lymphocytes that produce lymphokines (migration inhibition factor) when exposed to type I collagen (Figure 9). In addition, these circulating lymphocytes will lyse collagen-coated erythrocytes. Studies with antihuman T-cell antiserum showed that these cell-mediated phenomena require viable T-cells to show these effects. These experiments indirectly suggest that collagen has become "non-self" in patients with idiopathic pulmonary fibrosis, a possible result of the anatomic derangement of the alveolar interstitium. These findings also suggest that a possible pathogenic mechanism in idiopathic pulmonary fibrosis is the continued injury to the alveolar interstitium by secretory products of cells such as macrophages that aggregate to sites of alveolar inflammation by collagen-induced cell-mediated immune phenomena.

However, the finding that collagen becomes antigenic to persons with idiopathic pulmonary fibrosis does not answer the question as to what triggers the disease. Perhaps clues to future studies lie in the historical information from patients with the disease, 25% to 40% of whom clearly relate that their disease began after a viral syndrome accompanied by chest symptoms. This, together with the reported familial clusterings of idiopathic pulmonary fibrosis (188-194), and our recent finding* of relative increases in HLA-12 and HLA-29 in patients with no family history of the disorder suggest that there may be predispositions to the disease, perhaps associated with cell surface antigens that could be altered by lung injury.

Regardless of the trigger of idiopathic pulmonary fibrosis, we now have several lines of evidence that strongly suggest that therapeutic intervention should be directed toward stopping the inflammatory and immune process, rather than toward stopping the fibrotic process.

1. Histologic observations clearly show that early aspects of the disease are highly cellular, with alveolar inflammation predominating. This concurs with the suggestion by Scadding and Hinson (18) that patients with "cellular" biopsies respond better to corticosteroids than those with late stages of fibrosis, and the suggestion by Carrington and co-workers (195) that patients with "desquamative interstitial pneumonitis" (that is, early idiopathic pulmonary fibrosis) also respond better to therapy.

2. The radiographic features of the disease suggest inflammation early in the course, fibrosis later.

3. The uptake of ^{67}Ga by 67% of these patients strongly suggests the lung parenchyma has areas of active neutrophilic inflammation.

---

* Fulmer JD, Spasovska M, Mittal K, et al: Unpublished.

4. Bronchoalveolar lavage in these patients shows elevated levels of neutrophils and IgG.

5. There is clear evidence of T-cell-mediated processes directed against collagen in this disease (187).

6. There is no evidence of increased amounts of collagen or increased rates of collagen synthesis in the lung parenchyma of patients with idiopathic pulmonary fibrosis (143, 182, 183).

Thus, we have an ongoing study to attempt to intervene in the abnormal inflammatory and immune processes in idiopathic pulmonary fibrosis (112). All patients are treated with standard levels of corticosteroids (prednisone daily dose: initially 1 mg/kg for 6 weeks, decreased by 0.05 mg /kg · week until 0.25 mg/kg is reached), and, in a double-blind fashion, 50% of the patients also receive azathioprine (daily dose: 2.5 mg/kg). These patients are being followed at 3-month intervals with routine studies and, more importantly, with exercise studies to follow the fibrotic process; bronchoalveolar lavage to follow inflammatory cells and IgG levels; ^{67}Ga scans to follow inflammation; ventilation-perfusion studies to follow the status of the capillary bed, cystic lesions, and small airways; and dynamic compliance, maximum expiratory flow-volume curves, and maximum flow-static recoil curves to follow the status of the small airways.

In summary, this multidisciplinary approach to evaluating the same set of patients with idiopathic pulmonary fibrosis has allowed us to make inroads into the pathogenesis, diagnosis, pathophysiology, and therapy of this disorder. Most importantly, it has enabled us to define idiopathic pulmonary fibrosis as a characteristic and specific disease entity. Rather than a clinical diagnosis of exclusion, idiopathic pulmonary fibrosis has a clear set of criteria that distinguish it from other disorders. It is a disease that has protean manifestations to those affected, and all indications are that if therapy is to be successful early diagnosis and treatment are essential.

ACKNOWLEDGMENTS: Received 3 September 1976; accepted 7 October 1976.

► Requests for reprints should be addressed to Ronald G. Crystal, M.D.; Chief, Pulmonary Branch, National Heart, Lung, and Blood Institute, National Institutes of Health; Bethesda, MD 20014.

References

1. Hamman L, Rich AR: Fulminating diffuse interstitial fibrosis of the lungs. *Trans Am Clin Climatol Assoc* 51:154-163, 1935
2. Hamman L, Rich AR: Acute diffuse interstitial fibrosis of the lungs. *Bull Johns Hopkins Hosp* 74:177-212, 1944
3. Rubin EH, Lubliner R: The Hamman-Rich syndrome: review of the literature and analysis of 15 cases. *Medicine* 36: 397-463, 1957
4. Mitchum WR, Brady BM: Differential diagnosis of fibrosing lung lesions. *Radiology* 68:36-47, 1957
5. Anderson AE Jr, Foraker AG: Morphological aspects of interstitial pulmonary fibrosis. *Arch Pathol* 70:79-93, 1960
6. Scadding JG: Chronic diffuse interstitial fibrosis of the lungs. *Br Med J* 1:443-450, 1960
7. Holland RAB: Physiologic dead space in the Hamman-Rich syndrome. Physiologic and clinical implications. *Am J Med* 28:61-68, 1960
8. Gross P: The concept of the Hamman-Rich syndrome. A critique. *Am Rev Respir Dis* 85:828-832, 1962
9. Nahmias BB, Churchwell AG, Bowles FN: Diffuse interstitial pulmonary fibrosis (Hamman-Rich syndrome). *Am J Med* 31:154-162, 1961
10. Doctor L, Snider GL: Diffuse interstitial pulmonary fibrosis associated with arthritis. With comments on the definition of rheumatoid lung disease. *Am Rev Respir Dis* 85:413-422, 1962
11. Muschenheim C: Some observations on the Hamman-Rich disease. *Am J Med Sci* 241:279-288, 1961
12. Herbert FA, Nahmias BB, Gaensler EA, et al: Pathophysiology of interstitial pulmonary fibrosis. Report of 19 cases and follow-up with corticosteroids. *Arch Intern Med* 110:628-648, 1962
13. Livingstone JL, Lewis JG, Reid L, et al: Diffuse interstitial pulmonary fibrosis. *Q J Med* 33:71-103, 1964
14. Stack BHR, Grant IWB, Irvine WJ, et al: Idiopathic diffuse interstitial lung disease. *Am Rev Respir Dis* 92:939-948, 1965
15. Liebow AA, Steer A, Billingsley JG: Desquamative interstitial pneumonia. *Am J Med* 39:369-404, 1965
16. Gaensler EA, Goff AM, Prowse CM: Desquamative interstitial pneumonia. *N Engl J Med* 274:113-128, 1966
17. Marks A: Diffuse interstitial pulmonary fibrosis. *Med Clin North Amer* 51:439-457, 1967
18. Scadding JG, Hinson KFW: Diffuse fibrosing alveolitis (diffuse interstitial fibrosis of the lungs). *Thorax* 22:291-304, 1967
19. Spencer H: Interstitial pneumonia. *Annu Rev Med* 18:423-442, 1967
20. Spencer H: Chronic interstitial pneumonia, in *The Lung*, edited by Liebow AA, Smith DE. Baltimore, Williams & Wilkins, 1968, pp. 134-150
21. Liebow AA: New concepts and entities in pulmonary disease, in *The Lung*, edited by Liebow AA, Smith DE. Baltimore, Williams & Wilkins, 1968, pp. 332-365
22. Liebow AA, Carrington CB: Alveolar diseases. The interstitial pneumonias, in *Frontiers of Pulmonary Radiology*, edited by Simon M. New York, Grune & Stratton, 1967, pp. 102-141
23. Parr LH: Hamman-Rich syndrome. Idiopathic pulmonary interstitial fibrosis of the lung. *J Natl Med Assoc* 61:8-12, 1969
24. Hinson KFW: Diffuse pulmonary fibrosis. *Hum Pathol* 1: 275-288, 1970
25. DeRemee RA, Harrison EG Jr, Anderson HA: The concept of classical interstitial pneumonitis-fibrosis (CIP-F) as a clinicopathologic syndrome. *Chest* 61:213-220, 1972
26. Stack HR, Choo-Kang YFJ, Heard BE: The prognosis of cryptogenic fibrosing alveolitis. *Thorax* 27:535-542, 1972
27. McCombs RP: Diseases due to immunologic reactions in the lungs. *N Engl J Med* 286:1186-1194, 1972
28. Fraire AE, Greenberg SD, O'Neal RM, et al: Diffuse interstitial fibrosis of the lung. *Am J Clin Pathol* 59:636-647, 1973
29. Patchefsky AS, Israel HL, Hoch WS, et al: Desquamative interstitial pneumonia: relationship to interstitial fibrosis. *Thorax* 28:680-693, 1973
30. Scadding JG: Diffuse pulmonary alveolar fibrosis. *Thorax* 29: 271-281, 1974
31. Dill J, Ghose T, Landrigan P, et al: Cryptogenic fibrosing alveolitis. *Chest* 67:411-416, 1975
32. Rankin J, Chester EH: Diffuse interstitial diseases of the lung as a cause of pulmonary insufficiency. The alveolar-capillary block syndrome, in *Textbook of Pulmonary Disease*, edited by Baum GL. Boston, Little, Brown and Co., 1974, pp. 609-645
33. Tukiainen P: Needle biopsy in diffuse lung manifestations. An analysis of 145 consecutive cases. *Scand J Respir Dis [Suppl]* 94:1-110, 1975
34. Liebow AA: Definition and classification of interstitial pneumonias in human pathology, in *Progress in Respiration Research, vol. 8. Alveolar Interstitium of the Lung. Pathological and Physiological Aspects*, edited by Basset F, Georges R. New York, Karger, 1975, pp. 1-33
35. Heard BE: Pathology of interstitial lung diseases, with particular reference to terminology, classification and trephine lung biopsy. *Chest* 69(suppl):252-253, 1976
36. Diamond I: The Hamman-Rich syndrome in childhood. *Pediatrics* 22:279-288, 1958
37. Weingärtner L: [Diffuse interstitial progressive pulmonary fibrosis in childhood.] (Germ.) *Dtsch Med Wochenschr* 90: 511-516, 1965
38. Austrian R, McClement JH, Renzetti AD Jr, et al: Clinical and physiologic features of some types of pulmonary diseases with impairment of alveolar-capillary diffusion. The syndrome of "alveolar-capillary block." *Am J Med* 11:667-685, 1951
39. Finley TN, Swenson EW, Comroe JH Jr: The cause of arterial hypoxemia at rest in patients with "alveolar-capillary block syndrome." *J Clin Invest* 41:618-622, 1962
40. Wagner PD, Dantzker DR, Dueck R, et al: Distribution of ventilation-perfusion ratios in patients with interstitial lung disease. *Chest* 69 (suppl):256-257, 1976
41. Cudkowicz L, Madoff IM, Abelmann WH: Rheumatoid lung

disease. A case report which includes respiratory function studies and a lung biopsy. *Br J Dis Chest* 55:35-40, 1961
42. Tomasi TB Jr, Fudenberg HH, Finby N: Possible relationship of rheumatoid factors and pulmonary disease. *Am J Med* 33:243-248, 1962
43. Talbot JA, Calkins E: Pulmonary involvement in rheumatoid arthritis. *JAMA* 189(12):911-913, 1964
44. Brannan HM, Good A, Divertie MB, et al: Pulmonary disease associated with rheumatoid arthritis. *JAMA* 189(12): 914-918, 1964
45. Patterson CD, Harville WE, Pierce JA: Rheumatoid lung disease. *Ann Intern Med* 62:685-697, 1965
46. Petty TL, Wilkins M: The five manifestations of rheumatoid lung. *Dis Chest* 49:75-82, 1966
47. Walker WC, Wright V: Pulmonary lesions and rheumatoid arthritis. *Medicine* 47:501-520, 1968
48. Scadding JG: The lungs in rheumatoid arthritis. *Proc R Soc Med* 62:227-238, 1969
49. Popper MS, Bogdonoff ML, Hughes RL: Interstitial rheumatoid lung disease. A reassessment and review of the literature. *Chest* 62:243-250, 1972
50. Frank ST, Weg JG, Harkleroad LE, et al: Pulmonary dysfunction in rheumatoid disease. *Chest* 63:27-34, 1973
51. Gordon DA, Stein JL, Broder I: The extra-articular features of rheumatoid arthritis. A systematic analysis of 127 cases. *Am J Med* 54:445-452, 1973
52. Ellman P, Cudkowicz L: Pulmonary manifestations in the diffuse collagen diseases. *Thorax* 9:46-57, 1954
53. Sullivan MA, Miller DK: Pulmonary manifestations in collagen disease. *Arch Intern Med* 110:769-787, 1962
54. Divertie MB: Lung involvement in the connective-tissue disorders. *Med Clin N Am* 48(4):1015-1030, 1964
55. Huang CT, Lyons HA: Comparison of pulmonary function in patients with systemic lupus erythematosus, scleroderma, and rheumatoid arthritis. *Am Rev Respir Dis* 93:865-875, 1966
56. Laitinen O, Salorinne Y, Poppius H: Respiratory function in systemic lupus erythematosus, scleroderma, and rheumatoid arthritis. *Ann Rheum Dis* 32:531-535, 1973
57. Spain DM, Thomas AG: The pulmonary manifestations of scleroderma. An anatomic-physiological correlation. *Ann Intern Med* 32:152-161, 1950
58. Adhikari PK, Bianchi FA, Boushy SF, et al: Pulmonary function in scleroderma. Its relation to changes in the chest roentgenogram and in the skin of the thorax. *Annu Rev Respir Dis* 86:823-831, 1963
59. Wilson RJ, Rodnan GP, Robin ED: An early pulmonary physiologic abnormality in progressive systemic sclerosis (diffuse scleroderma). *Am J Med* 36:361-369, 1964
60. Masi AT, D'Angelo WA: Epidemiology of fatal systemic sclerosis (diffuse scleroderma). A 15-year survey in Baltimore. *Ann Intern Med* 66:870-883, 1967
61. DeMuth GR, Furstenburg NA, Dabich L, et al: Pulmonary manifestations of progressive systemic sclerosis. *Am J Med Sci* 255:94-104, 1968
62. D'Angelo WA, Fries JF, Masi AT, et al: Pathologic observations in systemic sclerosis (scleroderma). A study of fifty-eight autopsy cases and fifty-eight matched controls. *Am J Med* 46:428-440, 1969
63. Medsger TA Jr, Masi AT, Rodnan GP, et al: Survival with systemic sclerosis (scleroderma). A life-table analysis of clinical and demographic factors in 309 patients. *Ann Intern Med* 75:369-376, 1971
64. Colp CR, Riker J, Williams MH Jr: Serial changes in scleroderma and idiopathic interstitial lung disease. *Arch Intern Med* 132:506-515, 1973
65. Grace WJ, Kennedy RJ, Formato A: Therapy of scleroderma and dermatomyositis. *NY State J Med* 63:140-144, 1963
66. Brundin A: Pulmonary fibrosis in scleroderma and dermatomyositis. *Scand J Respir Dis* 51:160-170, 1970
67. Goldfischer J, Rubin EH: Dermatomyositis with pulmonary lesions. *Ann Intern Med* 50:194-206, 1959
68. Medsger TA Jr, Robinson H, Masi AT: Factors affecting survivorship in polymyositis. *Arthritis Rheum* 14:249-258, 1971
69. Sandbank M, Grunebaum M, Katzenellenbogen I: Dermatomyositis associated with subacute pulmonary fibrosis. *Arch Dermatol* 94:432-435, 1966
70. Pearson CM: Polymyositis. *Annu Rev Med* 17:63-82, 1966
71. Weaver AL, Brundage BH, Nelson RA, et al: Pulmonary involvement in polymyositis: report of a case with response to corticosteroid therapy. *Arthritis Rheum* 11:765-773, 1968
72. Bohan A, Peter JB: Polymyositis and Dermatomyositis. *N Engl J Med* 292:344-347, 403-407, 1975
73. Thompson PL, Mackay IR: Fibrosing alveolitis and polymyositis. *Thorax* 25:504-507, 1970
74. Thompson JE: Lung involvement in polymyositis. *Med J Aust* 1:1332-1333, 1971
75. Webb DR, Currie GD: Pulmonary fibrosis masking polymyositis. *JAMA* 222:1146-1149, 1972
76. Camp AV, Lane DJ, Mowat AG: Dermatomyositis with parenchymal lung involvement. *Br Med J* 1:155-156, 1972
77. Olsen GN, Swenson EW: Polymyositis and interstitial lung disease. *Am Rev Respir Dis* 105:611-617, 1972
78. Frazier AR, Miller RD: Interstitial pneumonitis in association with polymyositis and dermatomyositis. *Chest* 65:403-407, 1974
79. Duncan PE, Griffin JP, Garcia A, et al: Fibrosing alveolitis in polymyositis. A review of histologically confirmed cases. *Am J Med* 57:621-626, 1974
80. Schwarz MI, Matthay RA, Sahn SA, et al: Interstitial lung disease in polymyositis and dermatomyositis: analysis of six cases and review of the literature. *Medicine* 55:89-104, 1976
81. Hoffbrand BI, Beck ER: "Unexplained" dyspnoea and shrinking lungs in systemic lupus erythematosus. *Br Med J* 1:1273-1277, 1965
82. Huang C, Hennigar GR, Lyons HA: Pulmonary dysfunction in systemic lupus erythematosus. *N Engl J Med* 272:288-293, 1965
83. Gold WM, Jennings DB: Pulmonary function in patients with systemic lupus erythematosus. *Am Rev Respir Dis* 93:556-567, 1966
84. Gross M, Esterly JR, Earle RH: Pulmonary alterations in systemic lupus erythematosus. *Am Rev Respir Dis* 105:572-577, 1972
85. Eisenberg H, Dubois EL, Sherwin RP, et al: Diffuse interstitial lung disease in systemic lupus erythematosus. *Ann Intern Med* 79:37-45, 1973
86. Mackay IR, Ritchie B: Diffuse fibrosing alveolitis (diffuse interstitial fibrosis of the lungs): two cases with autoimmune features. *Thorax* 20:200-205, 1965
87. Gottlieb AJ, Spiera H, Teirstein AS, et al: Serologic factors in idiopathic diffuse interstitial pulmonary fibrosis. *Am J Med* 39:405-410, 1965
88. Turner-Warwick M, Doniach D: Auto-antibody studies in interstitial pulmonary fibrosis. *Br Med J* 1:886-891, 1965
89. Hobbs JR, Turner-Warwick M: Assay of circulating immunoglobins in patients with fibrosing alveolitis. *Clin Exp Immunol* 2:645-652, 1967
90. Nagaya H, Buckley CE III, Sieker HO: Positive antinuclear factor in patients with unexplained pulmonary fibrosis. *Ann Intern Med* 70:1135-1145, 1969
91. Turner-Warwick M, Haslam P: Antibodies in some chronic fibrosing lung diseases. I. Non-organ-specific antibodies. *Clin Allergy* 1:83-95, 1971
92. Turner-Warwick M, Haslam P: Antibodies in some chronic fibrosing lung diseases. II. Immunofluorescent studies. *Clin Allergy* 1:209-219, 1971
93. Nagaya H, Sieker HO: Pathogenic mechanisms of interstitial pulmonary fibrosis in patients with serum antinuclear factor. A histologic and clinical correlation. *Am J Med* 52:51-62, 1972
94. DeHoratius RJ, Abruzzo JL, Williams RC Jr: Immunofluorescent and immunologic studies of rheumatoid lung. *Arch Intern Med* 129:441-446, 1972
95. Nagaya H, Elmore M, Ford CD: Idiopathic interstitial pulmonary fibrosis. An immune complex disease? *Am Rev Respir Dis* 107:826-830, 1973
96. Kang KY, Yagura T, Sera Y, et al: Antinuclear factor in pneumoconioses and idiopathic pulmonary fibrosis. *Med J Osaka Univ* 23:249-256, 1973
97. Turner-Warwick M: Immunologic aspects of systemic diseases of the lungs. *Proc R Soc Med* 67:541-547, 1974
98. Haslam P, Turner-Warwick M, Lukoszek A: Antinuclear antibody and lymphocyte responses to nuclear antigens in patients with lung disease. *Clin Exp Immunol* 20:379-395, 1975
99. Rodnan GP, McEwen C, Wallace SL, editors: *Primer on the Rheumatic Diseases, Seventh Edition.* New York, The Arthritis Foundation, 1973, pp. 1-152
100. Winkelmann RK: Classification and pathogenesis of scleroderma. *Mayo Clin Proc* 46:83-91, 1971
101. Snider GL: Case records of the Massachusetts General Hospital. *N Engl J Med* 293:136-143, 1975
102. Rose GA, Spenser H: Polyarteritis nodosa. *Q J Med* 26:43-81, 1957
103. Wolff SM, Fauci AS, Horn RG, et al: Wegener's granulomatosis. *Ann Intern Med* 81:513-525, 1974
104. Davies D: Ankylosing spondylitis and lung fibrosis. *Q J Med* 41:395-417, 1972

105. MENDLOWITZ M: Clubbing and hypertrophic osteoarthropathy. *Medicine* 21:269-306, 1942
106. CUDKOWICZ L, WRAITH DG: An evaluation of the clinical significance of clubbing in common lung disorders. *Br J Tuberc* 51:14-31, 1957
107. BALCERZAK SP, BROMBERG PA: Secondary polycythemia. *Semin Hematol* 12:353-382, 1975
108. TURNER-WARWICK M: Fibrosing alveolitis and chronic liver disease. *Q J Med* 37:133-149, 1968
109. HAMER J: Cause of low arterial oxygen saturation in pulmonary fibrosis. *Thorax* 19:507-514, 1964
110. MCCARTHY D, CHERNIACK RM: Regional ventilation-perfusion and hypoxia in cryptogenic fibrosing alveolitis. *Am Rev Respir Dis* 107:200-208, 1973
111. BACHOFEN H, SCHERRER M: Lung tissue resistance in diffuse interstitial pulmonary fibrosis. *J Clin Invest* 46:133-140, 1967
112. FULMER JD, ROBERTS WC, CRYSTAL RG: Diffuse fibrotic lung disease: a correlative study. *Chest* 69(suppl):263-265, 1975
113. JONES NL, MCHARDY GJR, NAIMARK A, et al: Physiological dead space and alveolar-arterial gas pressure differences during exercise. *Clin Sci* 31:19-29, 1966
114. WASSERMAN K, WHIPP BJ: Exercise physiology in health and disease. *Am Rev Respir Dis* 112:219-249, 1975
115. MACKLEM PT: New tests to assess lung function. *N Engl J Med* 293:339-342, 1975
116. MACKLEM PT, BECKLAKE MR: The relationship between the mechanical and diffusing properties of the lung in health and disease. *Am Rev Respir Dis* 87:47-56, 1963
117. BACHOFEN M, WEIBEL ER: Basic pattern of tissue repair in human lungs following unspecific injury. *Chest* 65 (suppl):14S-19S, 1974
118. KUHN C: The cells of the lung and their organelles, in *The Biochemical Basis of Pulmonary Function,* edited by CRYSTAL RG. New York, Dekker, Marcel, Inc., 1976, pp. 3-48
119. CLEMENTS JA, KING RJ: Composition of the surface active material, in *The Biochemical Basis of Pulmonary Function,* edited by CRYSTAL RG. New York, Dekker, Marcel, Inc., 1976, pp. 363-387
120. SHORTLAND JR, DARKE CS, CRANE WAJ: Electron microscopy of desquamative interstitial pneumonia. *Thorax* 24:192-208, 1969
121. BASSET F, SOLER P, BERNAUBIN JF, et al: Contribution of electron microscopy to the study of interstitial pneumonias, in *Progress in Respiration Research, vol. 8. Alveolar Interstitium of the Lung, International Symposium,* edited by BASSET F, GEORGES R. New York, Karger, 1975, pp. 45-58
122. FARR GH, HARLEY RA, HENNIGAR GR: Desquamative interstitial pneumonia. An electron microscopic study. *Am J Pathol* 60:347-354, 1970
123. BREWER BD, HEATH D, ASQUITH P: Electron microscopy of desquamative interstitial pneumonia. *J Path* 97:317-323, 1969
124. GLANCY DL, FRAZIER PD, ROBERTS WC: Pulmonary parenchymal cholesterol-ester granulomas in patients with pulmonary hypertension. *Am J Med* 45:198-210, 1968
125. DAVIES D, MACFARLANE A, DARKE CS, et al: Muscular hyperplasia ("cirrhosis") of the lung and bronchial dilations as features of chronic diffuse fibrosing alveolitis. *Thorax* 21:272-289, 1966
126. KAPANCI Y, ASSIMACOPOULOS A, IRLE C, et al: "Contractile interstitial cells" in pulmonary alveolar septa: a possible regulator of ventilation/perfusion ratio? Ultrastructural, immunofluorescence, and *in vitro* studies. *J Cell Biol* 60:375-392, 1974
127. SEAL RME, HAPKE EJ, THOMAS GO, et al: The pathology of the acute and chronic stages of farmer's lung. *Thorax* 23:469-489, 1968
128. RÜTTNER JR, SPYCHER MA, STICHER H: The detection of etiologic agents in interstitial pulmonary fibrosis. *Hum Pathol* 4:497-512, 1973
129. WINKELMANN RK, DITTO WB: Cutaneous and visceral syndromes of necrotizing or "allergic" angiitis: a study of 38 cases. *Medicine* 43:59-89, 1964
130. THEROS EG: The value of radiologic-pathologic correlation in the education of the radiologist. *Am J Roentgenol* 107:235-257, 1969
131. JOHNSON TH JR: Radiology and honeycomb lung disease. *Am J Roentgenol* 104:810-821, 1968
132. GENEREUX GP: The end-stage lung. *Radiology* 116:279-289, 1975
133. BENSON MK, HUGHES DT: Serial pulmonary function tests in fibrosing alveolitis. *Br J Dis Chest* 66:33-44, 1972
134. BROWN CH, TURNER-WARWICK M: The treatment of cryptogenic fibrosing alveolitis with immunosuppressant drugs. *Q J Med* 40:289-302, 1971
135. SCHLUETER DP, IMMEKUS J, STEAD WW: Relationship between maximal inspiratory pressure and total lung capacity (coefficient of retraction) in normal subjects and in patients with emphysema, asthma, and diffuse pulmonary infiltration. *Am Rev Respir Dis* 96:656-665, 1967
136. TURNER JM, MEAD J, WOHL ME: Elasticity of human lungs in relation to age. *J Appl Physiol* 25:664-671, 1968
137. MCFADDEN ER JR, LYONS HA: Airway resistance and uneven ventilation in bronchial asthma. *J Appl Physiol* 25:365-370, 1968
138. HILL DJ, LANDAU LI, PHELAN PD: Small airway disease in asymptomatic asthmatic adolescents. *Am Rev Respir Dis* 106: 873-880, 1972
139. HECKSCHER T, BASS H, ORIOL A, et al: Regional lung function in patients with bronchial asthma. *J Clin Invest* 47:1063-1070, 1968
140. WOOLCOCK AJ, VINCENT NJ, MACKLEM PT: Frequency dependence of compliance as a test for obstruction in the small airways. *J Clin Invest* 48:1097-1106, 1969
141. GELB AF, ZAMEL N: Simplified diagnosis of small-airway obstruction. *N Engl J Med* 288:395-398, 1973
142. MEAD J, TURNER JM, MACKLEM PT, et al: Significance of the relationship between lung recoil and maximum expiratory flow. *J Appl Physiol* 22:95-108, 1967
143. FULMER JD, CRYSTAL RG: The biochemical basis of pulmonary function, in *The Biochemical Basis of Pulmonary Function,* edited by CRYSTAL RG. New York, Dekker, Marcel, Inc., 1976, pp. 419-466
144. OSTROW D, CHERNIACK RM: Resistance to airflow in patients with diffuse interstitial lung disease. *Am Rev Respir Dis* 108: 205-210, 1973
145. MISHKIN FS, BRASHEAR RE: Pulmonary and systemic blood pressure responses to large doses of albumin microspheres. *J Nucl Med* 12:251-252, 1971
146. TAPLIN GV, MACDONALD NS: Radiochemistry of macroaggregated albumin and newer lung scanning agents. *Semin Nucl Med* 1:132-152, 1971
147. WAGNER HN JR, TOW DE, LOPEZ-MAJANO V, et al: Factors influencing regional pulmonary blood flow in man. *Scand J Respir Dis* 62(suppl):59-72, 1966
148. WAGNER HN JR, SABISTON DC, IIO M: The diagnosis of pulmonary embolism by radioisotope scanning (abstract). *J Nucl Med* 5:345-346, 1964
149. DUGARD A, NAIMARK A: Effect of hypoxia on distribution of pulmonary blood flow. *J Appl Physiol* 23:663-671, 1967
150. WAGNER HN JR: The use of radioisotope techniques for the evaluation of patients with pulmonary disease. *Am Rev Respir Dis* 113:203-218, 1976
151. FRIEDMAN WF, BRAUNWALD E: Alterations in regional pulmonary blood flow in mitral valve disease studied by radioisotope scanning. A simple nontraumatic technique for estimation of left atrial pressure. *Circulation* 34:363-376, 1966
152. LOKEN MK, WESTGATE HD: Evaluation of pulmonary function using xenon 133 and the scintillation camera. *Am J Roentgenol* 100:835-843, 1967
153. DE ROO MJK, GORIS M, VAN DER SCHUEREN G, et al: Computerized dynamic scintigraphy of the lungs. *Respiration* 26: 408-424, 1969
154. LOKEN MK, MEDINA JR, LILLEHEI JP, et al: Regional pulmonary function evaluation using Xenon 133, a scintillation camera, and computer. *Radiology* 93:1261-1266, 1969
155. MACINTYRE WJ, INKLEY SR, ROTH E, et al: Spatial recording of disappearance constants of xenon-133 wash out from the lung. *J Lab Clin Med* 76:701-712, 1970
156. JOHNSON G, JONES AE, (eds.): Atlas of Gallium-67 Scintigraphy. New York, Plenum Press, 1973
157. GELRUD LG, ARSENEAU JC, JOHNSTON GS: Gallium-67 localization in experimental and clinical abscesses (abstract). *Clin Res* 20:881, 1972
158. KINOSHITA F, USHIO T, MAEKAWA A, et al: Scintiscanning of pulmonary diseases with ^{67}Ga-citrate. *J Nucl Med* 15:227-233, 1974
159. SIEMSEN JK, GREBE SF, SARGENT EN, et al: Gallium-67 scintigraphy of pulmonary diseases as a complement to radiography. *Radiology* 118:371-375, 1976
160. SWARTZENDRUBER DC, NELSON B, HAYES RL: Gallium-67 localization in lysosomal-like granules of leukemic and nonleukemic murine tissues. *J Natl Cancer Inst* 46:941-952, 1971
161. NELSON B, HAYES RL, EDWARDS CL, et al: Distribution of gallium in human tissues after intravenous administration. *J Nucl Med* 13:92-100, 1972
162. LARSON SM, MILDER MS, JOHNSTON GS: Interpretation of the ^{67}Ga photoscan. *J Nucl Med* 14:208-214, 1973

163. LINE BR, FULMER JD, JONES AE, et al: [67]Gallium scanning in idiopathic pulmonary fibrosis: correlation with histopathology and broncho-alveolar lavage. *Am Rev Respir Dis* 113(4):244, 1976
164. LANGHAMMER H, GLAUBITT G, GREBE SF, et al: [67]Ga for tumor scanning. *J Nucl Med* 13:25-30, 1972
165. REYNOLDS HY, NEWBALL HH: Analysis of proteins and respiratory cells obtained from human lungs by bronchial lavage. *J Lab Clin Med* 84:559-573, 1974
166. REYNOLDS HY, ATKINSON JP, NEWBALL HH, et al: Receptors for immunoglobulin and complement on human alveolar macrophages. *J Immunol* 114:1813-1819, 1975
167. REYNOLDS HY, NEWBALL HH: Fluid and cellular milieu of the human respiratory tract, in *Immunologic and Infectious Reactions in the Lungs*, edited by KIRKPATRICK CH, REYNOLDS HY. New York, Dekker, Marcel, Inc., 1976, pp. 3-27
168. REYNOLDS HY, FULMER JD, KAZMIEROWSKI JA, et al: Analysis of broncho-alveolar fluid in patients with hypersensitivity pneumonitis (HP) (abstract). *Clin Res* 24:388A, 1976
169. DAVIS GS, BRODY AR, LANDIS JH, et al: Quantitation of inflammatory activity in interstitial pneumonitis by bronchofiberscopic pulmonary lavage. *Chest* 69(suppl):254-255, 1976
170. KEIMOWITZ RI: Immunoglobins in normal human tracheobronchial washings. *J Lab Clin Med* 63:54-59, 1964
171. MCCOMBS RP: Diseases due to immunologic reactions in the lung. *N Engl J Med* 286:1186-1194, 1245-1252, 1972
172. KALTREIDER HB: Expression of immune mechanisms in the lung. *Am Rev Respir Dis* 113:347-379, 1976
173. BRADLEY K, MCCONNELL-BREUL S, CRYSTAL RG: Lung collagen heterogeneity. *Proc Natl Acad Sci USA* 71:2828-2832, 1974
174. BRADLEY K, MCCONNELL-BREUL S, CRYSTAL RG: Collagen in the human lung. Quantitation of rates of synthesis and partial characterization of composition. *J Clin Invest* 55:543-550, 1975
175. HANCE AJ, CRYSTAL RG: The connective tissue of lung. *Am Rev Respir Dis* 112:657-711, 1975
176. HANCE AJ, BRADLEY K, CRYSTAL RG: Lung collagen heterogeneity. Synthesis of type I and type III collagen by rabbit and human lung cells in culture. *J Clin Invest* 57:102-111, 1976
177. HANCE AJ, CRYSTAL RG: Collagen, in *The Biochemical Basis of Pulmonary Function*, edited by CRYSTAL RG. New York, Dekker, Marcel, Inc., 1976, pp. 215-271
178. SEYER JM, HUTCHESON ET, KANG AH: Collagen polymorphism in idiopathic chronic pulmonary fibrosis. *J Clin Invest* 57:1498-1507, 1976
179. MCLEES BD, SCHLEITER G, PINNELL SR: Isolation of type III collagen from human adult parenchymal lung tissue. *Biochemistry*, in press
180. GAY S, FIETZEK PP, REMBERGER K, et al: Liver cirrhosis: immunofluorescence and biochemical studies demonstate two types of collagen. *Klin Dtsch Med Wochenschr* 100: 205-207, 1975
181. POPPER H: Hepatic fibrosis and collagen metabolism in the liver, in *Collagen Metabolism in the Liver*, edited by POPPER H, BECKER K. New York, Stratton Corp., 1975, pp. 1-14
182. FULMER JD, BIENKOWSKI RS, COWAN MJ, et al: Comparison of collagen concentration, distribution, and synthesis in fibrotic and normal lungs (abstract). *Clin Res* 24:384A, 1976
183. HANCE AJ, HORWITZ AL, COWAN MJ, et al: Biochemical approaches to the investigation of fibrotic lung disease. *Chest* 69(2)(suppl):257-261, 1976
184. MCCULLAGH KA, BALIAN G: Collagen characterization and cell transformation in human atherosclerosis. *Nature* (Lond) 258:73-75, 1975
185. EPSTEIN EH JR, MUNDERLOH NH: Isolation and characterization of CNBr peptides of human $[\alpha 1(III)]_3$ collagen and tissue distribution of $[\alpha 1(I)]_2\alpha 2$ and $[\alpha 1(III)]_3$ collagens. *J Biol Chem* 250:9304-9312, 1975
186. EPSTEIN EH JR: $[\alpha 1(III)]_3$ human skin collagen. Release by pepsin digestion and preponderance in fetal life. *J Biol Chem* 249:3225-3231, 1974
187. KRAVIS TC, AHMED A, BROWN TE, et al: Pathogenic mechanisms in pulmonary fibrosis: collagen induced migration inhibition factor production and cytotoxicity mediated by lymphocytes. *J Clin Invest*, 58:1223-1232, 1976
188. HUGHES EW: Familial interstitial pulmonary fibrosis. *Thorax* 19:515-525, 1964
189. BONANNI PP, FRYMOYER JW, JACOX RF: A family study of idiopathic pulmonary fibrosis. A possible dysproteinemic and genetically determined disease. *Am J Med* 39:411-421, 1965
190. ADELMAN AG, CHERTKOW G, HAYTON RC: Familial fibrocystic pulmonary dysplasia: a detailed family study. *Can Med Assoc J* 95:603-610, 1966
191. SWAYE P, VAN ORDSTRAND HS, MCCORMACK LJ, et al: Familial Hamman-Rich syndrome. Report of eight cases. *Dis Chest* 55: 7-12, 1969
192. WAGLEY PF: A new look at the Hamman-Rich syndrome. *Johns Hopkins Med J* 131:412-424, 1972
193. SOLLIDAY NH, WILLIAMS JA, GAENSLER EA, et al: Familial chronic interstitial pneumonia. *Am Rev Respir Dis* 108:193-204, 1973
194. DAVIES BH, TUDDENHAM EGD: Familial pulmonary fibrosis associated with oculocutaneous albinism and platelet function defect. A new syndrome. *Q J Med* 45:219-232, 1976
195. CARRINGTON CB, GAENSLER EA, COUTU RE, et al: Usual and desquamative interstitial pneumonia. *Chest* 69(suppl):261-262, 1976

Analysis of Cellular and Protein Content of Broncho-Alveolar Lavage Fluid from Patients with Idiopathic Pulmonary Fibrosis and Chronic Hypersensitivity Pneumonitis

HERBERT Y. REYNOLDS, JACK D. FULMER, JOHN A. KAZMIEROWSKI, WILLIAM C. ROBERTS, MICHAEL M. FRANK, and RONALD G. CRYSTAL

From the Laboratory of Clinical Investigation, National Institute of Allergy and Infectious Disease; the Pulmonary Branch, National Heart and Lung Institute; and the Section of Pathology, National Heart and Lung Institute, National Institutes of Health, Bethesda, Maryland 20014

ABSTRACT To evaluate cellular and protein components in the lower respiratory tract of patients with idiopathic pulmonary fibrosis (IPF) and chronic hypersensitivity pneumonitis (CHP), limited broncho-alveolar lavage was done in 58 patients (19 IPF, 7 CHP, and 32 controls). Analysis of the cells and protein in the lavage fluids from patients with IPF revealed an inflammatory and eosinophilic response and a significant elevation of IgG in the lungs. With corticosteroid therapy, inflammation diminished but eosinophils remained. Lavage fluid from patients with CHP also had eosinophils and elevated levels of IgG. However, in contrast to IPF, lavage fluid from CHP patients contained IgM, fewer inflammatory cells, and a strikingly increased number (38–74%) of lymphocytes. Identification of lavage lymphocytes in CHP showed that T lymphocytes were significantly elevated and B lymphocytes were decreased compared to peripheral blood. These studies suggest that the lung in IPF and CHP may function as a relatively independent immune organ, and that analysis of cells and proteins in broncho-alveolar lavage fluid may be of diagnostic, therapeutic, and investigative value in evaluating patients with fibrotic lung disease.

This paper was presented in part at the American Federation for Clinical Research, Atlantic City, N. J., 2 May 1976. An abstract appeared in 1976 *Clin. Res.* **24**: 388.

Requests for reprints may be addressed to: Ronald G. Crystal, Room 6D06, Building 10, National Institutes of Health, Bethesda, Md. 20014.

Received for publication 14 June 1976 and in revised form 29 September 1976.

INTRODUCTION

The fibrotic lung diseases are a heterogeneous group of chronic, usually fatal disorders, characterized radiographically by a pattern of interstitial infiltration and physiologically by the loss of lung volume and a decrease in diffusing capacity. Histologically there is cellular infiltration of alveolar septa and an apparent increase in parenchymal collagen (1, 2).

Although some patients with pulmonary fibrosis can be grouped according to etiology (e.g., occupational, environmental, infectious, tumor, or drug) or by characteristic lung histology (e.g. eosinophilic granuloma), many can be classified only as having "idiopathic pulmonary fibrosis" (IPF).[1] Although the term 'IPF' implies that the etiology and pathogenesis of the disorder is unknown, there are clues which suggest that inflammatory and/or immune-mediated mechanisms are related to the continued activity of the disease (3).

In contrast to IPF, chronic hypersensitivity pneumonitis (CHP) is a group of fibrotic lung diseases in which the etiology is often known. With chronic inhalation of certain organic antigens, susceptible individuals develop a granulomatous interstitial disease which often leads to significant parenchymal fibrosis (4). Animal studies have suggested that in hypersensitivity

[1] *Abbreviations used in this paper*: CHP, chronic hypersensitivity pneumonitis; C4, C6, hemolytic complements; E, erythrocyte; FEV_1/FVC, forced expiratory volume (1 s)/forced vital capacity; IPF, idiopathic pulmonary fibrosis; PaO_2, mean resting arterial blood oxygen tension; PMN, polymorphonuclear leukocytes; SRBC, sheep red blood cells.

pneumonitis, local immune reactions in the lungs, involving both humoral and cellular mechanisms, are intimately related to the pathogenesis and activity of the disease process (5, 6).

Our understanding of these diseases, however, is restricted by limitations in the technologies available for their study. Lung tissue is not accessible for repeated studies and radiographical, physiological, and peripheral blood studies do not give a true assessment of the dynamic inflammatory and immune mechanisms operating in the local environment of the lung. The present study attempts to evaluate these mechanisms through an analysis of cellular and protein components in broncho-alveolar lavage fluid from a representative portion of the epithelial surface of the lower respiratory tract in patients with IPF and CHP.

METHODS

Study patients. A total of 26 patients, 19 with IPF and 7 with CHP, were included in this study. All underwent extensive clinical evaluation including bronchoscopy and 20 had open biopsies of the lung.

The mean age of the 19 patients with IPF was 50.0±3.5 yr;[2] 12 were men and 7 were women. All patients with IPF met the following criteria: an interstitial pattern on chest film, reduced total lung capacity, reduced lung compliance, reduced single breath diffusing capacity, resting hypoxemia which worsened with exercise, and a normal forced expiratory volume (1 s)/forced vital capacity (FEV_1/FVC). None had a significant environmental exposure, symptoms suggestive of hypersensitivity lung disease, left ventricular cardiac failure, or history of chronic pulmonary infections. 17 of the 19 patients with IPF had lung biopsies done within 2–11 mo before the broncho-alveolar lavage study. All biopsies showed septal fibrosis, septal cellular infiltration, and intra-alveolar cellularity. None had granuloma and none had refractile particles under polarized light microscopy. Seven patients currently smoked cigarettes. One patient had joint symptoms compatible with a collagen-vascular disease but had no supporting serologic evidence; one patient had a positive rheumatoid factor (titer 1:64) but no stigmata of joint disease; and one had positive antinuclear antibodies and was believed to have a mixed collagen-vascular disease.

Seven patients were untreated at the time of broncho-alveolar lavage; the other twelve were receiving prednisone (mean dose 24.4±4.0 mg daily). Peripheral blood values, including hemoglobin (14.0±0.5 g/100 ml), total leukocytes (8,300±747 cells/mm^3), and percentage of lymphocytes on peripheral smear (27.0±3.3%) were within normal limits for all 19 patients.

For untreated patients with IPF, the mean vital capacity was 64.0±5.0% of predicted normal values, functional residual capacity was 68.4±7.4% predicted, total lung capacity was 65.7±5.6% predicted, but FEV_1/FVC was normal. Carbon monoxide diffusing capacity was 48.3±6.9% predicted. The mean resting arterial blood oxygen tension (Pa_{O_2}) for this group was 71.6±5.0 mm Hg (on room air) and decreased to 49.0±2.5 mm Hg with exercise. The latter was done with a graded steady-state exercise protocol, each work level was for 6 min with arterial blood gases determined during the last 2 min.

For treated patients with IPF, these parameters were similar. The mean vital capacity was 66.7±4.2% predicted, functional residual capacity was 63.0±3.6% predicted, total lung capacity was 63.8±4.4% predicted, and the FEV_1/FVC was normal. The carbon monoxide diffusing capacity was 46.0±3.7% predicted, while the resting Pa_{O_2} was 73.3±4.2 mm Hg and decreased to 53.7±2.1 mm Hg with exercise.

Seven additional patients were referred to us as having IPF, but the episodic nature of the respiratory symptoms, serological studies, or histopathology of the lung biopsy suggested they had a form of hypersensitivity pneumonitis. All of the patients had a history of chronic intermittent respiratory and systemic symptoms related to their home or work environment. Four of the patients had acute episodes characterized by chills and fever accompanied by cough and dyspnea. The other three had a more insidious onset of cough and progressive dyspnea with no chills or fever. Four patients noted relief of symptoms when removed from their home or work environment and an exacerbation of symptoms with re-exposure to the apparent source of antigens. In four patients, the chest X-ray abnormalities have tended to persist even with removal from the apparent antigenic source. The mean physiologic data for these seven patients were: vital capacity, 82.1±6.4% predicted; functional residual capacity, 70.2±5.6% predicted; total lung capacity, 80.4±5.3% predicted; FEV_1/FVC normal (in all patients), carbon monoxide diffusing capacity, 66.1±6.4% predicted. The mean Pa_{O_2} was 76.1±6.4 mm Hg and decreased to 68.2±4.8 mm Hg with exercise. Additional clinical and laboratory information about individual patients with CHP is given in Table I.

Control patients. 32 patients (20 men, 12 women) with undiagnosed lesions limited to the right upper lung underwent broncho-alveolar lavage in the lingula or left lower lobe as part of the diagnostic bronchoscopy (7). 21 smoked cigarettes and 11 did not. None had evidence by physical examination or chest X ray of disease in the left lung and none were receiving drugs. The controls were age-matched for the IPF patients (nonsmokers 52.0±3.0 yr; smokers 48.0±2.4 yr).

Bronchoscopy and broncho-alveolar lavage. Informed consent was obtained from all patients. Patients were premedicated intramuscularly with atropine (0.6 mg) and diazepam (10 mg); topical lidocaine spray (2%) was used to obtain local anesthesia in the respiratory tract. Bronchoscopies were performed transnasally with a flexible fiberoptic instrument (model BFT 5B-2, Olympus Corporation of America, New Hyde Park, N. Y.). Bronchoscopy was done in the morning, approximately 3 h after prednisone was given to patients receiving this medication. The procedure was done with constant cardiac monitoring and with an intravenous infusion in place. If the resting arterial P_{O_2} on room air was below 70 mm Hg, the bronchoscopy was done with supplemental oxygen given by nasal prongs or face mask (with side port for the instrument).

After routine examination of the major airways, the bronchoscope was positioned in a segment of the lingula (B4 or 5). A total of 100 ml of sterile 0.9% saline (Abbott Laboratories, North Chicago, Ill.) was infused (30 ml twice and then 40 ml) and aspirated by suction after each infusion. The lavage fluid was immediately strained through a single layer of gauze to remove gross mucus and then centrifuged (500 g, 5 min) to separate cellular and protein components. The supernate was carefully decanted from the cell pellet for subsequent protein analysis.

Cellular analysis. The cell pellet was resuspended in modified Hank's balanced salt solution (without calcium and magnesium ions) and pelleted again with low-speed centrifugation. The cells were assayed for total number (model

[2] All data are presented as mean±SEM.

TABLE I

Clinical and Laboratory Features of Patients with Chronic Hypersensitivity Pneumonitis

Patient	Sex/age	Occupation	Symptoms	Duration of symptoms	Chest X ray	Lung biopsy histology	Precipitans: Serum	Precipitans: Lavage	Antigens	Therapy/comment
J. G.	M/47	Printer and farmer	Fever, exertional breathlessness, and exacerbation of fever at work	8 mo	Diffuse reticulonodular pattern	Granuloma, interstitial lymphocytes, and foamy macrophages	+	+	*Micropolyspora faeni*	No therapy, improved with avoidance of office air conditioner
R. B.	F/65	Housewife	Progressive exertional breathlessness	12 mo	Diffuse reticulonodular pattern	Granuloma, interstitial lymphocytes, and foamy macrophages	+	+	*Thermoactinomyces vulgaris* *Aureobasidium pullulans*	Prednisone, 60 mg/day when lavaged initially; dose was 17 mg/day when second lavage performed
W. C.	M/63	Retired engineer	Fever, cough, and breathlessness each winter	6 yr	Micronodular pattern	Bronchiolitis and peribronchial granuloma	+	+	*Thermoactinomyces vulgaris*	No therapy, improved after removal of humidifier from home
G. A.	F/54	Housewife	Recurrent fever, cough, and sputum	14 mo	Bibasilar reticular pattern	ND*	+	−	*Aureobasidium pullulans*	Prednisone discontinued 1 mo before lavage; improved when dehumidifier was removed from home; lung infiltrates cleared in several months
R. K.	M/40	Industrial worker	Progressive exertional breathlessness	10 mo	Diffuse reticular pattern	ND	+	−	*Aureobasidium pullulans* *Thermoactinomyces vulgaris*	No therapy, numerous exposures to synthetic fibers and chemicals, but definite antigen not found
N. M.	F/55	Schoolteacher	Fever, night sweating, and progressive breathlessness	9 mo	Diffuse reticular pattern	ND	−	−	—	Prednisone, 15 mg/day; six species of bacteria and fungi isolated from home dehumidifier
E. W.	F/54	Kitchen worker	Recurrent episodes of fever, night sweating, and breathlessness	5 yr	Diffuse reticular pattern	ND	−	−	—	No therapy, contact with flour or enzyme detergent exacerbated symptoms after several hours at work

* Not done.

TABLE II

General Characteristics of Lavage Fluid from Patients with IPF and from Controls

Groups	Number of patients	Recovery of infused lavage fluid	Total cells recovered	Cell viability	Concentration of protein in lavage fluid*	Concentration of albumin in lavage fluid
		%	$\times 10^7$	%	*mg/ml**	*mg/ml*
Control,						
Nonsmokers	11	48.3±6.3§ (30–80)	0.63±0.2‖ (0.1–1.1)	88.0±3.0	3.8±0.8 (1.3–7.6)	1.7±0.5 (0.5–3.0)
Smokers	21	43.0±4.0 (10–77)	1.44±0.4 (0.2–7.7)	82.2±3.5	2.5±0.3 (0.7–5.2)	1.0±0.1 (0.3–1.9)
IPF,						
No therapy‡	7	31.0±8.0 (15–65)	2.61±1.0‖ (1.3–7.0)	90.7±2.3	3.9±0.9 (1.6–8.1)	1.2±0.4 (0.3–2.8)
On therapy‡	12	41.0±4.2 (20–74)	1.33±0.4 (0.3–3.6)	87.3±3.1	2.8±0.4 (0.7–4.3)	0.9±0.2 (0.3–2.0)
Nonsmokers	12	41.7±4.3 (15–74)	1.85±0.6 (0.2–8.0)	84.0±5.0	3.4±0.6 (1.1–8.0)	1.0±0.2 (0.3–2.6)
Smokers	7	33.8±7.0 (15–65)	1.36±0.4 (0.2–3.6)	87.4±3.2	2.9±0.8 (0.8–7.5)	1.1±0.4 (0.2–2.8)
CHP	7**	48.1±3.8 (30–66)	1.83±0.27 (1.0–3.7)	92.2±2.1	15.2±2.2¶ (7.0–26.0)	2.8±0.5¶ (0.8–6.3)

* Broncho-alveolar lavage was concentrated to a 1.0-ml volume.

‡ Includes nonsmokers and smokers.

§ Mean±SEM, range for the group observed given in parentheses.

‖ The difference in total cells recovered in IPF (no therapy) and control (nonsmokers) was significantly different (Student's t test, $P < 0.05$).

¶ The concentration of protein and albumin in lavage fluid of patients with CHP was significantly greater than that in all other groups ($P < 0.05$ all cases).

** 10 lavages in seven patients; repeat lavages after general clinical improvement, generally showed a decrease in total protein concentration (J. G. 23.0–8.2 mg/ml; R. B. 26.0–8.9 mg/ml; W. C. 17.0–7.0 mg/ml).

FN, Coulter Electronics, Hialeah, Fla.), viability (8) and differential counts. The latter were made from cytocentrifuge smears stained with Wright-Giemsa.

For patients with CHP, the relative proportions of bone marrow-derived (B) and thymus-derived (T) lymphocytes were determined in lavage and peripheral blood. Lymphocytes were separated from the respiratory cell pellet or from heparinized blood with a two-step procedure (9). First, mononuclear cells were banded by density gradient centrifugation with Hypaque-Ficoll (Pharmacia Fine Chemicals, Inc., Piscataway, N. J.) (10) and subsequently washed three times in Eagle's minimum essential medium (Grand Island Biological Co., Grand Island, N. Y.). Secondly, columns of Sephadex G-10 (Pharmacia Fine Chemicals, Inc.) were used to deplete the cell preparations of monocytes or alveolar macrophages (11, 12). For respiratory cells, a column of 10 ml Sephadex gel was equilibrated with Eagle's minimum essential medium containing 10% fetal calf serum, 10^7 cells were washed into the column and the nonadherent cells were eluted with Eagle's minimum essential medium at room temperature. For blood cells the column was made with 30 ml of Sephadex and 10^8 cells were used. This column method consistently yielded a 95–98% pure population of lymphocytes with viability of at least 95%. The net recovery of total lymphocytes from the original cell pellet was 85.0±4.0%. Comparison of the original cell pellet and the postcolumn purified lymphocytes showed no change in the relative proportion of T and B lymphocytes (12). The percentage of T lymphocytes were defined as those forming erythrocyte (E) rosettes with sheep red blood cells (SRBC) (13). The percentage of B lymphocytes was defined as those forming rosettes with SRBC (E)-rabbit IgM-anti-SRBC antibody (A)-mouse serum complement (C) complexes (EAC rosettes) (14, 15). Details of these reagents and procedures have been described elsewhere (16).

Protein analysis. The supernate from the initial centrifugation was concentrated at 4°C to a final volume of 1.0 ml with a combination of positive pressure ultrafiltration (Diaflo, UM-10 membrane, Amicon Corp., Scientific Sys. Div., Lexington, Mass.) and negative pressure dialysis. Quantitative measurements in this concentrated lavage included: total protein by the Lowry method (17); albumin and immunoglobins G and M by radial immunodiffusion in agar (Behring Diagnostics, American Hoechst, Somerville, N. J.); IgE with a radioimmunoabsorbent method (Pharmacia Laboratories Inc.); and hemolytic complement (C4 and C6 titers) (18, 19).

Similar methods were used to quantitate serum protein values.

When initial studies of lavage fluid from patients with IPF indicated that approximately 25% of the total IgA was monomeric (7S) and 75% was polymeric (11S), it was apparent that radial immunodiffusion precipitation, using a single IgA standard protein, would not accurately quantitate the two populations of IgA present. To obviate this problem, 0.3 ml of the concentrated lavage fluid was sedimented in 10–40% linear sucrose density gradients (20); the 7S and 11S IgA fractions were selectively pooled, dialyzed to remove residual sucrose, and quantitated using human monomeric IgA and secretory IgA standards, respectively (7). The 11S component was identified as secretory IgA by size, immunoreactivity with secretory component antiserum and the presence of J-chain. Total IgA was calculated from the sum of the monomeric and secretory values and extrapolated to a 1-ml volume.

Specific precipitating antibodies against a variety of antigens[3] known to cause CHP were assayed by Ouchterlony radial immunodiffusion in the laboratories of F. Wenzel at the Marshfield Clinic, Marshfield, Wis.; similar assays were done in our laboratories using antigens obtained from Hollister-Stier Labs, Spokane, Wash. (lot 089701) and Greer Labs, Lenoir, N. C. (lot K5B-8).

Statistical comparisons. Group data are expressed as a mean±SEM; mean values were compared with Student's *t* test (two-tailed) analysis.

RESULTS

61 lavage procedures were performed in 58 patients (19 IPF, 7 CHP, and 32 controls). Lavage required 5–10 min to complete. It was well tolerated by patients and did not add to the discomfort or morbidity of bronchoscopy.

Since prior studies have demonstrated in normal subjects that cigarette smoking can significantly influence the recovery of respiratory cells (7, 21–23), results from patients with IPF are also segregated as to smoking status (Table II). The percentage of lavage fluid recovered from patients with IPF on no therapy tended to be less than from other groups, particularly the nonsmoking controls ($P = 0.08$) (Table II).

Analysis of cells in IPF lavage. The total number of cells recovered from lavage of patients with untreated IPF was significantly greater than from nonsmoking controls ($P < 0.05$) but not significantly different than from smoker controls ($P > 0.1$). Recovery of cells from IPF patients on therapy appeared to be less than from those untreated, but this difference was not significant ($P > 0.1$). Smoking status did not influence the total number of cells recovered from patients with IPF. The viability of lavage fluid cells was similar between all groups (Table II).

Of patients with IPF (nontreated and treated), 73%

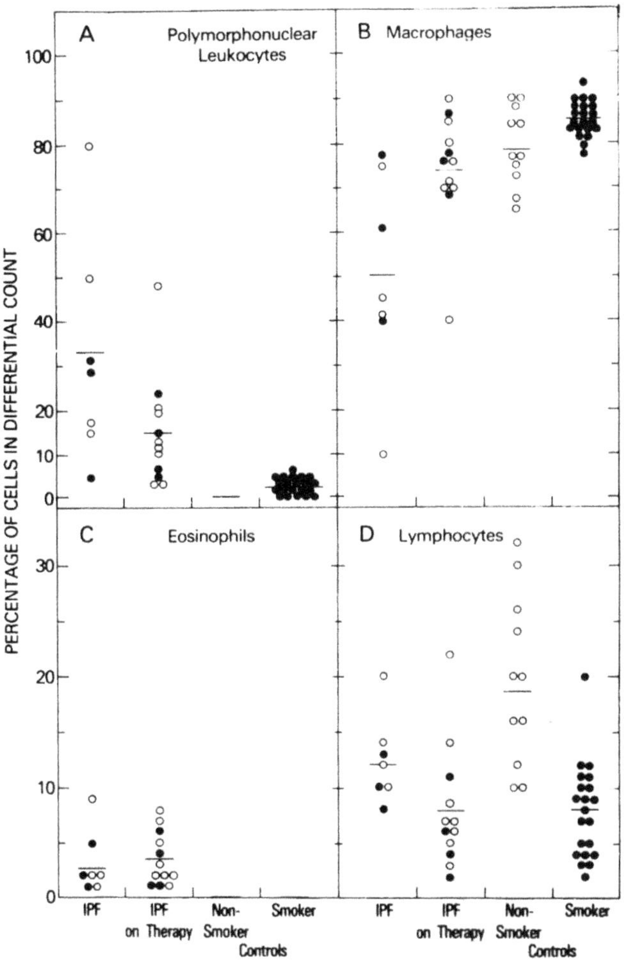

FIGURE 1 Percentage of cells identified in the differential count of lavage fluid is shown for patients with untreated IPF, patients with treated IPF, nonsmoker controls, and smoker controls. A horizontal line represents the mean for the group. Nonsmokers (○) and smokers (●) are designated. In nonsmoking controls, there were no PMNs found; in nonsmoking controls and smoking controls no eosinophils were present.

had a greater percentage of polymorphonuclear leukocytes (PMN) in their lavage differential count than did controls (Fig. 1A). Although there was a broad range which overlapped, the mean percentage of PMNs in treated IPF (14.0±4.0%) was significantly lower ($P < 0.05$) than that in untreated IPF (33.0±8.0%). In the smoking controls, PMNs were infrequent (3.0±0.4%) and in the nonsmoking controls they were absent. There was no significant difference in the percentage of PMNs in lavage from IPF nonsmokers and smokers.

The percentage of macrophages (Fig. 1B) found in control groups and for treated IPF patients were not significantly different. The lower percentage of macrophages in the untreated IPF group ($P < 0.05$) was

[3] Antigens used included: *Micropolyspora faeni*, *Thermoactinomyces vulgaris*, *T. viridis*, *T. sacchari*, *Aspergillus fumigatus*, *Asp. sydowi*, *Asp. glaucus*, *Asp. niger*, pigeon sera, pigeon droppings, *Cryptostroma corticale*, and *Aureobasidium pullulans*.

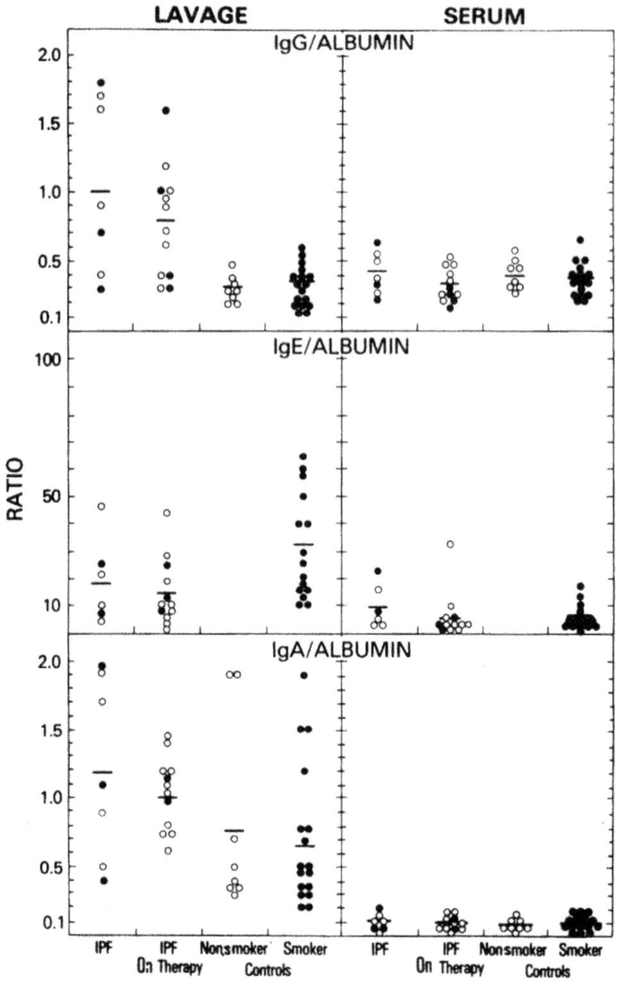

FIGURE 2 A comparison of immunoglobulin levels in lavage fluid and serum is shown for patients with untreated IPF, IPF patients under treatment, nonsmoker controls, and smoker controls. The immunoglobulin data are presented as a ratio to the respective albumin level in the same sample (Results). A horizontal line denotes the mean for the group. Nonsmokers (○), smokers (●) are designated. IgG/albumin and IgA/albumin ratios are expressed as milligram per milligram. IgE/albumin ratios are in nanogram per milligram; these levels are not available for the nonsmoker controls.

probably secondary to the relative increase in PMNs in these patients.

The percentage of eosinophils (Fig. 1C) in the IPF cell differentials was significantly higher ($P < 0.001$) than for control subjects in whom eosinophils were not detected. Eosinophils persisted in IPF despite anti-inflammatory therapy. The number of eosinophils in the peripheral blood of these patients was not elevated except for mildly increased absolute circulating eosinophil counts in 3 of the 19 IPF patients (718 ±46 eosinophils/mm^3 for the 3 patients).

The percentage of lymphocytes in IPF lavage fluid (Fig. 1D) was neither increased compared with controls nor altered appreciably by therapy. Erythrocytes in the respiratory cell pellets generally were less than 3%.

Protein analysis in IPF. Quantitative analysis of proteins recovered from the lower respiratory tract of human subjects is difficult, since the broncho-alveolar bathing fluid can only be recovered by "washing" it out. Two approaches can be used to obviate this problem.

First, a standardized lavage procedure (100 ml infusion) was used. Although a variable amount of lavage fluid was recovered from individual patients, the mean volumes recovered from the different patient groups were not significantly different (Table II), and quantitative measurements of lavage proteins can be expressed as units per milliliter of concentrated lavage fluid. For example, there were no significant differences between the total protein concentrations found in lavage fluid of all groups analyzed (Table II).

Secondly, lavage protein values can be expressed in relation to a reference protein in the lavage. Albumin was chosen as this reference standard (24) because it is not synthesized in the lung and its presence in broncho-alveolar fluid reflects transudation from the intravascular compartment. In addition, the relative amounts of albumin in lavage analyses were not significantly different in the various patient groups (Table II). Likewise, albumin values in serum were comparable for the various groups (data not shown). The ratio of a specific protein (milligram per milliliter) to albumin (milligram per milliliter) in lavage fluid could be compared directly to the ratio of these proteins in serum. Thus, the ratio of a specific protein to albumin in lavage should be the same as that in serum if proteins are present in the lower respiratory tract secondary to transudation from serum. A high ratio of a specific protein to albumin in lavage was taken as evidence of a relative increase of that protein in the lower respiratory tract compared to serum. This second method was found to be much more useful, and all of the data are presented in this manner. The mean concentrations of each protein (amount per milliliter) in lavage can be calculated from the protein to albumin ratios by using the mean albumin concentrations for each group (Table II).

Serum IgG to albumin ratios were similar in all patients; the individual ratios were always less than 0.65 (Fig. 2). In control subjects, lavage IgG/albumin ratios, likewise, were always less than 0.65. In IPF patients, however, lavage IgG/albumin ratios were greater than 0.65 in 63% (12 of 19) patients. The mean ratios for lavage fluid in untreated IPF (1.06 ±0.24) and treated IPF (0.78±0.12) were significantly higher than those for controls ($P < 0.01$ all comparisons). The elevated lavage IgG/albumin levels in IPF were not dependent upon the smoking status of the patient (Fig. 2).

In general, patients on treatment for IPF had lower ratios of lavage IgE/albumin than smoker controls ($P < 0.025$) despite considerable variation in the control values. 50% of the untreated IPF patients also had lower lavage IgE/albumin values than controls, but the mean for this group was not significantly lower than controls ($P > 0.1$). Unfortunately, data were not available for nonsmoker controls, but results obtained in nonsmoking volunteers demonstrate lavage IgE/albumin values comparable to those found in the smoker controls (7). Serum levels of IgE/albumin were similar in all groups. Lavage IgE/albumin for some IPF patients tended to be higher than that in serum; for controls the lavage values were significantly higher than serum values ($P < 0.001$) (Fig. 2). One subject (A. R.) in the untreated IPF group was excluded because of a history of atopic disease. Interestingly, his serum IgE level was 3,000 ng/ml (IgE albumin ratio of 100) while his lavage IgE was 24 ng/ml (IgE/albumin ratio of 9).

IgA/albumin values in the serum of all patients were in a narrow range (ratio 0.05–0.2 in all cases) while the IgA/albumin values in lavage fell broadly over a 10-fold range (0.2–2.0). As expected in all groups, lavage IgA/albumin was significantly higher than serum values, but there were no significant differences in lavage values between groups (Fig. 2). In controls, 9% of lavage IgA was monomeric (7) while in IPF 25–30% of lavage IgA was in the monomeric form. Interestingly, the use of IgA/albumin ratios to analyze IPF serum values obscured the fact that serum IgA levels were increased (>3.5 mg/ml) in 71% of the untreated IPF group but only in 25% of the treated IPF patients.

With double-diffusion immunoprecipitation analysis of lavage fluid, IgM was detected in only 15% of specimens from IPF patients (sensitivity of the IgM assay was 0.1 mg/ml). Likewise, this immunoglobulin was found in approximately 5% of control specimens (7). Serum IgM values were within the normal range for our laboratory (0.9–1.7 mg/ml) for IPF patients on no therapy (1.5±0.3 mg/ml) and for those on treatment (1.7±0.3 mg/ml). Serum values for control nonsmokers (1.8±0.2 mg/ml) and smokers (1.5±0.3 mg/ml) were comparable.

C4 hemolytic complement titers in lavage, expressed as a ratio to albumin, were the same for the IPF groups and for smoker controls (Fig. 3). However, mean ratios in lavage fluid were significantly lower ($P < 0.01$) than corresponding serum ratios for the IPF group on therapy and for smoker controls. Likewise, mean lavage values of C6/albumin were comparable in all groups, but were also significantly lower than respective serum ratios ($P < 0.01$). In addition, mean serum C6/albumin values in the IPF groups were significantly greater ($P < 0.01$) than those of smoker controls.

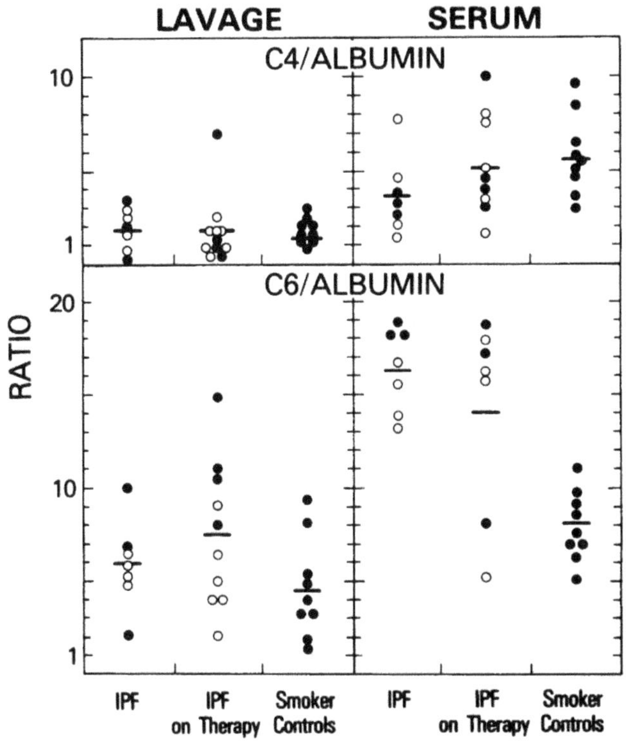

FIGURE 3 A comparison of complement levels in lavage fluid and serum is shown for patients with untreated IPF, patients with IPF under treatment and smoker controls. The mean value for each group is given by a horizontal bar. Nonsmokers (○), smokers (●) are designated. The C4 data are calculated as 10^{-3} hemolytic titer per milligram albumin; the C6 data are calculated as hemolytic titer per milligram albumin.

Cell and protein analysis in CHP. The mean recovery of the lavage fluid from patients with CHP (about 48%) was generally better than in the IPF groups but the total cell recovery was comparable (Table II). PMNs represented an average of 8.5% of respiratory cells in CHP (Fig. 4). (A higher percentage was noted for patient R. K. and for the second analysis in R. B. and W. C.; both of these latter patients had an episode of bronchitis 3–4 wk before the second lavage study.) Eosinophils represented 0.5–2% of all respiratory cells of patients with CHP while approximately 29% of the lavage cells were alveolar macrophages with distinctive foamy macrophages constituting about 10% of the macrophage population.

In striking contrast to patients with IPF and to controls, lymphocytes accounted for approximately 62% of the lavage cells in CHP. When lavage lymphocytes were characterized by sheep erythrocyte (T cells) and complement (B cells) rosette techniques (Fig. 4), the

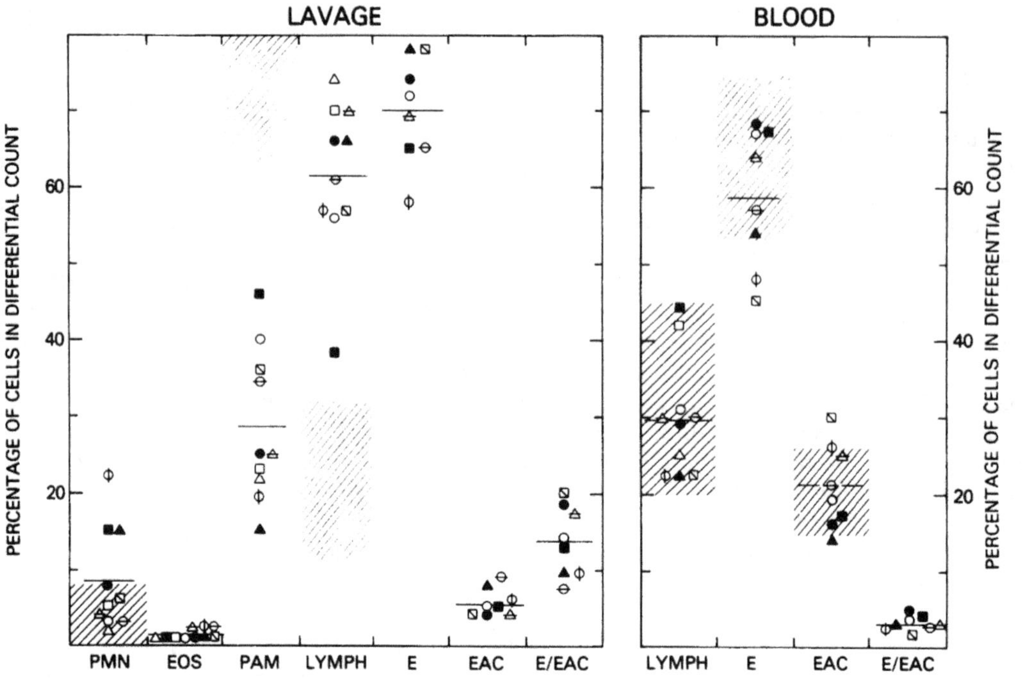

FIGURE 4 Percentage of cells identified in the differential count of lavage fluid of seven patients with chronic hypersensitivity pneumonitis. There were 10 lavages done in 7 patients. A single symbol is used for each patient described in Table I: J. G. first lavage (○); J. G. lavage 7 mo later (●); R. B. first lavage (□); R. B. lavage 11 mo later (■); W. C. first lavage (△); W. C. lavage 11 mo later (▲); N. M. (⧅); E. W. (⊖); R K. (⦶); G. A. (⧋). (PMN, polymorphonuclear leukocytes; EOS, eosinophils; PAM, pulmonary alveolar macrophages; LYMPH, lymphocytes; E, T lymphocytes; EAC, B lymphocytes; E/EAC, ratio of T to B lymphocytes.) A horizontal line represents a mean for the group. For the lavage data, shaded areas represent the range of values found in lavage of controls (nonsmokers and smokers) given in Fig. 1. In normals, no eosinophils are found in lavage and the range for macrophages is 63–92%. For the blood data, the shaded areas represent the control values established for peripheral blood lymphocytes from young adults (n = 15). All of the data in this figure is expressed as a percentage of total cells in a differential count except for the E/EAC column (lavage and blood) which is presented as the ratio of percentage E to percentage EAC.

vast majority of respiratory lymphocytes were identified as T lymphocytes (mean 70±2.5%) and only about 6% could be identified as B lymphocytes. The mean ratio of E/EAC (T/B cells) was about 14. Approximately 24% of the respiratory lymphocytes were unidentified with our immune reagents and were considered null cells.

In contrast, values for peripheral blood leukocytes and lymphocytes were within the normal range in all patients with CHP. Analysis of the blood lymphocytes demonstrated that 59% were T cells and 21% were B cells, giving a blood T to B mean ratio of 3:1. The percentage of T lymphocytes in lavage was significantly greater ($P < 0.025$) than in blood and the percentage of B lymphocytes in lavage was significantly less ($P < 0.005$). The resulting T to B ratios in lavage compared with those in blood were also significantly different ($P < 0.005$).

The mean total protein concentration present in the concentrated lavage fluid from these patients (15.2 ±2.2 mg/ml) was significantly higher than that found in IPF groups or controls ($P < 0.01$) (Table II). This was not due simply to more transudation of serum, since the ratio of albumin to total protein in CHP (mean 0.14±0.02) was much less than in IPF (0.32 ±0.03) or controls (0.44±0.07) ($P < 0.01$ for all comparisons). Repeat lavages in three CHP patients, done at times when there had been general clinical improvement, yielded less total protein (Table II).

Part of the excess broncho-alveolar protein in CHP was IgG. With the exception of the second analysis of R. B., the ratios of lavage IgG/albumin were ≥1.1 in all cases of CHP. These ratios were higher than those found in 75% of the IPF patients and higher than any controls (Fig. 5 vs. Fig. 2). In contrast, the corresponding serum ratios in CHP (mean 0.42±0.03) were similar to IPF and controls. IgG-rich fractions recovered from sucrose gradient fractionation of lavage and serum of patients J. G. and R. B. contained precipitating antibody to thermophylic actinomycetes (*M. faeni*) antigens when assayed by double-diffusion immunoprecipitation in agar.

IgM was measurable in all lavage specimens in CHP; its mere detection made it unusual in comparison with IPF (15% had lavage IgM) or controls (5% had lavage IgM). The IgM/albumin levels in lavage vs. serum (Fig. 5) indicated a proportionally greater amount in the bronchoalveolar fluid than in serum. No precipitating antibodies were detected in lavage or serum IgM fractions recovered from sucrose gradients.

IgE/albumin levels in CHP lavage were higher than those found in serum. The lavage and serum ratios, however, were normal compared to the smoker controls (Fig. 5 vs. Fig. 2). Total IgA/albumin in CHP lavage was elevated compared with serum but was similar to controls. As found in IPF and controls, C4/albumin and C6/albumin levels were lower in CHP lavage fluid as compared with serum.

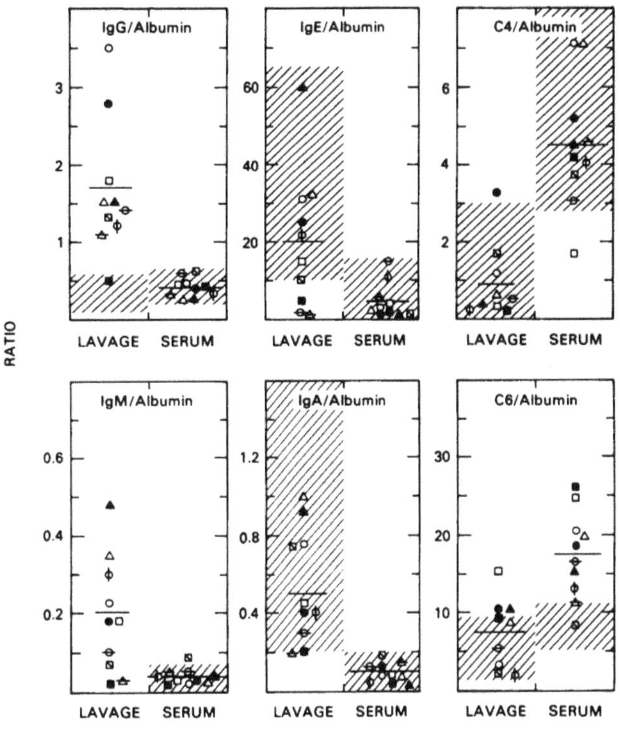

FIGURE 5 Quantitation of proteins in broncho-alveolar lavage and serum from patients with chronic hypersensitivity pneumonitis. The symbols for the patients are as in Fig. 4: J. G. first lavage (○); J. G. lavage 7 mo later (●); R. B. first lavage (□); R. B. lavage 11 mo later (■); W. C. first lavage (△); W. C. lavage 11 mo later (▲); N. M. (⧅); E. W. (⊖); R. K. (⌽); G. A. (◬). The immunoglobulin data (lavage and serum) are presented as a ratio to the respective albumin level in the same sample: IgG/albumin (milligrams per milligram), IgE/albumin (nanograms per milligram), IgM/albumin (milligrams per milligram), IgA/albumin (milligrams per milligram). C4 data are presented as 10^{-3} hemolytic titer per milligram albumin; C6 data are presented as hemolytic titer per milligram albumin. Shaded areas are the range of values for control (nonsmokers and smokers) given in Fig. 2 and 3. For control lavage IgM/albumin is <0.01 and, IgA/albumin is 0.3 to 1.8. For control blood, C4/albumin is 2.8–9.8.

DISCUSSION

Limited lavage of the lower respiratory tract is a simple extension of routine fiber-optic bronchoscopy. While routine measurements, such as chest films and pulmonary function studies, monitor general lung function, analysis of broncho-alveolar lavage fluid is a direct attempt to evaluate specific mechanisms which may contribute to the continued activity of lung disease. Quantitation of cells and proteins in lavage of patients with IPF and CHP has demonstrated that the epithelial surface of the lower respiratory tract is involved in inflammatory and immunologic reactions that would not be suspected from analysis of blood alone. In addition, comparison of lavage cells and immunoglobulins from IPF and CHP show a number of similarities and differences which may be important in understanding these disorders.

Analysis of the lavage fluid from patients with IPF indicates that these patients have a local inflammatory process which was not seen in controls. How the presence of polymorphonuclear leukocytes relates to the fibrotic process is not known, but these studies suggest that when patients with IPF are treated, this inflammatory response tends to diminish.

In addition to the local accumulation of PMNs, the lower respiratory tract in IPF has a striking increase in IgG compared with serum IgG and with control lavage IgG. Since the IgG/albumin levels in the lavage fluid of these patients are significantly higher than their serum IgG/albumin levels, it is unlikely that the elevated IgG is secondary to transudation resulting from the inflammatory process. It is probable that in IPF there is local pulmonary production of IgG (25, 26) and/or the mechanisms of IgG catabolism or removal are faulty. It is thus possible that part of the pathogenesis of IPF is secondary to IgG antibody being formed in the lung parenchyma in response to as yet unidentified antigen(s) resulting in local antibody-antigen complexes.

In CHP, the local accumulation of IgG is even more impressive. This finding is consistent with the concept that the pathogenesis of hypersensitivity pneumonitis is associated with a type III immune reaction in lung (3). In accord with this concept, two of the CHP patients (J. G. and R. B.) had broncho-alveolar IgG precipitins against thermophylic actinomycetes antigens. The lavage fluid from the CHP patients also contained significant quantities of IgM (compared to serum) further emphasizing the possible role of humoral immunity in this disease.

While the elevated levels of respiratory IgG in IPF and IgG and IgM in CHP suggest local type III immune reactions, both IPF and CHP patients also had eosinophils present in their lavage fluid. This finding is interesting in several respects: (*a*) in general, patients with IPF and CHP did not have blood eosinophilia; (*b*) controls had no eosinophils in their lavage fluid; and (*c*) therapy with corticosteroids did not influence the local eosinophil accumulation. Although these findings suggest that a localized allergic reaction might be occurring in the lung parenchyma of these patients, the generally low levels of IgE/albumin in lavage fluid from patients with IPF and CHP argue against the classic type type I reagin-mediated lung reaction being important (3, 27–29). Thus disease mechanisms in IPF and CHP are probably not associated with combined type I and III immune reactions found in a disorder such as allergic bronchopulmonary aspergillosis (3).

In both IPF and CHP, the total IgA/albumin levels in lavage were normal. However, in both disorders, the relative proportion of monomeric IgA in the broncho-alveolar fluid was increased compared with controls. The reason for this finding is not clear although it is possible that the monomeric IgA represents transudation from the intravascular compartment. Alternatively, inflammation enhanced proteolytic degradation of locally produced secretory IgA could explain this finding. Irrespective of the cause of increased monomeric IgA in the lower respiratory tract in IPF and CHP, neither disorder appears to be associated with a local abnormality of secretory IgA.

There is no direct evidence in these studies that either IPF of CHP are associated with local complement-mediated reactions. Although C4/albumin levels in the broncho-alveolar fluid tended to be lower than serum (Figs. 3, 5), there was no difference between IPF, CHP, or controls. The lower values of complement activity in all lavage analyses may be more apparent than biologically significant. Although complement titers were promptly assayed, its activity is known to be labile and undoubtedly some activity is lost in the lung washout and concentrating procedures. The elevated levels of serum C6 in IPF and CHP may be due to C6 acting as an acute phase reactant in these patients.

While the eosinophils, IgG, IgA, IgE, C4, and C6 levels in the lavage fluid of IPF an CHP are quite similar, analysis of other cellular and protein contents of the broncho-alveolar fluid in CHP provides a striking contrast to that in IPF and controls. Lavage fluid of these patients contained alveolar macrophages with foamy cytoplasm which are considered to be characteristic of the histology found in the hypersensitivity lung disorders (4). Such cells were not noted in IPF or controls. In 10 lavage analyses from 7 patients with CHP, the average percentage of broncho-alveolar lymphocytes was 62% compared to about 10% in IPF (treated and untreated), 8% in smoker controls and 18% in nonsmoker controls. Even though all patients with CHP had elevated broncho-alveolar IgG and IgM, and two had IgG precipitating antibodies in the lavage fluid against a specific fungal antigen, the exaggerated broncho-alveolar lymphocyte response in CHP is not one of B lymphocytes, as might be expected, but rather one of T lymphocytes. This finding suggests, as in experimental animal models of hypersensitivity pneumonitis (5, 6), that cell-mediated mechanisms may also be important in CHP. Thus, in human hypersensitivity disease, there is preliminary evidence of localized humoral and cellular immunity in the pathogenesis of the disorder. The consequences of this T-cell accumulation in CHP are unknown, although it is possible that activation of these cells to liberate local mediators may provide a stimulus for granuloma formation, eosinophil accumulation and/or cell injury.

Based on the high ratio of T/B lymphocytes found in CHP lavage fluid compared to blood (Fig. 4), T cells appeared to be sequestered in affected pulmonary tissue. This finding was even more striking when compared to the recent studies of Daniele et al. (30) who noted that in normal humans, broncho-alveolar T/B ratios were the same as in blood. These lymphocyte results together with the immunoglobulin data in both IPF and CHP suggest that the lung can function partially independent of systemic humoral- and cell-mediated immune systems.

Lung biopsies were available from 17 of the IPF patients and from 3 of the CHP patients. In most, the biopsy was done some months before the lavage study. Nevertheless, in 17 of the 20 patients in whom biopsy was performed, the cells in the alveoli and small airways were similar and in same relative proportions as found in cell differential counts obtained from broncho-alveolar lavage. Thus, our findings corroborate those of Davis et al. (31) who found cell content of lavage to be similar to alveolar cellular content in patients with interstitial pneumonitis.

It is doubtful that analysis of broncho-alveolar lavage fluid can ever give as much information about parenchymal pathology in lung disease as can an open lung biopsy specimen. However, whereas open lung biopsy is usually done only once to establish a diagnosis, broncho-alveolar lavage does permit periodic assessment of the disease process with little risk and discomfort to the patient. Thus, analysis of lavage fluid from patients with fibrotic lung disease adds another dimension to evaluation of these disorders. Lavage fluid represents the epithelial milieu of the lung parenchyma and therefore gives further insight into local phenomena causing the lung disease. It may prove useful in following the effect of therapy on these disorders. Most importantly, the differences between the cellular analyses in CHP compared to IPF and controls indicate that broncho-alveolar lavage could be useful diagnostically in categorizing patients with pulmonary fibrosis even when specific organic antigens cannot be readily identified.

ACKNOWLEDGMENTS

We thank Doctors Norton Elson, Joel Moss, and Edward Stool who did the lavage procedures; Dr. Fritz Wenzel of the Marshfield Clinic for serologic studies; Dr. Anthony S. Fauci and Dr. Charles H. Kirkpatrick for their advice; Ms. Thelma Gaither, Ms. Patricia A. Johnson, and Mr. Geoffrey Hudson for technical help; Dr. David W. Alling for help with the statistical analysis; and Mrs. Nancy Wyne, Mrs. Joy Barchers, and Mrs. Kristen Cook for their editorial assistance.

REFERENCES

1. Liebow, A. A., and C. B. Carrington, 1968. The interstitial pneumonias. *In* Frontiers of Pulmonary Radiology. M. Simon, E. J. Potchen, and M. Lemay, editors. Grune & Stratton, Inc. New York. 102–141.
2. Fulmer, J. D., and R. G. Crystal. 1976. The biochemical basis of pulmonary function. *In* The Biochemical Basis of Pulmonary Function. R. G. Crystal, editor. Marcel Dekker, Inc., New York. 419–466.
3. McCombs, R. P. 1972. Diseases due to immunologic reactions in the lungs. *N. Engl. J. Med.* **286:** 1186–1194, 1245–1252.
4. Fink, J. N., 1976. Hypersensitivity pneumonitis. *In* Immunologic and Infectious Reactions in the Lung. C. H. Kirkpatrick, and H. Y. Reynolds, editors. Marcel Dekker, Inc., New York 229–241.
5. Hensley, G. T., J. N. Fink, and J. J. Barboriak. 1974. Hypersensitivity pneumonitis in the monkey. *Arch. Pathol.* **97:** 33–38.
6. Moore, V. L., G. T. Hensley, and J. N. Fink. 1975. An animal model of hypersensitivity pneumonitis in the rabbit. *J. Clin. Invest.* **56:** 937–944.
7. Reynolds, H. Y., and H. H. Newball. 1974. Analysis of proteins and respiratory cells obtained from human lungs by bronchial lavage. *J. Lab. Clin. Med.* **84:** 559–573.
8. Hanks, J. H., and J. H. Wallace. 1958. Determination of cell viability. *Proc. Soc. Exp. Biol. Med.* **98:** 188–192.
9. Kazmierowski, J. A., A. S. Fauci, and H. Y. Reynolds. 1976. Characterization of lymphocytes in bronchial lavage fluid from monkeys. *J. Immunol.* **116:** 615–618.
10. Böyum, A. 1968. Isolation of mononuclear cells and granulocytes from human blood. *Scand. J. Clin. Invest.* **21** (Suppl. 97): 77–89.
11. Ly, I. A., and R. I. Mishell. 1974. Separation of mouse spleen cells by passage through columns of Sephadex G-10. *J. Immunol. Methods.* **5:** 239–247.
12. Schwartz, R. H., A. R. Bianco, B. S. Handwerger, and C. R. Kahn. 1975. Demonstration that monocytes rather than lymphocytes are the insulin-binding cells in preparations of human blood mononuclear leukocytes; implications for studies of insulin-resistant states in man. *Proc. Natl. Acad. Sci. U. S. A.* **72:** 474–478.
13. Weiner, M. S., C. Bianco, and V. Nussenzweig. 1973. Enhanced binding of neuraminidase-treated sheep erythrocytes to human T lymphocytes. *Blood.* **42:** 939–946.
14. Bianco, C., R. Patrick, and V. Nussenzweig. 1970. A population of lymphocytes bearing a membrane receptor for antigen-antibody-complement complexes. I. separation and characterization. *J. Exp. Med.* **132:** 702–720.
15. Frank, M. M., and T. Gaither. 1970. The effect of temperature on the reactivity of guinea pig complement with γG and γM haemolytic antibodies. *Immunology.* **19:** 967–974.
16. Reynolds, H. Y., J. P. Atkinson, H. H. Newball, and M. M. Frank. 1975. Receptors for immunoglobulin and complement on human alveolar macrophages. *J. Immunol.* **114:** 1813–1819.
17. Lowry, O. H., N. J. Rosebrough, A. L. Farr, and R. Randall. 1951. Protein measurement with the Folin phenol reagent. *J. Biol. Chem.* **193:** 265–275.
18. Gaither, T. A., D. W. Alling, and M. M. Frank. 1974. A new one step method for the functional assay of the fourth component (C_4) of human and guinea pig complement. *J. Immunol.* **113:** 574–583.
19. May, J. E. and M. M. Frank. 1972. Complement-mediated tissue damage: contribution of the classical and alternate complement pathways in the Forssman reaction. *J. Immunol.* **108:** 1517–1525.
20. Reynolds, H. Y., and J. S. Johnson. 1971. Structural units of canine serum and secretory immunoglobulin A. *Biochemistry.* **10:** 2821–2827.
21. Harris, J. O., E. W. Swenson, and J. E. Johnson, III. 1970. Human alveolar macrophages: comparison of phagocytic ability, glucose utilization, and ultrastructure in smokers and nonsmokers. *J. Clin. Invest.* **49:** 2086–2096.
22. Sharp, P. M., G. A. Warr, and R. R. Martin. 1973. Effects of smoking on bronchial immunoglobulins. *Clin. Res.* **21:** 672. (Abstr.)
23. Cantrell, E. T., G. A. Warr, D. L. Busbee, and R. R. Martin. 1973. Induction of aryl hydrocarbon hydroxylase in human pulmonary alveolar macrophages by cigarette smoking. *J. Clin. Invest.* **52:** 1881–1884.
24. Keimowitz, R. I. 1964. Immunoglobulins in normal human tracheobronchial washings. A qualitative and quantitative study. *J. Lab. Clin. Med.* **63:** 54–59.
25. Van Furth, R., and F. Aiuti. 1969. Immunoglobulin synthesis by tissue of the gastro-intestinal and respiratory tracts. *Protides Biol. Fluids Proc. Colloq. Bruges.* **16:** 479–484.
26. Martinez-Tello, F. J., D. G. Braun, and W. A. Blanc. 1968. Immunoglobulin production in bronchial mucosa and bronchial lymph nodes, particularly in cystic fibrosis of the pancreas. *J. Immunol.* **101:** 989–1003.
27. Ishizaka, K., and R. W. Newcomb. 1970. Presence of IgE in nasal washings and sputum from asthmatic patients. *J. Allergy.* **46:** 197–204.
28. Waldman, R. H., C. Virchow, and D. S. Rowe. 1973. IgE levels in external secretions. *Int. Arch. Allergy Appl. Immunol.* **44:** 242–248.
29. Patterson, R., J. N. Fink, J. J. Pruzansky, C. Reed, M. Roberts, R. Slavin, and C. R. Zeiss. 1973. Serum immunoglobulin levels in pulmonary allergic aspergillosis and certain other lung diseases, with special reference to immunoglobulin E. *Am. J. Med.* **54:** 16–22.
30. Daniele, R. P., M. D. Altose, and D. T. Rowlands, Jr. 1975. Immunocompetent cells from the lower respiratory tract of normal human lungs. *J. Clin. Invest.* **56:** 986–995.
31. Davis, G. S., A. R. Brody, J. N. Landis, W. G. B. Graham, J. E. Craighead, and G. M. Green. 1976. Quantitation of inflammatory activity in interstitial pneumonitis by bronchofiberscopic pulmonary lavage. *Chest.* **69**(Suppl.): 265–266.

Small Airways in Idiopathic Pulmonary Fibrosis

COMPARISON OF MORPHOLOGIC AND PHYSIOLOGIC OBSERVATIONS

JACK D. FULMER, WILLIAM C. ROBERTS, EDWYNA R. VON GAL, and RONALD G. CRYSTAL

From the Pulmonary Branch and the Pathology Branch, National Heart, Lung, and Blood Institute, National Institutes of Health, Bethesda, Maryland 20014

ABSTRACT 18 patients with idiopathic pulmonary fibrosis were studied to determine if they had morphologic evidence of small airways disease and if physiologic testing could predict morphologic findings. In the presence of normal airway function by standard physiologic studies (forced expiratory volume in 1 s/forced vital capacity and airway resistance by plethysmography), dynamic compliance, maximum expiratory flow-volume curves, and maximum flow-static recoil curves were measured to detect physiologic alterations consistent with small airways abnormalities. These physiologic data were then compared with estimates of small airways diameter made in lung biopsy specimens.

94% (17 of 18) of the patients had peribronchiolar fibrosis or peribronchiolar inflammation or bronchiolitis. 67% (12 of 18) had an overall estimate of small airways diameter of "narrowed," whereas 33% (6 of 18) had airways that overall were "not narrowed." 59% (10 of 17) had frequency-dependent dynamic compliance, 50% (9 of 18) had abnormal maximum expiratory flow-volume curves, and 39% (7 of 18) had abnormal maximum flow-static recoil curves. Comparisons between morphologic and physiologic data revealed a significant correlation between the results of dynamic compliance and the overall estimate of small airways diameter ($P = 0.001$), and the results of maximum flow-volume curves and the overall estimate of small airways diameter ($P = 0.009$); there was no significant correlation between the results of maximum flow-static recoil curves and the overall estimate of small airways diameter ($P = 0.1$).

The results of this study suggest that: (*a*) idiopathic pulmonary fibrosis is a disease of small airways as well as alveoli; (*b*) dynamic compliance and the maximum expiratory flow-volume curve can predict the overall status of small airways diameter in idiopathic pulmonary fibrosis; and (*c*) whereas the maximum flow-static recoil curve predicts the overall estimate of small airways diameter in most patients with this disease, it is the least sensitive of these three monitors of small airways.

Reprint requests may be addressed to Dr. Fulmer, Room 6N260, Bldg. 10, National Institutes of Health, Bethesda, Md. 20014.

Received for publication 13 October 1976 and in revised form 11 April 1977.

INTRODUCTION

Idiopathic pulmonary fibrosis (IPF)[1] is a well-defined subgroup of the fibrotic lung disorders, characterized by distinct clinical, radiographic, physiologic, and morphologic features (1–16). These patients usually have exertional breathlessness, a diffuse interstitial infiltrate on chest X ray, decreased lung volumes, decreased diffusing capacity, and hypoxemia which worsens with exercise. Although the hypoxemia in IPF was initially thought to result from a diffusion barrier to oxygen (17), current data suggest that it mostly results from a ventilation-perfusion imbalance (18, 19).

In general, the most likely cause of hypoxemia secondary to a ventilation-perfusion imbalance is maldistribution of ventilation resulting either from airways disease or alterations in regional compliance or both. Because IPF has been considered to be a disease of alveoli and not of airways, maldistribution of ventilation in this disorder has previously been attributed to alterations in regional compliance (18). However, recent studies in disorders other than IPF (e.g. asthma)

[1] *Abbreviations used in this paper*: Cdyn, dynamic compliance; Cstat, static compliance; D_{LCO}, carbon dioxide diffusing capacity; $FEV_1\%$, forced expiratory volume in 1 s/forced vital capacity; FRC, functional residual capacity; IPF, idiopathic pulmonary fibrosis; MEFV, maximum expiratory flow volume; MFSR, maximum flow static recoil; P_L, transpulmonary pressure; Pst, static transpulmonary pressure; Raw, airway resistance; RV, residual volume; TLC, total lung capacity; VC, vital capacity; $\dot{V}_{max}$, maximum expiratory flow.

have demonstrated that hypoxemia can result from the maldistribution of ventilation due to narrowing of small (<2 mm) airways, an obstruction which is not detected by standard physiologic studies (20, 21).

In light of these newer concepts of small airways disease, the present study was designed to: (*a*) evaluate the morphology of small airways in IPF; (*b*) determine if patients with IPF have physiologic alterations consistent with small airways disease; and (*c*) attempt to correlate these morphologic and physiologic findings. To do so, we chose a group of patients with IPF who had normal airway function by standard physiologic studies and who had undergone lung biopsy within close proximity to a physiologic evaluation of small airways function. The results demonstrate that we must expand the concepts of IPF to consider it a disorder of small airways as well as alveoli.

METHODS

Patient population

Over an 18-mo period, 150 patients were referred to the Pulmonary Branch, National Heart, Lung, and Blood Institute for evaluation of interstitial lung disease. From this group, patients were determined to have IPF if they fit the following criteria (14–16).

Clinical. History of exertional breathlessness; no history of exposure to inorganic, organic, gaseous, physical, or pharmacologic agents known to cause pulmonary fibrosis; no history suggestive of an allergic pulmonary disorder; no history of chronic pulmonary infection; and no historical or physical evidence of left ventricular failure. All patients underwent fiberoptic bronchoscopy (B2F, Olympus Corporation of America, New Hyde Park, N. Y.) and were demonstrated to have normal airways within limits of the procedure.

Roentgenographic. The presence of a diffuse infiltrative pattern (reticular, reticulonodular, or ground glass) on a routine posterior-anterior chest film and no evidence of left ventricular disease.

Physiologic. Reduced lung volumes or reduced diffusing capacity or both; mild to moderate hypoxemia at rest which worsened with exercise, and a static volume-pressure curve consistent with fibrotic disease (see below for physiologic methods).

Morphologic. Lung biopsy showing varying degrees of alveolar septal fibrosis and inflammation with interstitial and intra-alveolar inflammatory cells (predominantly mononuclear cells, but often accompanied by neutrophils and eosinophils); no granuloma, no vasculitis, no evidence of inorganic material by polarized light microscopy, and negative cultures for bacteria and fungi.

Patients were included in the current study if they met all of the diagnostic criteria for IPF, and had no evidence of airways disease by standard criteria (forced expiratory volume in 1 s/forced vital capacity and airway resistance). In addition, they had to have had a recent lung biopsy demonstrating airways of <2 mm in diameter and be able to participate in measurement of at least two of three monitors of small airways (see below).

From the initial group of 150 patients, 50 had the diagnosis of IPF and 18 of these fit all of the criteria to be included in this study. Patients who were excluded from the study were done so largely because of failure to have a recent biopsy or because of advanced disease and inability to participate in physiologic studies. 15 had no evidence of a collagen vascular disease, two (M. C., V. J.) had rheumatoid arthritis, and one (O. N.) had an overlap connective tissue syndrome. Eight patients had open lung biopsy at our institution with physiologic testing performed within 2 wk before biopsy. The remaining 10 patients had lung biopsies performed at an outside institution with physiologic testing performed at our institution 3–18 mo (average 4 mo) after biopsy.

Airway morphology

Morphological observations were made by one of us (W. C. R.) without knowledge of the results of the physiological testing. All observations were made on surgical specimens fixed in formalin, processed in alcohols and xylene, imbedded in paraffin, sectioned at 6 μm intervals, and then stained with hematoxylin and eosin. Serial sections were evaluated whenever possible. Airways of 2-mm diameter or less which had nearly perpendicular cuts were selected for evaluation. Each biopsy contained an average of 7.7±0.7[2] airways which were suitable for study.

The following histologic features of small airways were noted if present: peribronchiolar fibrosis, peribronchiolar inflammation, and bronchiolitis. In addition, the diameters of small airways were graded as to whether they were normal, narrowed, or dilated by the following criteria: (*a*) comparing the diameter of the bronchiolar lumen to the diameter of the lumen of the accompanying pulmonary artery (the bronchiolar lumen should be as large or larger than the lumen of the artery); (*b*) comparing the diameter of the bronchiolar lumen in the biopsy to the bronchiolar lumen of noninflated normal lung with comparable sized bronchioles and pulmonary arteries; and (*c*) comparing the thickness of the bronchiolar wall to the thickness of the wall of comparably sized airways of noninflated normal lungs. Changes in pulmonary artery diameter associated with pulmonary hypertension were quantitated to adjust lumen diameter to a normal size and prevent over estimation of airway diameter. If an airway was normal or dilated, but on serial section was shown to be narrowed at some point, it was graded as narrowed.

To facilitate comparison of morphologic and physiologic studies, an overall estimate of the diameter of the small airways in each biopsy was made using the following criteria: if 60% or more airways in the biopsy were narrowed, airways diameter was considered "narrowed," independent of status of the other airways; if 70% or more of the airways in the biopsy were normal or dilated (i.e. 30% or less were narrowed), airways diameter was considered "not narrowed," independent of the status of the other airways. If 31–59% of the airways in the biopsy were narrowed, the morphologic data for that patient were not used for statistical comparison with the physiologic data.

Lung volumes, timed expiratory maneuver, and diffusing capacity

Lung volumes, timed expiratory maneuver and diffusing capacity were measured on a computerized lung analyzer (Warren E. Collins, Inc., Braintree, Mass.). Vital capacity (VC), forced vital capacity, forced expiratory volume in 1 s, and inspiratory capacity were done in the standing position. Functional residual capacity (FRC) was done in the sitting

[2] All data will be presented as mean±SEM.

position utilizing a closed circuit helium equilibration technique (22). Expiratory reserve volume was subtracted from FRC to obtain residual volume (RV) and VC was added to RV to obtain observed total lung capacity (TLC). Predicted values for VC, forced expiratory volume in 1 s, and forced expiratory volume in 1 s/forced vital capacity ($FEV_1\%$) were obtained from the data of Morris et al. (23). Predicted FRC and RV were obtained from the normals of Goldman and Becklake (24). Predicted TLC was obtained by adding predicted VC to predicted RV. The lower limit of lung volumes was considered to be −20% of the predicted value. The lower limit for $FEV_1\%$ was considered to be equal to the predicted $FEV_1\%$−5% (25).

Single-breath carbon monoxide diffusing capacity (D_{LCO}) was performed by the method of Ogilvie et al. (26). The program was modified so that alveolar volume was determined by a single-breath helium dilutional technique. Alveolar gas was quantitated after absorption of CO_2; gas concentrations were then adjusted by 6% for CO_2 removal (6% is the usual alveolar CO_2 concentration). The results were compared to the predicted values of Gaensler and Wright (27).

Airway resistance

Airway resistance (Raw) was determined by modification of the method of Dubois et al. (28) using a constant volume plethysmograph (Warren E. Collins, Inc.). Statham differential transducers (Pm 6 and 15, Gould, Inc., Oxnard, Calif.) were interfaced with carrier amplifiers (model 8805 B, Hewlett-Packard Co., Palo Alto, Calif.). Flow was measured with a heated number 3 Fleisch pneumotachograph (Medical Products, Blue Bell, Pa.). All transducers had a frequency response within ±5% up to 6 cycles/s. The Fleisch pneumotachograph was linear from 0.1–6 liters/s. Data were recorded on a storage oscilloscope (Tektronix, Inc., Beaverton, Oreg.) and either traced directly on cellulose paper or photographed. Raw was measured by the slope of where the loop crossed a flow of 1 liter/s. The resistance of the pneumotachograph, shutter assembly, and mouth piece (0.35 cm H_2O/liter per s) was subtracted from the total Raw. Normal Raw was considered to be $\leqq$ 2.5 cm H_2O/liter per s (28).

Maximum expiratory flow-volume relationship

The relationship between maximum expiratory flow and volume (MEFV) was determined in the sitting position utilizing a wedge spirometer (570, Med-Science Electronics, Inc., St. Louis, Mo.) connected to a rapidly responding (1,500 in/s^2) XY recorder (model 7046A, Hewlett-Packard Co.). The apparatus was calibrated electronically and checked manually utilizing a 1-liter syringe (Warren E. Collins, Inc.) and a 0–10-liter/s flow meter (Vol-O-Flow, National Institute Laboratories Inc., Rockville, Md.). Calibration of flow was accomplished by incorporating a low resistance three-way valve (Warren E. Collins, Inc.) between a flow generator (vacuum cleaner) and flow meter and spirometer so that flow rate and time could be controlled; flow was linear from 0.1 to 10 liters/s.

A minimum of three MEFV curves were performed at each sitting and most patients had four to six curves done during their evaluation. The two most reproducible curves with the best flow rates and volumes within ±5% of VC (as quantitated by standard water spirometry) were accepted. Final MEFV curves were constructed from these data using the highest flow rates at all volumes.

The final MEFV data were analyzed by three methods: (*a*) with flow (liters/second) plotted against volume (observed VC); (*b*) with flow (liters/second) plotted against volume (percent observed TLC); and (*c*) with flow divided by observed TLC (liters/second per liter) plotted against volume (percent observed VC remaining). Because of the wide variation in lung volumes in the patient population, method *c* was found to be most useful; these data were compared to the normal values of Gelb et al. (29).

Static compliance, dynamic compliance, and isovolume pressure-flow curves

These data were obtained in the sitting position utilizing a wedge spirometer for quantitation of volume and flow rates. Transpulmonary pressure (P_L) was measured as the difference between mouth and esophageal pressure utilizing a Sanborn 268-B differential strain gauge and carrier preamplifier (Hewlett-Packard Co.). Volume, flow, and P_L signals were recorded on a Brush model 480, eight channel universal recorder (Gould, Inc.). The esophageal pressure signal was transmitted by a 10 cm, thin-walled, latex balloon (Young Rubber Co., Trenton, N.J.) positioned in the lower third of the esophagus by first passing it into the stomach and observing for a positive defection, then withdrawing the balloon approximately 10 cm so that the pressure signal was maximum and artifact free. Balloon volume was corrected by the methods of Milic-Emili et al. (30) or Lemen et al. (31); the latter technique was simpler and closely agrees with the former.

The wedge spirometer was calibrated electronically and checked manually utilizing a 1-liter syringe and a 0–10 liter/s flow meter. Using a sine wave generator, the frequency response of the spirometer was ±5% at 6 cycles/s and flow was linear from 0.1 to 10 liters/s. The Sanborn 268-B differential strain gauge was linear between 0–100 cm H_2O and had a frequency response which was ±5% at 6 cycles/s. Evaluation of phase lag between signals of flow, volume, and esophageal balloon pressure was performed by inserting the balloon inside the wedge spirometer and applying a sine wave (using a 500-ml pump) to the system. These signals were in phase (<5° shift) up to 3 cycles/s.

A constant volume history was assured by having the patient hyperventilate and then inspire to TLC three times (32). Static transpulmonary pressure (Pst) was measured at TLC and during deflation as the pressure difference between mouth and esophageal pressure with glottis open and flow being interrupted by a solenoid-operated shutter.

Static volume-pressure curves were constructed utilizing a mean of four deflation maneuvers with 12–14 points per maneuver. Volume was converted to body temperature and pressure saturated and required to be ±5% of VC (as recorded on standard spirometry). Because of the marked variability of Pst below 50% observed TLC, static volume-pressure curves were constructed from TLC to 50% observed TLC. Volume was expressed both as a percentage of observed and predicted TLC and compared to the predicted data of Turner et al. (32).

Data for generation of isovolume pressure-flow curves were obtained by having the patient exhale from TLC to RV at varying efforts from maximum flow to 0.5 liter/s. From simultaneously recorded flow, volume, and P_L data, isovolume pressure-flow curves were constructed at 70, 50, and 30% VC according to the method of Hyatt et al. (33).

Dynamic compliance (Cdyn) was measured by having the patient first hyperventilate, inspire to TLC three times, and then breathe at a constant tidal volume at increasing frequencies up to 100 breaths/min. Flow, volume, and P_L were simultaneously recorded while a constant resting end expiratory point and resting end inspiratory point were maintained by having the patient observe his breathing pattern (volume) on a time base oscilloscope. For each frequency, Cdyn was calculated by dividing the volume change by the change in pressure at points of zero flow over 10 or more breaths and averaging the results. Cdyn was expressed as a percentage of initial Cdyn (Cdyn/initial Cdyn) and plotted against respiratory frequency. A frequency dependent decrease in Cdyn/ initial Cdyn of > 20% was considered to be abnormal (34, 35).

To determine the effect of bronchodilators on Cdyn, these maneuvers were repeated immediately after 0.5 ml of 1% isoetherine was administered as an aerosol inhalant.

Maximum flow-static recoil relationship

The relationship between maximum flow and static recoil (MFSR) was determined by plotting maximum expiratory flow ($\dot{V}_{max}$; obtained from the MEFV curve from 80 to 50% observed TLC) against Pst (derived from the static volume-pressure curve) at the same lung volumes (36). These data were also plotted utilizing $\dot{V}_{max}$ and Pst expressed as percentage of predicted lung volume. Predicted MFSR curves were obtained by plotting $\dot{V}_{max}$ predicted by the data of Cherniack and Raber (37) against Pst at the same lung volume predicted by the data of Turner et al. (32). The prediction curves were grouped by age range from 25 to 45 yr and greater than 45 yr. These curves compare favorably to the normal curves of Mead et al. (36) and Ostrow and Cherniack. (38).

Statistical analysis of data

Three statistical methods were used for data analysis: Spearman rank correlation, two-tailed Student's *t*-test, and Fisher's exact test. To facilitate discussion of the analysis, the data were grouped as follows: "clinical data" include age, sex, duration of symptoms, smoking history, and drug therapy; "standard physiologic studies" include VC, FRC, TLC, RV/TLC, and D_{LCO}; "physiologic monitors of small airways" include Cdyn, MEFV curves, and MFSR curves; and "overall estimate of small airways diameter" refers to the rating ("narrowed" or "not narrowed") given to each biopsy as defined by the criteria listed above.

The choice of a statistical method for comparisons among clinical, physiologic, and morphologic data was dictated by the form of the data. Spearman rank correlation (39) was used when one variable was ranked and the other variable was ranked or continuous. The two-tailed Student's *t* test (40) was used when the mean values for a continuous variable could be determined for each of two ranked groups. Fisher's exact (41) test was used when both variables could be ranked in two categories and a contingency table could be constructed. In certain comparisons, more than one statistical comparison was used. A standard Pearson correlation was not used because it assumes a normal distribution for both variables and in all comparisons made at least one variable was ranked.

Utilizing these criteria, the following statistical comparisons were made:

(*a*) Spearman rank correlation of clinical data vs. overall estimate of small airways diameter; standard physiologic studies vs. overall estimate of small airways diameter; clinical data vs. physiologic monitors of small airways; and standard physiologic studies vs. physiologic monitors of small airways; (*b*) two-tailed Student's *t* test of standard physiologic studies vs. overall estimate of small airways diameter; and (*c*) Fisher's exact test of physiologic monitors of small airways vs. overall estimate of small airways diameter; and RV/TLC, MEFV curves and MFSR curves vs. Cdyn.

RESULTS

Clinical data. The 18 study patients ranged in age from 27 to 67 yr, 12 were male and 6 were female (Table I). Six patients never smoked; an additional three were light cigarette smokers (<10 pack yr) and one was a cigar smoker. The remaining eight patients were either moderate (10–25 pack yr) or heavy smokers (>25 pack yr) and none had a history of sputum production. The duration of symptoms (before study at National Institutes of Health) ranged from 0.5 to 10 yr, but was ≤ 2 yr in all but one patient (W. L.). Eight patients were taking prednisone at the time of evaluation; one was taking phenylbutazone, and none was taking sympathomimetic agents or xanthines.

Morphologic evaluation of small airways in IPF. A total of 138 small airways were suitable for evaluation in the lung biopsies of the 18 patients (Table II). The most frequently observed morphologic abnormality was peribronchiolar fibrosis, either alone or together with peribronchiolar inflammation and bronchiolitis (Fig. 1). No airway was seen with bronchiolitis alone. Only one patient (W. L. S.) had completely normal airways.

Each biopsy was graded an average of three times. Using the grading criteria for airway diameter, the mean intraobserver coefficient of variation was 9.1 ±0.2%; the mean interobserver error was 10%. Of the total airways evaluated, 19% were of normal diameter, 27% were dilated, and 54% were narrowed (Table II). The dominant histologic abnormality accompanying narrowed airways was peribronchiolar fibrosis with infolding and stenosis (Fig. 1 B); seen less frequently was peribronchiolar fibrosis or inflammation and bronchiolitis (Fig. 1 C). The presence of histologic abnormalities of small airways did not necessarily mean the airway would be narrowed; peribronchiolar inflammation and peribronchiolar fibrosis were associated with airways that were of normal diameter (Fig. 1 A) or dilated (Fig. 1 D).

Using the criteria listed in Methods, overall estimates of small airways diameter revealed that 12 of the 18 patients (67%) had "narrowed" airways (i.e. in these patients, 60% or more of the small airways evaluated were narrowed) and the remaining 6 patients (33%) had "not narrowed" airways (i.e. in these patients, 70% or more of the airways evaluated were normal or dilated).

Standard physiologic studies and routine monitors of airways. The lung volumes were variable in the 18 patients with IPF, but the mean predicted values were significantly reduced (Table III). Although patients with histologically proven IPF are generally considered to have reduced volumes, one (E. B.) had a TLC within the normal range. Likewise, although almost all of the patients had a reduced D_{LCO} (mean 52.7% predicted), one patient (B. T.) had a D_{LCO} within the normal range. Thus, all of the patients had either a reduced TLC or D_{LCO}, and 89% had both. The average RV/TLC was 31.8%; 10 patients had normal RV/TLC (<30% observed).

TABLE I
Clinical Data of 18 Patients with IPF

Patient	Age	Sex	Height	Weight	Smoking history*	Duration of symptoms	Drugs‡
	yr		*cm*	*kg*		*yr*	
E. B.	48	M	195	100	Heavy	1.5	None
M. C.	57	F	158	76	Nonsmoker	0.5	Phenylbutazone
R. C.	66	M	172	68	Nonsmoker	0.5	Prednisone
N. C.	27	M	174	53	Light	2.0	Prednisone
A. D.	67	M	164	65	Medium§	0.5	Prednisone
G. F.	51	M	183	76	Medium§	2.0	Prednisone
A. H.	26	F	178	62	Light§	2.0	None
W. H.	41	M	183	84	Light§	2.0	None
V. J.	27	F	162	48	Nonsmoker	0.5	None
W. L.	67	M	179	86	Heavy§	10.0	None
O. N.	27	F	171	63	Nonsmoker	1.5	Prednisone
P. R.	31	F	175	88	Medium	0.5	Prednisone
J. C. S.	61	M	172	77	Heavy§	1.5	None
W. E. S.	66	M	173	85	Cigars§	1.0	None
R. S.	52	M	186	66	Nonsmoker	2.0	Prednisone
J. K. S.	46	M	182	80	Medium§	2.0	Prednisone
W. L. S.	58	M	171	72	Medium§	1.0	None
B. T.	47	F	163	83	Nonsmoker	0.5	None
Mean±SEM	48.1±3.6		174.5±2.2	74.6±3.1		1.7±0.5	

* Light, <10 pack-yr; moderate, 10–25 pack-yr; heavy, >25 pack-yr.
‡ Only anti-inflammatory agents are listed; none of the patients was taking xanthines or sympathomimetics.
§ Stopped smoking >6 mo before study.

Routine monitors of airways (FEV_1%, Raw) were normal in all patients tested. Four patients (G. F., W. L., J. K. S., R. S.) were unable to perform the necessary maneuvers to measure Raw because of marked resting breathlessness.

Volume-pressure relationship. Most patients exhibited increased elastic recoil at lung volumes above FRC with a shift of the volume-pressure curve downward and to the right when volume was expressed as a percentage of predicted TLC (Fig. 2). One patient (E. B.) had a borderline shift in the volume-pressure curve to the left of the predicted normal curve for his age. When volume was expressed as a percentage of measured TLC (Fig. 3), five patients (A. H., P. R., G. F., R. C., W. L.) had curves which were similar to normal except at high lung volumes.

Physiologic monitors of small airways. Cdyn, performed in 17 patients, was frequency independent in 7 and frequency dependent in 10 (Fig. 4). Three patients (G. F., P. R., and B. T.) exhibited Cdyn which was less frequency dependent after nebulized bronchodilators. In no case did the use of bronchodilators cause the Cdyn to become independent of frequency (data not shown).

Nine patients had abnormal MEFV curves with reduced flows at low lung volumes and nine had normal to increased flows at all lung volumes (Fig. 5). All three methods of analysis of the MEFV data (see Methods) give comparable results.

Seven patients had reduced flow rates for a given P_{st} with a shift of the MFSR curve to the right of the normal range. The remaining 11 patients had normal to increased flow rates for a given P_{st} (Fig. 6). Both methods of analysis (see Methods) gave comparable results.

Obtaining meaningful MEFV and MFSR curves depends upon achieving maximum flow. To verify that maximum flow was achieved in these studies, isovolume pressure-flow curves were constructed. 15 patients achieved maximum flow and effort independence at 50% VC (data not shown). The remaining three patients (M. C., G. F., W. E. S.) were not able to perform the necessary maneuvers to construct isovolume pressure-flow curves because of breathlessness and inability to perform sustained expiratory maneuvers at variable flow rates.

Comparison of clinical, physiologic, and morphologic studies. Of the 17 patients[3] whose clinical and physiologic data were used for statistical comparisons

[3] One patient (R. C.) was excluded from the statistical comparisons with the overall estimate of small airway diameter because the lung biopsy was a drill biopsy which contained only one airway.

TABLE II

Morphologic Evaluation of Small Airways in Lung Biopsy Specimens of 18 Patients with IPF

Patient	Biopsy site*	Number of airways examined	Histology‡ Peri-bronchiolar fibrosis	Peri-bronchiolar inflammation	Bronchiolitis	Small airway diameter Normal	Dilated	Narrowed	Overall estimate of small airway diameter§
						Number (%)			
E. B.	LUL	6	+	0	0	2 (33)	0 (0)	4 (67)	Narrowed
M. C.	LLL	8	+	+	0	0 (0)	1 (13)	7 (87)	Narrowed
R. C.	RLL	1	0	+	0	0 (0)	0 (0)	1 (100)	Narrowed
N. C.	LLL	6	+	+	+	0 (0)	2 (33)	4 (67)	Narrowed
A. D.	LLL	11	+	0	0	1 (9)	7 (63)	3 (27)	Not narrowed
G. F.	LLL	2	+	0	0	0 (0)	0 (0)	2 (100)	Narrowed
A. H.	LUL	10	+	0	0	1 (10)	0 (0)	9 (90)	Narrowed
W. H.	LLL LUL	10	+	0	0	7 (70)	0 (0)	3 (30)	Not narrowed
V. J.	RLL	5	0	+	0	3 (60)	1 (20)	1 (20)	Not narrowed
W. L.	RLL	9	+	+	+	1 (11)	2 (22)	6 (67)	Narrowed
O. N.	LUL	9	0	+	0	1 (11)	6 (67)	2 (22)	Not narrowed
P. R.	LLL	7	+	+	+	2 (29)	0 (0)	5 (71)	Narrowed
J. C. S.	LLL	6	+	0	0	2 (33)	0 (0)	4 (67)	Narrowed
W. E. S.	RUL RLL RML	10	+	0	0	0 (0)	4 (40)	6 (60)	Narrowed
R. S.	RLL	10	+	0	0	1 (10)	2 (20)	7 (70)	Narrowed
J. K. S.	LLL	12	+	0	0	0 (0)	10 (83)	2 (17)	Not narrowed
W. L. S.	RLL	5	0	0	0	5 (100)	0 (0)	0 (0)	Not narrowed
B. T.	LLL	11	0	+	+	1 (9)	1 (9)	9 (82)	Narrowed
Total		138				27 (19)‖	36 (27)‖	75 (54)‖	

* LUL, left upper lobe; LLL, left lower lobe; RUL, right upper lobe; RML, right middle lobe; RLL, right lower lobe.

‡ +, present; 0, not present.

§ The overall estimate of small airway diameter was narrowed if ≥60% of the airways in the biopsy were narrowed, independent of the status (normal or dilated) of the other airways; the overall estimate of small airway diameter was not narrowed if ≤30% of the airways were narrowed, independent of the status (normal or dilated) of the other airways; if 31–59% of the airways were narrowed, the morphologic data was not used for statistical comparisons with the physiologic data. Patient R. C. had a needle biopsy with only one airway present; this data was not used for statistical comparisons.

‖ Percent total.

FIGURE 1 Examples of small airways in open lung biopsies of patients with IPF. A. Small airway of normal diameter in a 27-yr-old female (V. J.) demonstrating peribronchiolar inflammation (×130). B. Narrowed small airway in a 26-yr-old female (A. H.) demonstrating peribronchiolar fibrosis with infolding and stenosis (×220). C. Narrowed small airway in a 47-yr-old female (B. T.) demonstrating peribronchiolar inflammation and bronchiolitis (×130). D. Dilated small airway in a 67-yr-old male (A. D.) demonstrating peribronchiolar fibrosis (×80). All sections were stained with hematoxylin and eosin.

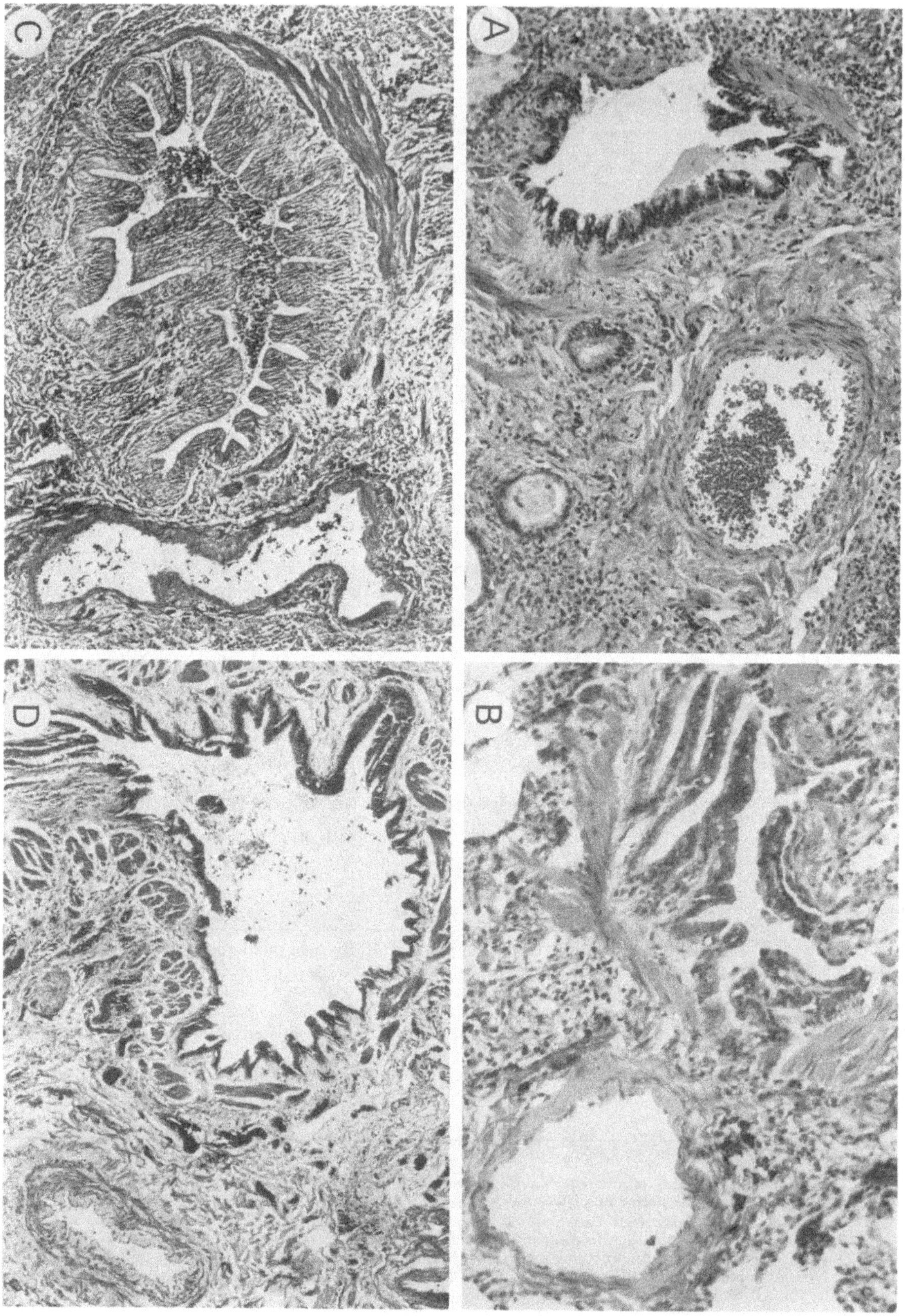
A
B
C
D

Table III
Standard Physiologic Studies of 18 Patients with IPF

Patient	VC Liters	VC % Predicted	FRC Liters	FRC % Predicted	TLC Liters	TLC % Predicted	RV/TLC % Observed	Diffusing capacity* ml CO/mm Hg/min	Diffusing capacity* % Predicted	FEV_1% % Observed	FEV_1% % Predicted	Raw cm H_2O/liter/s
E. B.	4.84	83	3.53	73	7.17	86	31	16.3	48	72	96	1.16
M. C.	2.02	73	1.25	60	2.81	70	28	11.1	53	83	104	1.80
R. C.	2.98	71	2.14	60	4.17	64	28	8.9	42	78	109	2.38
N. C.	1.50	28	2.11	60	3.10	44	52	17.3	74	90	112	2.50
A. D.	2.19	59	1.85	63	3.52	61	37	11.8	49	86	122	1.60
G. F.	3.56	71	2.71	65	5.33	71	31	9.4	33	70	98	ND‡
A. H.	3.46	75	2.73	76	4.81	72	29	17.2	66	76	97	0.68
W. H.	2.85	50	1.93	43	3.66	46	25	12.6	52	83	113	0.99
V. J.	1.95	50	1.65	60	2.71	50	27	12.7	71	93	114	1.28
W. L.	2.90	65	2.43	61	4.35	62	33	7.0	31	74	109	ND‡
O. N.	1.86	45	1.73	54	2.62	43	29	9.5	57	98	125	2.12
P. R.	2.55	60	2.76	81	4.24	67	47	11.5	47	81	102	1.68
J. C. S.	2.34	55	1.42	55	4.02	74	41	12.7	57	77	109	1.50
W. E. S.	2.30	35	1.62	42	3.22	49	28	11.8	58	72	104	1.36
R. S.	1.41	33	1.49	34	2.57	33	29	5.0	25	96	120	ND‡
J. K. S.	3.42	65	2.91	85	4.70	68	27	8.3	30	91	123	ND‡
W. L. S.	3.32	78	1.91	53	4.32	67	24	14.8	60	32	114	0.82
B. T.	1.62	48	1.77	62	3.56	50	37	14.4	96	85	112	1.14
Mean	2.67	56.0	2.10	60.4	3.93	59.8	31.8	11.7	52.7	82.4	110.0	1.54
±SEM	±0.21	±3.7	±0.14	±2.9	±.27	±3.2	±1.7	±0.8	±4.2	±2.1	±2.1	±0.17

* Single-breath carbon monoxide diffusing capacity.
‡ ND, not done.

with the overall estimate of small airways diameter, 11 had "narrowed" airways and 6 had "not narrowed" airways. The overall estimate of small airway diameter did not correlate with age, sex, smoking history, duration of symptoms, drugs (on or off anti-inflammatory medications), lung volumes (VC, FRC, TLC), or diffusing capacity (Tables IV, V). There was, however, a significant association between RV/TLC and the over-

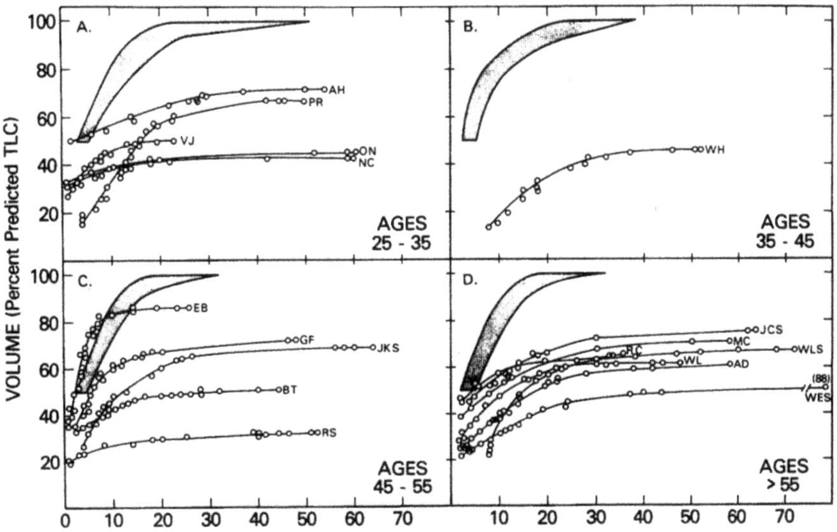

Figure 2 Static deflation volume-pressure curves for 18 patients with IPF grouped by age. Lung volume is expressed as percent predicted TLC. Pst is expressed in cm H_2O. Shaded area is the normal range established by Turner et al. (32).

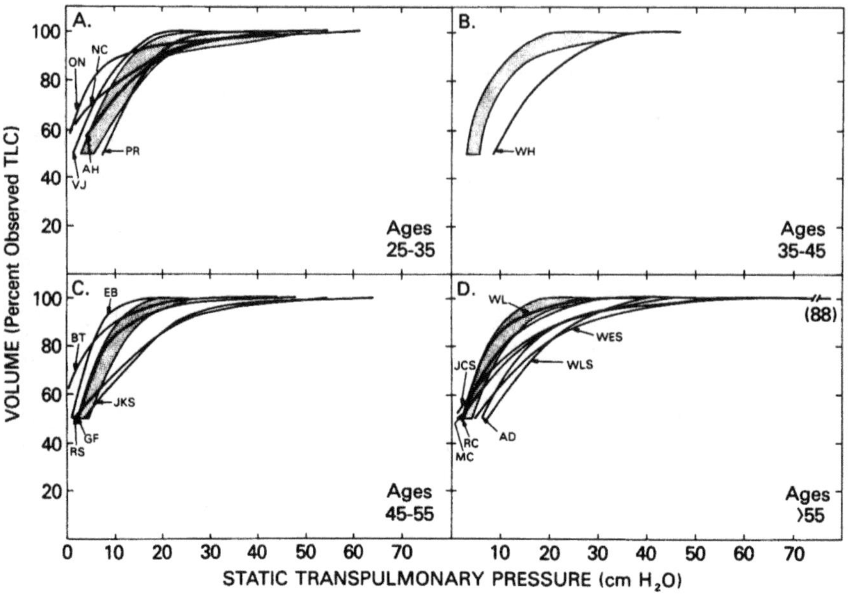

FIGURE 3 Static deflation volume-pressure curves for 18 patients with IPF grouped by age. Lung volume is expressed as percentage of observed (measured) TLC. Pst is expressed in cm H_2O. Shaded area is the normal range established by Turner et al. (32).

all estimate of small airways diameter whether the comparison was done by Spearman rank correlation ($P = 0.017$, Table IV) or Student's t test ($P = 0.046$, Table V). In general, patients with narrowed airways had elevated RV/TLC; in no case was an increased RV/TLC (>30% observed) associated with small airways whose overall status were not narrowed.

By entrance criteria for the study, all patients had normal $FEV_1\%$ and Raw, and thus there was no possible correlation between these monitors of large and

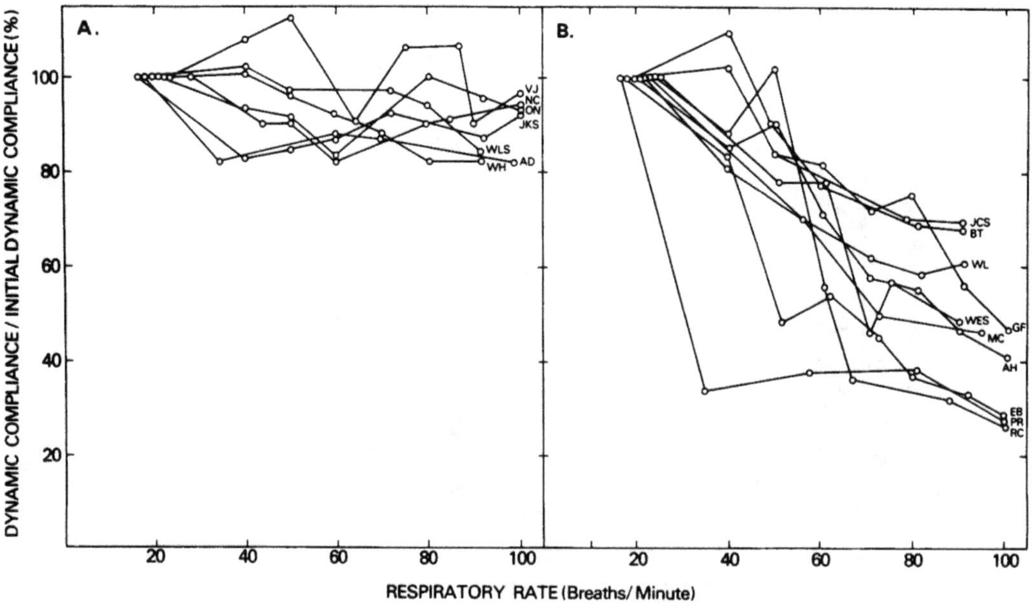

FIGURE 4 Cdyn in 17 patients with IPF expressed as a percentage of initial Cdyn. Respiratory rate is in breaths per minute. A. In seven patients Cdyn was independent of frequency. B. In 10 patients Cdyn was frequency dependent.

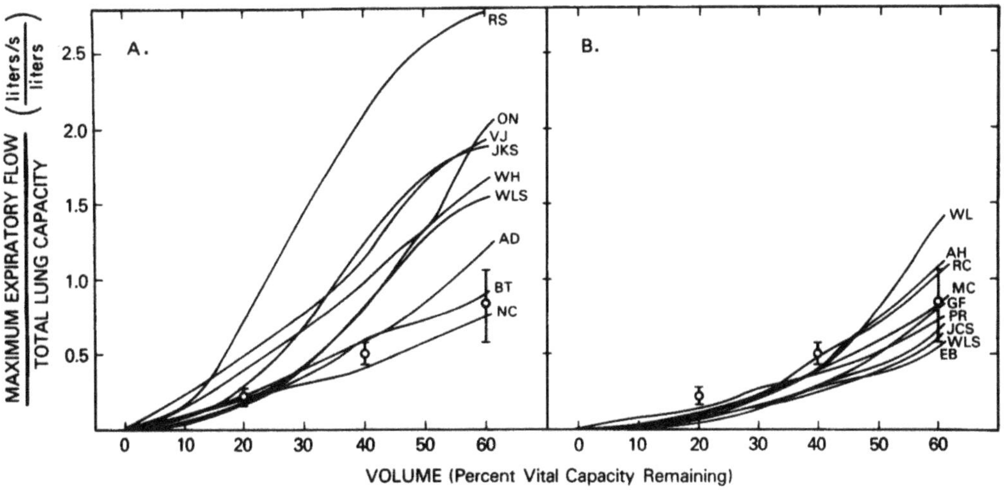

FIGURE 5 MEFV curves of 18 patients with IPF. Flow is expressed in liters per second/observed TLC; volume is expressed as percent VC remaining (60–0%). Open circles with error bars are the mean±SEM established by Gelb et al. (29).

medium airways and the morphologic evidence of narrowed small airways. In comparison, two of the physiologic tests of small airways function (Cdyn, MEFV curves) could predict the overall estimate of small airways diameter in open lung biopsy specimens.

Cdyn was the most sensitive predictor of the diameter of small airways ($P = 0.001$, Table VI); 9 of the 10 patients in whom airways were narrowed had frequency-dependent Cdyn and all 6 patients with not narrowed airways had normal Cdyn. Only one patient who had narrowed airways exhibited normal Cdyn; in no case was Cdyn frequency dependent in a patient who had airways of normal diameter.

The next most sensitive predictor of small airways diameter was the MEFV curve ($P = 0.009$, Table VI). 8 of the 11 patients in whom airways were narrowed had abnormal MEFV curves, whereas all 6 patients in whom airways were considered not narrowed had normal MEFV curves. However, three patients with narrowed small airways had normal MEFV curves. Like Cdyn, in no case was the MEFV curve abnormal in a patient who had airways that were considered not narrowed.

The third physiologic monitor of small airways, the MFSR relationship, was abnormal in 7 of the 11 patients with narrowed airways, and normal in all 6 patients with airways that were not narrowed (Table VI). However, four patients with narrowed airways had MFSR curves within the normal range. Like the other monitors of small airways, the MFSR curve was never

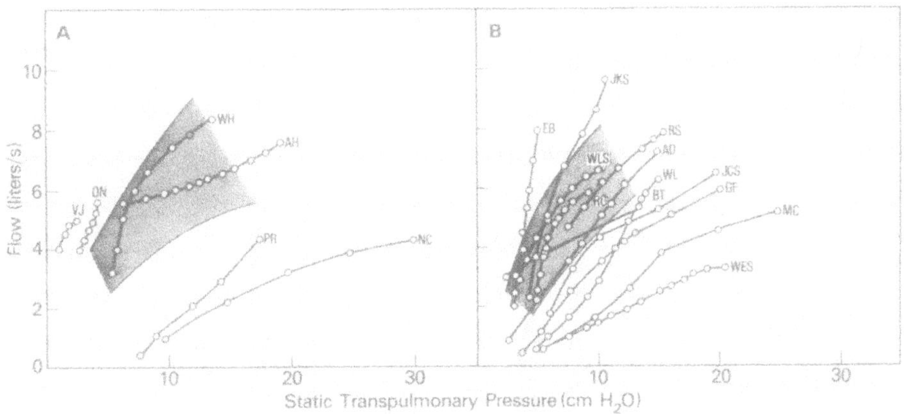

FIGURE 6 MRSR curves in 18 patients with IPF grouped by age. Flow is expressed in liters/second and Pst is expressed in cm H_2O. The shaded normal range is derived by plotting $\dot{V}_{max}$ predicted by the data of Cherniack and Raber (37) against Pst at the same lung volume predicted by the data of Turner et al. (32).

TABLE IV

Comparison of Clinical and Standard Physiologic Studies with the Overall Estimate of Small Airways Diameter of Patients with IPF

Comparison*	r value	P value
Clinical data‡ vs. overall estimate of small airways diameter§		
Age	0.139	0.601
Sex	0.030	0.904
Smoking history	−0.052	0.836
Duration of symptoms	0.144	0.588
Drugs	−0.044	0.862
Standard physiologic studies‖ vs. overall estimate of small airways diameter§		
VC	0.013	0.961
FRC	0.126	0.635
TLC	0.277	0.282
RV/TLC	0.568	0.017
Diffusing capacity	−0.050	0.842

* Comparison is by Spearman rank correlation.
‡ Data from Table I.
§ Data from Table II.
‖ Data from Table III.

TABLE V

Comparison of Standard Physiologic Studies between Groups of Patients with Overall Estimate of Small Airways that are Narrowed to Groups of Patients with Overall Estimate of Small Airways that Are Not Narrowed

Physiologic parameter	Mean value of physiologic parameter in each group of patients*: Those with airways that are narrowed‡	Those with airways that are not narrowed‡	P value§
VC	58.1	59.7	0.750
TLC	61.6	55.8	0.480
FRC	60.8	59.7	0.870
RV/TLC	35.5	28.2	0.046
Diffusing capacity	53.4	43.2	0.980

* Data from Table III; percent predicted values are used for all physiologic parameters except RV/TLC for which percent observed is used.
‡ Grouped according to the overall estimate of small airway diameter; see Table II.
§ Two-tailed Student's *t* test.

abnormal in a patient whose airways were considered not narrowed. Even so, the lack of a significant association between the MFSR curve and the overall estimate of small airways diameter suggested that the MFSR curve is not as sensitive as Cdyn or the MEFV curve in detecting narrowed small airways in patients with IPF.

There was no significant correlation between age, sex, smoking history, duration of symptoms, VC, FRC, RV/TLC, D_{LCO}, and the physiologic monitors of small airways (Table VII). However, there was a significant negative correlation between TLC and Cdyn and between TLC and the MEFV curves; patients with smaller total lung capacities tended to have normal Cdyn and normal MEFV curves, whereas those with larger total lung capacities tended to have frequency-dependent Cdyn and abnormal MEFV curves.

Although comparison of the physiologic data with the overall estimate of small airways diameter suggests that RV/TLC (Tables IV, V), Cdyn, and MEFV curves (Table VI) can predict narrowed small airways, only the results of the MEFV curves correlated with the results of Cdyn (the most sensitive predictor of the overall estimate of small airways diameter, Table VIII), suggesting a divergence in the physiologic functions monitored by some of these tests.

DISCUSSION

Although narrowing and stenosis of small airways were noted in the original description of IPF by Hamman and Rich (1), subsequent morphologic reports have largely concentrated on the alveoli and alveolar interstitium (3, 4, 8–10, 13); perhaps because the significance of small airways abnormalities in the pathophysiology of some chronic pulmonary disorders has only recently been recognized (42, 43). The data presented in this investigation indicate that morphologic and physiologic abnormalities of small airways are present

TABLE VI

Comparison between the Physiologic Monitors of Small Airways and the Overall Estimate of Small Airways Diameter in Patients with IPF

Physiologic study	Results*	Number of patients	Overall estimate of small airways diameter‡: Narrowed	Not narrowed	P value§
Cdyn	Normal	7	1	6	0.001
	Abnormal	9‖	9	0	
MEFV curve	Normal	9	3	6	0.009
	Abnormal	8‖	8	0	
MFSR curve	Normal	10‖	4	6	0.100
	Abnormal	7	7	0	

* Data from Figs. 4–6.
‡ Data from Table II.
§ Fisher's exact test.
‖ One patient (R. C.) was not included in the statistical analysis because the biopsy showed only one airway.

Table VII
Comparison of the Clinical Data and Standard Physiologic Studies with the Physiologic Monitors of Small Airways in Patients with IPF

	Physiologic monitors of small airways*					
	Cdyn		MEFV curve		MFSR	
	r value§	*P* value§	*r* value§	*P* value§	*r* value§	*P* value§
Clinical data‡						
Age	0.274	0.305	0.253	0.328	0.106	0.689
Sex	0.163	0.553	0.044	0.862	0.0635	0.803
Smoking history	0.042	0.870	0.250	0.665	0.219	0.598
Duration of symptoms	0.028	0.914	0.063	0.806	0.274	0.288
Standard physiologic studies‖						
VC	−0.3011	0.256	−0.047	0.055	−0.237	0.639
TLC	−0.5611	0.023	−0.663	0.004	−0.066	0.797
FRC	−0.261	0.332	0.289	0.259	−0.132	0.619
RV/TLC	−0.371	0.156	−0.266	0.303	−0.371	0.140
Diffusing capacity	−0.151	0.584	−0.217	0.592	−0.184	0.515

* Data from Figs. 4–6.
‡ Data from Table I.
§ Comparisons made using Spearman rank correlation.
‖ Data from Table III.

in IPF. The patients studied were representative of patients with IPF; the duration of symptoms and lung biopsy were typical of patients in mid-course (3–13). None had morphologic findings consistent with "end stage" lung (44).

Morphologic evaluation of small airways in IPF. Only one patient had completely normal airways; in the remainder, the majority of the small airways had peribronchiolar fibrosis or peribronchiolar inflammation or both; a smaller number of airways had coexisting bronchiolitis. Our data base does not allow for definitive conclusions as to whether these abnormalities are part of the same process that involves the alveolar interstitium; however, the localization of most of the airway pathology in the peribronchiolar tissue suggests that the inflammation and fibrosis of the small airways is secondary to the interstitial process. The dominant small airways abnormalities (peribronchiolar fibrosis, peribronchiolar inflammation, or both) were observed in all nonsmokers (M. C., R. C., V. J., O. N., R. S., B. T.) and all smokers (E. B., N. C., A. D., G. F., A. H., W. H., W. L., P. R., J. C. S., W. E. S., J. K. S.) except one (W. L. S.; Tables I, II). Thus, even though bronchiolar fibrosis and inflammation have been described in smokers (45–47), the lack of correlation of airway abnormalities and smoking history (Table IV, $P = 0.836$) suggests smoking was not the causative agent in these patients with IPF. In addition, there was no evidence that the airway abnormalities were secondary to intercurrent infection, because all bacterial, mycobacterial, fungal, and viral cultures of open lung biopsies done at our institution were negative.

Some degree of bronchiolectasis was present in approximately one-fourth of all airways evaluated. Although there is no correlation between the morphologic assessment of the severity of disease and airway diameter, it is our impression that small airways in IPF progress through stages beginning with peribronchiolar inflammation leading to peribronchiolar fibrosis. With progressive fibrosis, it is probable that some air-

Table VIII
Comparison of the Results of RV/TLC, MEFV Curve, and MFSR Curve with the Results of Cdyn in Patients with IPF

Physiologic study	Results	Number of patients	Cdyn* Normal	Cdyn* Abnormal	*P* value‡
RV/TLC*§	Normal	10	4	6	0.500
	Abnormal	7‖	2	5	
MEFV curve¶	Normal	8‖	7	1	0.001
	Abnormal	9	0	9	
MFSR curve**	Normal	10‖	6	4	0.310
	Abnormal	7	1	6	

* Data from Fig. 4.
‡ Fisher's exact test.
§ Data from Table III.
‖ One patient (R. S.) was excluded because he was unable to do Cdyn.
¶ Data from Fig. 5.
** Data from Fig. 6.

ways stenose, whereas others become distorted and ectatic (44). However, this would be difficult to prove.

Even though almost all of the patients had morphologic abnormalities of small airways, these do not necessarily imply airways dysfunction. If intrinsic small airways abnormalities contribute significantly to airways dysfunction, the feature which should be compared to the physiologic studies is airway diameter (e.g. narrowed or not narrowed). 12 of the 18 patients had an overall estimate of small airways diameter of narrowed; the morphologic data, therefore, suggest that these patients have physiologic alterations consistent with obstruction of small airways.

It may be argued that biopsy specimens are not representative of the disease and that multiple samples, available only at autopsy, are necessary to fully evaluate IPF; or that biopsy specimens present special problems in the evaluation of airways diameter because it is not possible to "physiologically" inflate and fix an open lung biopsy as can be done with postmortem lung. However, it is critical that evaluation of small airways in IPF be done with biopsy (rather than postmortem) material because: (*a*) patients with IPF often die from a generalized pulmonary infection, a process which in itself may alter the morphology and diameter of small airways; (*b*) those who die without respiratory infection usually have "end-stage" lung, in which the disease is too far advanced to allow for rational morphologic analysis; and (*c*) to compare airway morphology with airway function (i.e. with physiologic studies), it is necessary to make the interval between the two as short as possible; a situation which is impossible when relying on postmortem lung.

Thus, to study small airway morphology in IPF in mid-course, it is mandatory that only biopsy material be used. To attempt to minimize errors in estimating airway diameter, detailed diameter grading was not attempted, only categories of narrowed, normal, or dilated were used. In addition, three independent criteria were used to estimate airway diameter; all done without knowledge of the physiologic data. Each method of diameter estimate gave similar results. In addition, to attempt to provide "representative" biopsies, the specimens were taken in areas appearing "average" on the chest roentgenogram.

Physiologic evaluation of small airways in IPF. None of the study patients had evidence of increased resistance to airflow by standard monitors of airway function (FEV_1%, Raw). However, a significant number had abnormalities in physiologic tests considered to be monitors of small airways function. 59% had frequency-dependent Cydn (a decrease in Cdyn/initial Cdyn of greater than 20% with increasing respiratory rates). The remaining patients had normal Cdyn (a change of no more than 20% of Cdyn/initial Cdyn at increasing respiratory rates). In addition, 50% of the patients had abnormal MEFV curves and 39% had abnormal MEFV curves.

When the Cdyn data were plotted as percent of static compliance (Cstat) as described by Woolcock et al. (56), five of the seven patients (W. H., W. L. S., O. N., N. C., J. C. S.) with normal Cdyn (Fig. 3, group A.) had Cdyn/Cstat of < 80% at initial breathing frequencies (data not shown). This subgroup of patients did not, however, exhibit a progressive fall in Cdyn with increasing respiratory rates regardless of the method of analysis (Cdyn/initial Cdyn or Cdyn/Cstat). Four of these patients have been restudied at 3–6 mo intervals and exhibit identical reductions in Cdyn/Cstat at initial breathing frequencies without frequency dependence. Reduced Cdyn/Cstat at initial respiratory rates have been previously noted in fibrotic lung disease (49, 50). The reason for this is not clear, although alterations in surface forces which result in increased hysteresis are possible (49). In our patients, analysis of physiologic and morphologic data did not reveal significant differences between this subgroup of patients compared to those whose Cdyn/Cstat were > 80% at initial respiratory rates. The former did, however, tend to have more severe fibrosis.

Other physiologic studies have suggested that patients with IPF have small airways abnormalities. In a study of airway function in pulmonary fibrosis, Ostrow and Cherniack (38) included patients with "cryptogenic fibrosing alveolitis" whose physiologic features were similar to our patients. Like our study group, their patients had normal airway function by standard criteria, yet a significant number had physiologic evidence of increased resistance to airflow in small airways. A similar study by Yernalt et al. (49) also demonstrated that many of these patients have evidence of increased small airways resistance. In contrast, Schofield et al. (51) measured upstream conductance in patients with fibrotic lung disease (three with IPF), and found that these patients had normal upstream conductance. However, it is likely that those patients fall into the group of our patients (61%) that also had normal MFSR curves.

Recent studies have suggested that closing volume and closing capacity might be useful monitors of small airways in fibrotic lung disease (52, 53). In our group of 18 patients, we have performed more than 200 determinations of closing volume and closing capacity using the methods of Buist and Ross (54, 55). These tests were quite variable, even when performed on the same patient on consecutive days of the same hospitalization (data not shown). Thus, we do not find these to be useful in patients with IPF. Although closing volume and closing capacity may be useful for the detection of small airways abnormalities in patients with normal elastic recoil, they are less useful when recoil is increased as in patients with IPF. In addition, although the phase III data of the single breath nitrogen test was highly reproducible in these patients, there was no correlation between the slope of phase III (ΔN_2/liter) and any of the clinical, physiologic or morphologic parameters under study.

Comparison of clinical, physiologic, and morphologic data in IPF. Although it is generally accepted that MFSR curves can detect airflow obstruction in the presence of increased elastic recoil (48), it must be remembered that the use of Cdyn and MEFV curves as monitors of small airways function has been established only in the presence of normal lung resistance and normal elastic recoil (56–58). Inasmuch as patients with IPF have elevations of both (50, 59), it is possible that these physiologic abnormalities are secondary to alterations in regional compliance produced by the alveolar disease. To establish the valid use of these studies in IPF, it is necessary to demonstrate an association between these monitors of small airways function and the actual morphologic evidence of narrowed small airways.

The correlative data (Table VI) strongly suggest that Cdyn and MEFV curves detect, with a high degree of reliability, which patients with IPF have narrowed airways and which have not narrowed airways. These statistical comparisons are important because it could be argued that because both Cdyn and MEFV curves detect alterations in mechanical (resistance × compliance) time constants (56–58, 60), it is possible that abnormalities in these tests reflect abnormalities in regional compliance as well as airway resistance. However, if regional compliance abnormalities alone were responsible for making these tests abnormal in IPF, we would expect the results of Cdyn and MEFV curves to be randomly distributed, rather than yielding significant correlations with the morphologic estimates of small airways diameter. In addition, if volume pressure data are plotted with volume expressed as a percentage of measured TLC (Fig. 3) as Gibson and Pride have suggested (61), five patients who exhibited frequency-dependent Cdyn have curves which are similar to normals. This would suggest that there is uniform involvement of parenchyma and would favor the fact that frequency-dependent Cdyn is related to airways disease.

Even though 39% of the patients had abnormal MFSR curves, these data did not correlate with the morphologic assessment of airway narrowing ($P = 0.10$, Table VI). This lack of significant correlation occurred because although patients with not narrowed airways always had a normal MFSR curve, 4 of the 11 patients with narrowed airways also had normal MFSR studies. Thus, of the three physiologic methods (Cdyn, MEFV, MFSR) used in this study to test small airway function, the MFSR curve is the least sensitive. This may be due to the complexity of the volume-pressure curve in this disease, particularly at low lung volumes. Although almost all of our patients had increased elastic recoil near TLC, some had reduced recoil near FRC (Fig. 2 and 3). Similar volume-pressure curves were observed by Ostrow and Cherniack (38) and Yernalt et al. (49). The reduction in elastic recoil near FRC may result from a multitude of factors (e.g. rearrangements of connective tissue, increased tissue rigidity, destructive lesions), all of which may modify the usefulness of relying on measurement of upstream resistance as a monitor of small airways narrowing in IPF.

In comparison to Cdyn and MEFV curves, there were no significant associations among VC, FRC, and D_{LCO}, and the overall estimate of small airways diameter. Even though TLC correlated significantly with Cdyn and MEFV curves (Table VII), there was no correlation between TLC and overall estimate of small airways diameter. Thus, TLC cannot be used as a predictor of small airways disease in these patients. There was, however, a significant association between RV/TLC and airways diameter, suggesting that narrowing of small airways may account for the commonly observed increased RV/TLC seen in IPF (6, 7, 16). Although statistically significant, there was only a small difference in RV/TLC between patients grouped according to the estimate of airways diameter. Therefore, we do not believe that RV/TLC is a predictor of small airways diameter in IPF.

If we use frequency dependency of Cdyn as the best criterion for small airways dysfunction in IPF (Cdyn correlates best with the overall estimates of airway diameter, Table VI), it is interesting to note that results of MEFV curves correlate well with Cdyn, but the MFSR and RV/TLC results do not (Table VIII). These results are similar to that found by Martin et al. (62) and Gelb et al. (57) in evaluating these studies for use in patients with isolated small airways disease. Thus, Cdyn remains as the most sensitive and valid monitor of small airways disease, even in disorders as diverse as asthma (63) and IPF.

Inasmuch as age, sex, duration of symptoms, drugs, and smoking history could possibly modulate small airways disease, it was important to determine whether there were associations between these parameters and the morphologic assessment of small airways diameter or the physiologic monitors of small airways function. However, no significant correlates were found (Tables IV, V, VII).

Significance of small airways disease in IPF. The demonstration of morphologic and physiologic evidence of small airways abnormalities in IPF may have significant clinical implications. First, the detection of small airways dysfunction in IPF may be useful for staging this disease. Second, the hypoxemia may be, in part, secondary to ventilation-perfusion mismatching resulting from increased resistance to airflow in small airways. In our patient group, a small number of patients under therapy have demonstrated improvement of small airways function with lessening of hypoxemia with exercise. Thus, as suggested by Ostrow and Cherniack (38), small airways dysfunction may respond to therapeutic intervention which may significantly improve the level of oxygenation of patients with IPF.

ACKNOWLEDGMENTS

We thank Doctors Norton Elson and Byron McLees for their advice; Dr. David DeMetts for his help with the statistical analysis; Edwyna von Gal and Filippina Giacometti for their expert technical assistance; and Kirsten Cook and Nancy Wyne for their editorial assistance.

REFERENCES

1. Hamman, L., and A. R. Rich. 1944. Acute diffuse interstitial fibrosis of the lungs. *Bull. Johns Hopkins Hosp.* **74:** 177–212.
2. Rubin, E. H., and R. Lubliner. 1957. The Hamman-Rich syndrome: review of the literature and analysis of 15 cases. *Medicine (Baltimore).* **36:** 397–463.
3. Anderson, A. E., Jr., and A. G. Foraker. 1960. Morphological aspects of interstitial pulmonary fibrosis. *Arch. Pathol.* **70:** 79–93.
4. Scadding, J. G. 1960. Chronic diffuse interstitial fibrosis of the lungs. *Br. Med. J.* **1:** 443–450.
5. Herbert, F. A., B. B. Nahmias, E. A. Gaensler, and H. E. MacMahon. 1962. Pathophysiology of interstitial pulmonary fibrosis: report of 19 cases and follow-up with corticosteroids. *Arch. Intern. Med.* **110:** 628–648.
6. Livingstone, J. L., J. G. Lewis, L. Reid, and K. E. Jefferson. 1964. Diffuse interstitial pulmonary fibrosis: clinical, radiological, and pathological study based on 45 patients. *Q. J. Med.* **33:** 71–103.
7. Marks, A. 1967. Diffuse interstitial pulmonary fibrosis. *Med. Clin. North Am.* **51:** 439–457.
8. Scadding, J. G., and K. F. W. Hinson. 1967. Diffuse fibrosing alveolitis (diffuse interstitial fibrosis of the lungs): correlation of histology at biopsy with prognosis. *Thorax.* **22:** 291–304.
9. Liebow, A. A., and C. B. Carrington. 1967. Alveolar diseases: the interstitial pneumonias. *In* Frontiers of Pulmonary Radiology. M. Simon, E. J. Potchen, and M. LeMay, editors. Grune & Stratton, Inc., New York. 102–141.
10. Liebow, A. A. 1968. New concepts and entities in pulmonary disease. *In* The Lung. A. A. Liebow and D. E. Smith, editors. Williams and Wilkins, Baltimore. 332–365.
11. DeRemee, R. A., E. G. Harrison, Jr., and H. A. Andersen. 1972. The concept of classical interstitial pneumonitis-fibrosis (CIP-F) as a clinicopathologic syndrome. *Chest.* **61:** 213–220.
12. Stack, B. H. R., Y. F. J. Choo-Kang, and B. E. Heard. 1972. The prognosis of cryptogenic fibrosing alveolitis. *Thorax.* **27:** 535–542.
13. Scadding, J. G. 1974. Diffuse alveolar pulmonary fibrosis. *Thorax.* **29:** 271–281.
14. Kravis, T. C., A. Ahmed, T. E. Brown, J. D. Fulmer, and R. G. Crystal. 1976. Pathogenic mechanisms in pulmonary fibrosis: collagen-induced migration inhibition factor production and cytotoxicity mediated by lymphocytes. *J. Clin. Invest.* **58:** 1223–1232.
15. Reynolds, H. Y., J. D. Fulmer, J. A. Kazmierowski, W. C. Roberts, M. M. Frank, and R. G. Crystal. 1977. Analysis of cellular and protein content of broncho-alveolar lavage fluid from patients with idiopathic pulmonary fibrosis and chronic hypersensitivity pneumonitis. *J. Clin Invest.* **59:** 165–175.
16. Crystal, R. G., J. D. Fulmer, W. C. Roberts, M. L. Moss, B. R. Line, and H. Y. Reynolds. 1976. Idiopathic pulmonary fibrosis: clinical, histologic, radiographic, physiologic, scintigraphic, cytological, and biochemical aspects. *Ann. Intern. Med* **85:** 769–788.
17. Austrian, R., J. H. McClement, A. D. Renzetti, Jr., K. W. Donald, R. L. Riley, and A. Cournand. 1951. Clinical and physiologic features of some types of pulmonary diseases with impairment of alveolar-capillalry diffusion: the syndrome of "alveolar-capillary block." *Am. J. Med.* **11:** 667–685.
18. Finley, T. N., E. W. Swenson, and J. H. Comroe, Jr. 1962. The cause of arterial hypoxemia at rest in patients with "alveolar-capillary block syndrome." *J. Clin. Invest.* **41:** 618–622.
19. Wagner, P. D., D. R. Dantzker, R. Dueck, J. L. DePolo, K. Wasserman, and J. B. West. 1976. Distribution of ventilation-perfusion ratios in patients with interstitial lung disease. *Chest.* **69**(Suppl.): 256–257.
20. McFadden, E. R., Jr., and H. A. Lyons. 1968. Airway resistance and uneven ventilation in bronchial asthma. *J. Appl. Physiol.* **25:** 365–370.
21. Heckscher, T., H. Bass, A. Oriol, B. Rose, N. R. Anthonisen, and D. V. Bates. 1968. Regional lung function in patients with bronchial asthma. *J. Clin. Invest.* **47:** 1063–1070.
22. Meneely, G. R., and N. L. Kaltreider. 1949. The volume of the lung determined by helium dilution: description of method and comparison with other procedures. *J. Clin. Invest.* **28:** 129–139.
23. Morris, J. F., A. Koski, and L. C. Johnson. 1971. Spirometric standards for healthy nonsmoking adults. *Am. Rev. Respir. Dis.* **103:** 57–67.
24. Goldman, H. I., and M. R. Becklake. 1959. Respiratory function tests: normal values at medium altitudes and the predicition of normal results. *Am. Rev. Tuberc. Pulm. Dis.* **79:** 457–467.
25. Macdonald, J. B., T. J. Cole, and A. Seaton. 1975. Forced expiratory time—its reliability as a lung function test. *Thorax.* **30:** 554–559.
26. Ogilvie, C. M., R. E. Forster, W. S. Blakemore, and J. W. Morton. 1957. A standard breath holding technique for the clinical measurement of the diffusing capacity of the lung for carbon monoxide. *J. Clin. Invest.* **36:** 1–17.
27. Gaensler, E. A., and G. W. Wright. 1966. Evaluation of respiratory impairment. *Arch. Environ. Health* **12:** 146–189.
28. Dubois, A. B., S. Y. Botelho, and J. H. Comroe, Jr. 1956. A new method for measuring airway resistance in man using a body plethysmograph: values in normal subjects and in patients with respiratory disease. *J. Clin. Invest.* **35:** 327–335.
29. Gelb, A. F., W. M. Gold, R. R. Wright, H. R. Bruch, and J. A. Nadel. 1973. Physiologic diagnosis of subclinical emphysema. *Am. Rev. Respir. Dis.* **107:** 50–63.
30. Milic-Emili, J., J. Mead, J. M. Turner, and E. M. Glauser. 1964. Improved technique for estimating pleural pressure from eosphageal balloons. *J. Appl. Physiol.* **19:** 207–211.
31. Lemen, R., M. Benson, and J. G. Jones. 1974. Absolute pressure measurements with hand-dipped and manufactured esophageal balloons. *J. Appl. Physiol.* **37:** 600–603.

32. Turner, J. M., J. Mead, and M. E. Wohl. 1968. Elasticity of human lungs in relation to age. *J. Appl. Physiol.* **25:** 664–671.
33. Hyatt, R. E., D. P. Schilder, and D. L. Fry. 1958. Relationship between maximum expiratory flow and the degree of lung inflation. *J. Appl. Physiol.* **13:** 331–336.
34. Seaton, Anthony, N. LeRoy Lapp, and W. K. C. Morgan. 1972. Lung mechanics and frequency dependence of compliance in coal miners. *J. Clin. Invest.* **51:** 1203–1211.
35. Blair, H. Thomas, S. B. Greenberg, P. M. Stevens, P. A. Bilunos, and R. B. Couch. 1976. Effects of rhinovirus infection on pulmonary function of healthy human volunteers. *Am. Rev. Respir. Dis.* **114:** 95–102.
36. Mead, J., J. M. Turner, P. T. Macklem, and J. B. Little. 1967. Significance of the relationship between lung recoil and maximum expiratory flow. *J. Appl. Physiol.* **22:** 95–108.
37. Cherniack, R. M., and M. B. Raber. 1972. Normal standards for ventilatory function using an automated wedge spirometer. *Am. Rev. Respir. Dis.* **106:** 38–46.
38. Ostrow, D., and R. M. Cherniack. 1973. Resistance to airflow in patients with diffuse interstitial lung disease. *Am. Rev. Respir. Dis.* **108:** 205–210.
39. Snedecor, G. W., and W. G. Cochran. 1967. Statistical Methods. Iowa State University Press, Ames, Iowa. 6th edition. 194.
40. Snedecor, G. W., and W. G. Cochran. 1967. Statistical Methods. Iowa State University Press, Ames, Iowa. 6th edition. 59–61.
41. Brownlee, K. A. 1960. Statistical Theory and Methodology in Science and Engineering. John Wiley & Sons, Inc., New York. 123–125.
42. Hogg, J. C., P. T. Macklem, and W. M. Thurlbeck. 1968. Site and nature of airway obstruction in chronic obstructive lung disease. *N. Engl. J. Med.* **278:** 1355–1360.
43. Despas, P. J., M. Leroux, and P. T. Macklem. 1972. Site of airway obstruction in asthma as determined by measuring maximal expiratory flow breathing air and a helium-oxygen mixture. *J. Clin. Invest.* **51:** 3235–3243.
44. Heppleston, A. G. 1956. The pathology of honeycomb lung. *Thorax.* **11:** 77–93.
45. Niewoehner, D. E., J. Kleinerman, and D. B. Rice. 1974. Pathological changes in the peripheral airways of young cigarette smokers. *N. Engl. J. Med.* **291:** 755–758.
46. Thurlbeck, W. M. 1973. Disease of small airways, with particular reference to lesions found in asymptomatic chronic bronchitis without emphysema. *Chest.* **63** (Suppl.): 70S–71S.
47. Zamel, N., J. Hogg, and A. Gelb. 1976. Mechanisms of maximal expiratory flow limitation in clinically unsuspected emphysema and obstruction of peripheral airways. *Am. Rev. Respir. Dis.* **113:** 337–345.
48. Macklem, P. T. 1975. Tests of lung mechanics. *N. Engl. J. Med.* **293:** 339–342.
49. Yernalt, J. C., M. DeJonghe, A. DeCoster, and M. Englert. 1975. Pulmonary mechanics in diffuse fibrosing alveolitis. *Bull. Physio-pathol. Respir.* **11:** 231–244.
50. Macklem, P. T., and M. R. Becklake. 1963. The relationship between the mechanical and diffusing properties of lung in health and disease. *Am. Rev. Respir. Dis.* **87:** 47–56.
51. Schofield, N. M., R. J. Davies, I. R. Cameron, and M. Green. 1976. Small airways in fibrosing alveolitis. *Am. Rev. Respir. Dis.* **113:** 729–735.
52. Levinson, R. S., L. F. Metzger, N. N. Stanley, J. S. Brody, and N. S. Cherniack. 1973. Airway function in interstitial disease. *Am. Rev. Respir. Dis.* **107:** 1105. (Abstr.)
53. Levinson, R. S., L. F. Metzger, N. N. Stanley, S. G. Kelsen, M. D. Altose, N. S. Cherniack, and J. S. Brody. 1977. Airway function in sarcoidosis. *Am. J. Med.* **62:** 51–59.
54. Buist, A. S., and B. B. Ross. 1973. Predicted values for closing volumes using a modified single breath nitrogen test. *Am. Rev. Respir. Dis.* **107:** 744–752.
55. Buist, A. Sonia. 1975. The single-breath nitrogen test. *N. Engl. J. Med.* **293:** 438–440.
56. Woolcock, A. J., N. J. Vincent, and P. T. Macklem. 1969. Frequency dependence of compliance as a test for obstruction of the small airways. *J. Clin. Invest.* **48:** 1097–1106.
57. Gelb, A. F., and N. Zamel. 1973. Simplified diagnosis of small-airway obstruction. *N. Engl. J. Med.* **288:** 395–398.
58. Gelb, A. F., and B. J. MacAnally. 1973. Early detection of obstructive lung disease by analysis of maximal expiratory flow-volume curve. *Chest.* **64:** 749–753.
59. Bachofen, H., and M. Scherrer. 1967. Lung tissue resistance in diffuse interstitial fibrosis. *J. Clin. Invest.* **46:** 133–140.
60. Otis, A. B., C. B. McKerrow, R. A. Bartlett, J. Mead, M. B. McIlroy, N. J. Selverstone, and E. P. Radford. 1956. Mechanical factors in distribution of pulmonary ventilation. *J. Appl. Physiol.* **8:** 427–443.
61. Gibson, A. J., and N. B. Pride. 1976. A reappraisal of lung mechanics in fibrosing alveolitis. *Chest.* **69**(Suppl.): 256.
62. Martin, R. R., D. Lindsay, P. Despas. D. Bruce, M. Leroux, N. R. Anthonisen, and P. T. Macklem. 1975. The early detection of airway obstruction. *Am. Rev. Respir. Dis.* **111:** 119–125.
63. Hill, D. J., L. I. Landu, and P. D. Phelan. 1972. Small airway disease in asymptomatic asthmatic adolescents. *Am. Rev. Respir. Dis.* **106:** 873–880.

Fibrosing Mediastinitis Causing Pulmonary Arterial Hypertension Without Pulmonary Venous Hypertension

Clinical and Necropsy Observations

ERNEST N. ARNETT, M.D.*
Bethesda, Maryland

JAMES M. BACOS, M.D.
ABE M. MACHER, M.D.†
H. BRANDIS MARSH, M.D.
Washington, D.C.

DANIEL D. SAVAGE, M.D., Ph.D.
JACK D. FULMER, M.D.
WILLIAM C. ROBERTS, M.D.
Bethesda, Maryland

Clinical and morphologic observations are described in two patients with severe pulmonary arterial hypertension without pulmonary venous hypertension from fibrosing mediastinitis. In one patient, both main pulmonary arteries and one major pulmonary vein were severely narrowed by dense fibrous tissue; in the second patient, only the right main pulmonary artery was severely narrowed. Both patients had normal intrapulmonary arteries and normal pulmonary parenchyma. Of nine previously described necropsy patients with pulmonary hypertension due to fibrosing mediastinitis, seven had severe narrowing of multiple large pulmonary veins and in six of them the pulmonary hypertension was entirely due to pulmonary venous obstruction. In one other patient, the pulmonary hypertension was due to obstruction of one main pulmonary artery and several large pulmonary veins. Each of these seven previously described patients had severe changes in the small intrapulmonary arteries. Of the other two previously described patients with pulmonary hypertension from fibrosing mediastinitis, one had severe narrowing of only the main right pulmonary artery, and the other, of both main pulmonary arteries. Thus, although pulmonary arterial hypertension in patients with fibrosing mediastinitis is usually due to obstruction of multiple large pulmonary veins and to severe secondary changes in small intrapulmonary arteries, fibrosing mediastinitis can cause severe pulmonary hypertension by obstructing the right or both main pulmonary arteries.

Fibrosing mediastinitis, an uncommon condition, is a rare cause of severe pulmonary hypertension. When occurring in patients with fibrosing mediastinitis, pulmonary hypertension usually is due to obstruction of multiple large pulmonary veins and to severe secondary narrowings of small intrapulmonary arteries. A rare cause of pulmonary hypertension in patients with fibrosing mediastinitis is extraluminal obstruction of major extrapulmonary pulmonary arteries. Recently, we studied two patients with severe pulmonary arterial hypertension without pulmonary venous hypertension secondary to obstruction of one or both main pulmonary arteries by fibrosing mediastinitis. Observations in them are described herein.

From the Pathology, Cardiology and Pulmonary Branches, National Heart, Lung and Blood Institute, National Institutes of Health, Bethesda, Maryland; and the Division of Cardiology, Department of Medicine, Washington Hospital Center, Washington, D.C. Requests for reprints should be addressed to Dr. William C. Roberts, Building 10A, Room 3E-30, National Institutes of Health, Bethesda, Maryland 20014. Manuscript accepted October 8, 1976.

* Present address: Department of Medicine, The Johns Hopkins Hospital, Baltimore, Maryland 21205.

† Present address: Laboratory of Clinical Investigation, National Institute of Allergy and Infectious Diseases, National Institutes of Health, Bethesda, Maryland 20014.

CASE REPORTS

Case 1. A 35 year old black woman, who was found to have a positive tuberculin skin test at age 14 years, was in good health until age 33 (25 months before death) when she coughed blood and for several days thereafter noted intermittent pleuritic chest pain. Chest roentgenogram showed an infiltrate in the upper lobe of the left lung, and fiberoptic bronchoscopy disclosed inflammation of the bronchus in the upper lobe of the left lung. Results of cytologic examination and cultures of bronchial washings were negative for tumor cells and for acid-fast organisms. Despite the negative cultures, the patient was treated with isoniazid for 18 months and with ethambutol for six months. She remained asymptomatic after the episode of hemoptysis until seven months before death when she noted the onset of exertional dyspnea which increased over the ensuing three months.

Four months before death, examination disclosed a precordial systolic murmur; an electrocardiogram showed right axis deviation and right ventricular hypertrophy. Chest roentgenograms showed mild cardiac enlargement, a "fibronodular" infiltrate in the upper lobe of the left lung and a pleural effusion in the right lung. Lung scan showed multiple perfusion defects and almost total lack of flow to the upper lobe of the right lung. Right-sided cardiac catheterization revealed the following pressures: mean pulmonary capillary wedge, 7 mm Hg; pulmonary artery, 85/25 mm Hg (mean 45 mm Hg); right ventricle 85/17 mm Hg and right atrium (mean) 17 mm Hg. Superior vena cavagram disclosed marked narrowing at the level of the carina. Pulmonary angiography revealed narrowed main right and left pulmonary arteries, and their branches at the hila of the lungs, with normal appearing intralung arteries. Examination 67 days before death disclosed her to be thin. The blood pressure was 120/90 mm Hg; pulse rate 110 beats/min, and respiratory rate 23 breaths/min. Percussion sound was dull, and auscultation disclosed egophony at the base of the right lung. A third heart sound was heard at the lower left sternal border. The first heart sound was normal, but the pulmonic component of the second heart sound was loud. A grade 3/6 holosystolic murmur which increased in intensity with inspiration was present at the lower left sternal border. The liver was enlarged and pulsatile, but no subcutaneous edema was present. An electrocardiogram (Figure 1) revealed right axis deviation and right ventricular hypertrophy. Chest roentgenograms (Figure 2) revealed cardiomegaly, a wide mediastinal shadow, an infiltrate in the upper lobe of the left lung, calcified right paratracheal lymph nodes and a pleural effusion in the right lung. The blood hematocrit value was 32 per cent; white blood cell count $9{,}800/mm^3$ and erythrocyte sedimentation rate 24 mm in 1 hour. Tests for antinuclear factor, rheumatoid factor and lupus erythematosus cells yielded negative results. Histoplasma complement fixation test results were negative. Multiple cultures for acid-fast organisms in sputum, urine, bone marrow aspirate and pleural fluids were negative, and pleural biopsy specimens revealed no granulomas. Superior vena cavagram revealed discrete narrowing at the level of the innominate vein. Catheterization (nine days before death) disclosed the following pressures: peripheral right pulmonary artery, 10/0 mm Hg (mean 4 mm Hg) and pulmonary trunk, 70/11 mm Hg (mean 32 mm Hg). Pulmonary angiography disclosed no flow to the upper lobe of the right lung, severely diminished flow to the upper lobe of the left lung, and marked constriction of both right and left main pulmonary arteries at the hila.

Four days before death, thoracotomy disclosed extensive amounts of dense fibrous tissue in the mediastinum, surrounding both pulmonary arteries and the superior vena cava. The right pulmonary artery and the superior vena cava were dissected free: the main right pulmonary artery was widened with a Teflon® graft and the superior vena cava was widened with a pericardial patch. Postoperatively, the pressure in the pulmonary trunk and distal right pulmonary artery remained increased (60 to 70 mm Hg systolic). A chest roentgenogram, obtained 24 hours postoperatively, showed opacification of the entire upper lobe of the right lung; reexploration disclosed infarction of that lobe, and it was excised. The patient remained hypotensive, however, and she died three days later.

At necropsy (A76-223), dense fibrous tissue surrounded the great vessels, superior vena cava, major bronchi and lower trachea (Figures 3 and 4). The fibrous tissue caused marked narrowing of the lumens of the superior vena cava, both main right and left pulmonary arteries, and the lower left pulmonary vein (Figure 5). Although its grafted portion was widely patent (Figure 4), the main right pulmonary artery was still severely narrowed just distal to the distal attachment of the graft. The pericardial sac was free of excess fluid or fi-

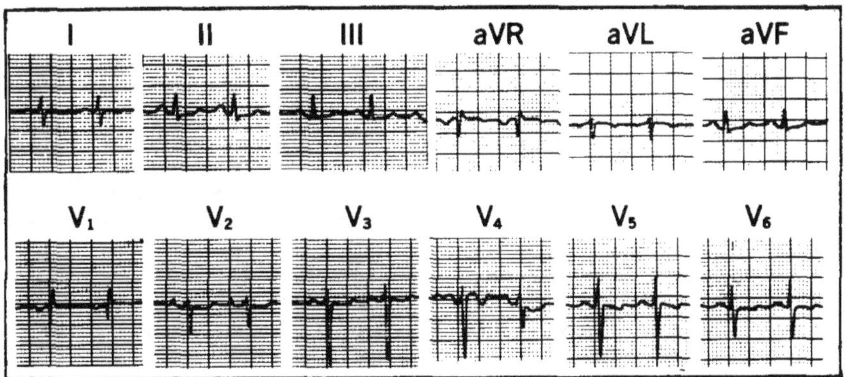

Figure 1. *Case 1. Electrocardiogram 67 days before death showing right axis deviation, right ventricular hypertrophy and incomplete right bundle branch block.*

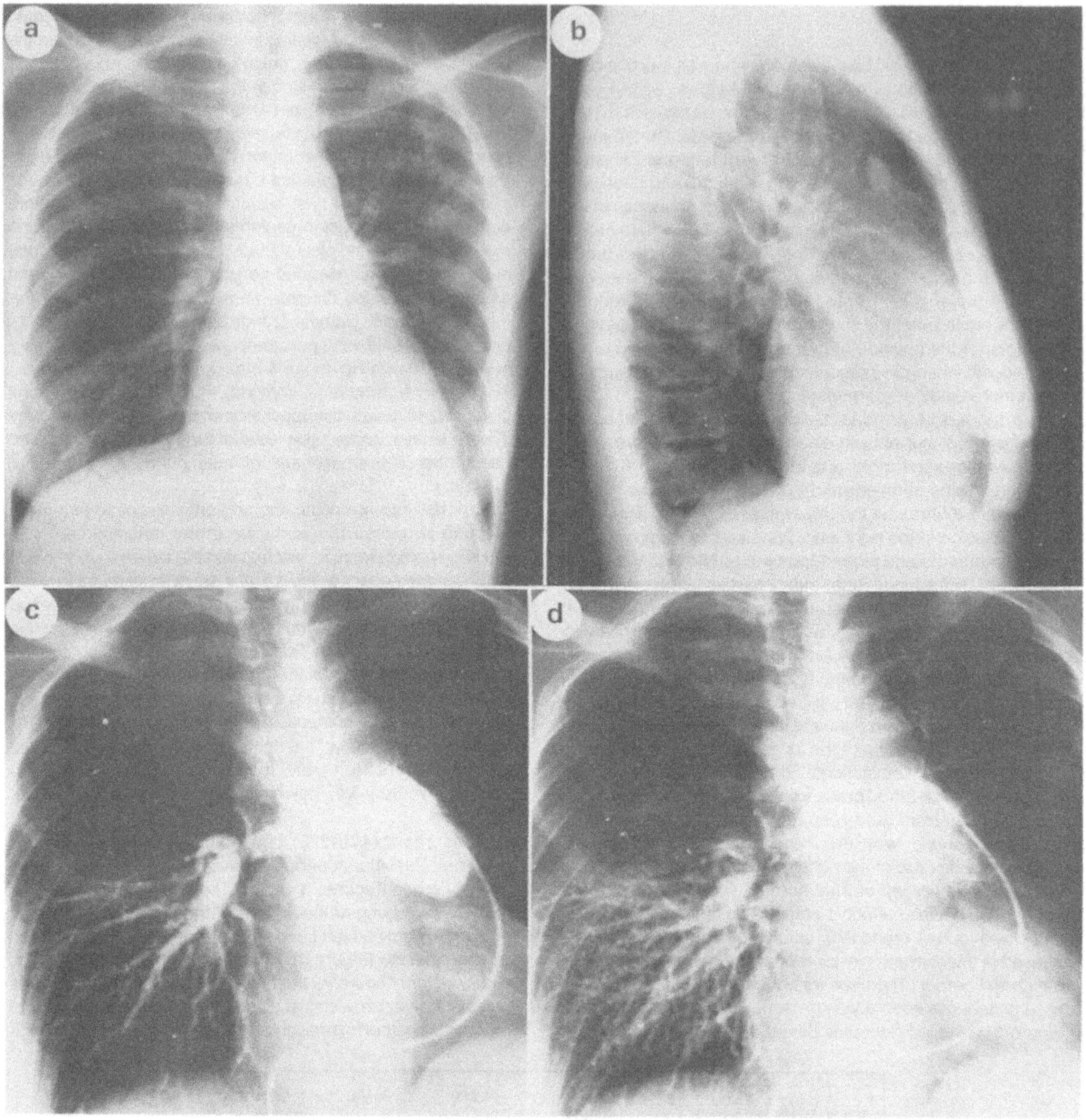

Figure 2. *Case 1.* ***a*** *and* ***b,*** *posteroanterior and lateral chest roentgenograms 67 days before death. The cardiac and mediastinal silhouettes are widened, the pulmonary trunk is prominent, and a coarse reticular infiltrate is present in the left upper lobe. A focal calcific deposit is present in the anterior mediastinum on the lateral film.* ***c*** *and* ***d,*** *pulmonary arteriograms nine days before death, 2.5 and 3.7 seconds, respectively, after injection of contrast material into the dilated pulmonary trunk. There is discrete narrowing of the main right pulmonary artery at the hilum and poststenotic dilatation of the branches to the right, middle and lower lobes. The arteries to the upper lobe of the right lung and to the entire left lung are totally obstructed.*

brous tissue. Histologic sections of the dense mediastinal tissue showed only a few scattered foci of mononuclear cells in addition to the scar. No granulomas were found in remnants of mediastinal lymph nodes, and no acid-fast bacilli or fungi were seen. The heart weighed 300 g; the wall of the right ventricle was hypertrophied, and both right-sided cardiac chambers were dilated (Figure 3). Histologic sections revealed focal interstitial scar and thromboembolic material in the lumen of a rare small muscular pulmonary artery in the upper lobe of the left lung.

Case 2. A 70 year old black woman was well until age 64 years when exertional dyspnea, dizziness, arthralgias of large joints, anorexia and weight loss were noted. Six months later,

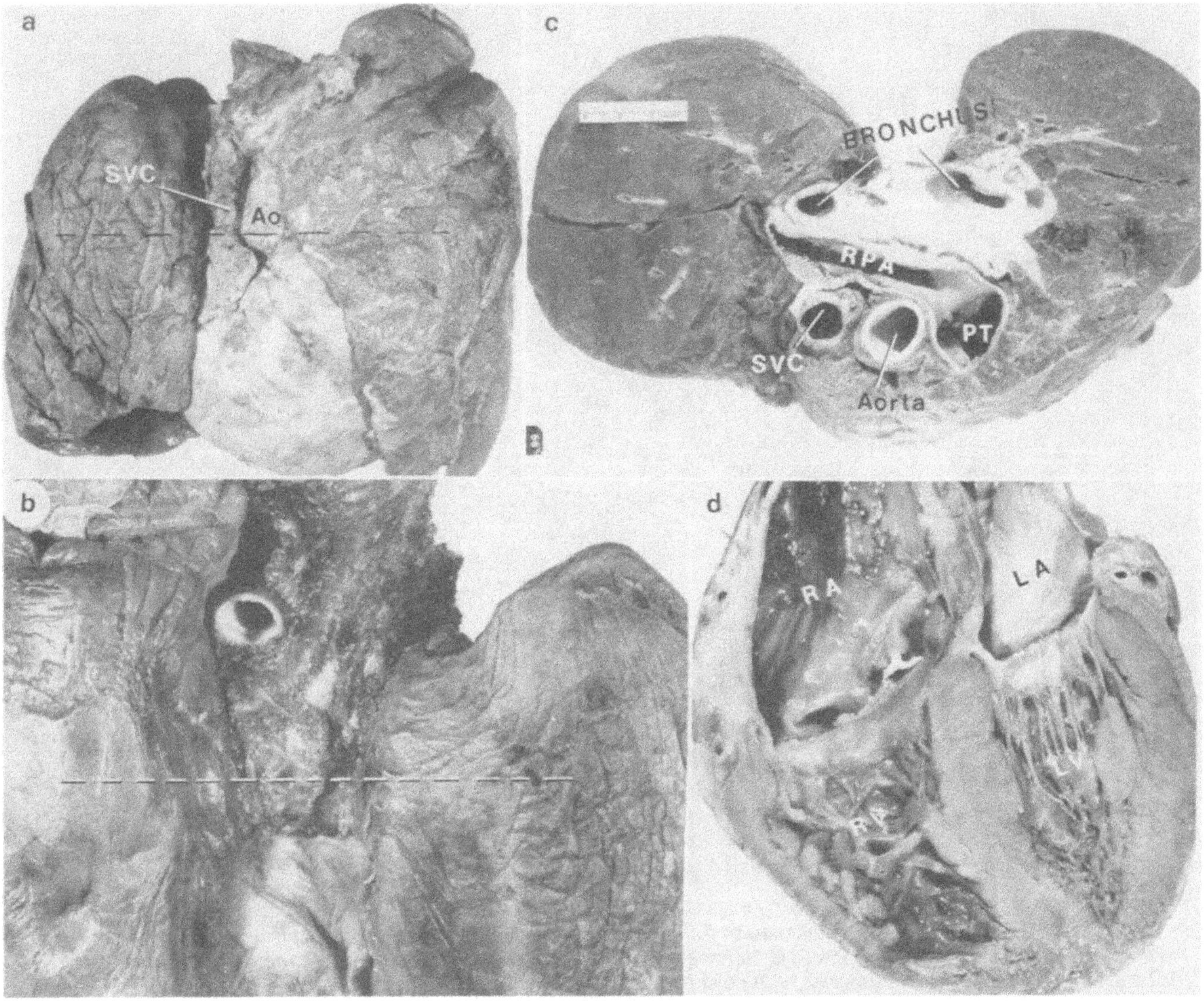

Figure 3. *Case 1. Heart and lungs.* ***a,*** *anterior view of the enblock heart and lungs. Dense fibrous tissue surrounds the cephalad portion of the superior vena cava (SVC), as well as the transverse portion of aorta (Ao) and its branches. The upper lobe of the right lung is absent.* ***b,*** *posterior view of the enblock heart and lungs. The superior and posterior mediastinal spaces are totally obliterated by dense fibrous tissue.* ***c,*** *transverse cut through the mediastinum and both lungs at the level indicated by dashed lines in* ***a*** *and* ***b.*** *PT = pulmonary trunk; RPA = right pulmonary artery.* ***d,*** *longitudinal cut of the heart. The right ventricular (RV) wall is thick, and both right ventricle and right atrium (RA) are dilated. The left ventricle (LV) and left atrium (LA) are of normal size.*

persistent frontal headache, blurred vision and photophobia of the right eye appeared. Examination revealed severe episcleritis and an enlarged tender right temporal artery. The hematocrit value was 32 per cent, erythrocyte sedimentation rate 38/mm in 1 hour, the results of the test for rheumatoid factor were weakly positive and of the tuberculin skin test negative. Chest roentgenogram and electrocardiogram disclosed no abnormalities. Biopsy of the right temporal artery revealed "atherosclerosis." Corticosteroid eye drops were prescribed. Prednisone therapy (60 mg/day) was started 65 months before death, marked symptomatic improvement followed, and seven months later administration of this drug was discontinued. Several months later, however, exertional dyspnea, dizziness and arthralgia recurred, and they were followed by cough, night sweats, exertional chest pain and dysphagia for solid foods. Examination 34 months before death disclosed a loud pulmonic component of the second sound and a systolic murmur which increased in intensity with inspiration and radiated into the right anterior precordium, right axilla and back. A chest roentgenogram showed marked enlargement of the cardiac silhouette, and an electrocardiogram showed right ventricular hypertrophy. Lung scan showed a large perfusion defect in the right lung, and pulmonary arteriography disclosed severe narrowing of the right main pulmonary artery and severely diminished flow to the right lung. The right-sided cardiac pressures were pulmonary artery wedge (mean) 8 mm Hg, a wave 8 mm Hg, v wave 12 mm Hg; pulmonary trunk 45/12 mm Hg (mean 23 mm Hg); right ventricle 45/8 mm Hg; and right atrium (mean) 7 mm Hg. The systolic pressure in the right pulmonary artery distal to

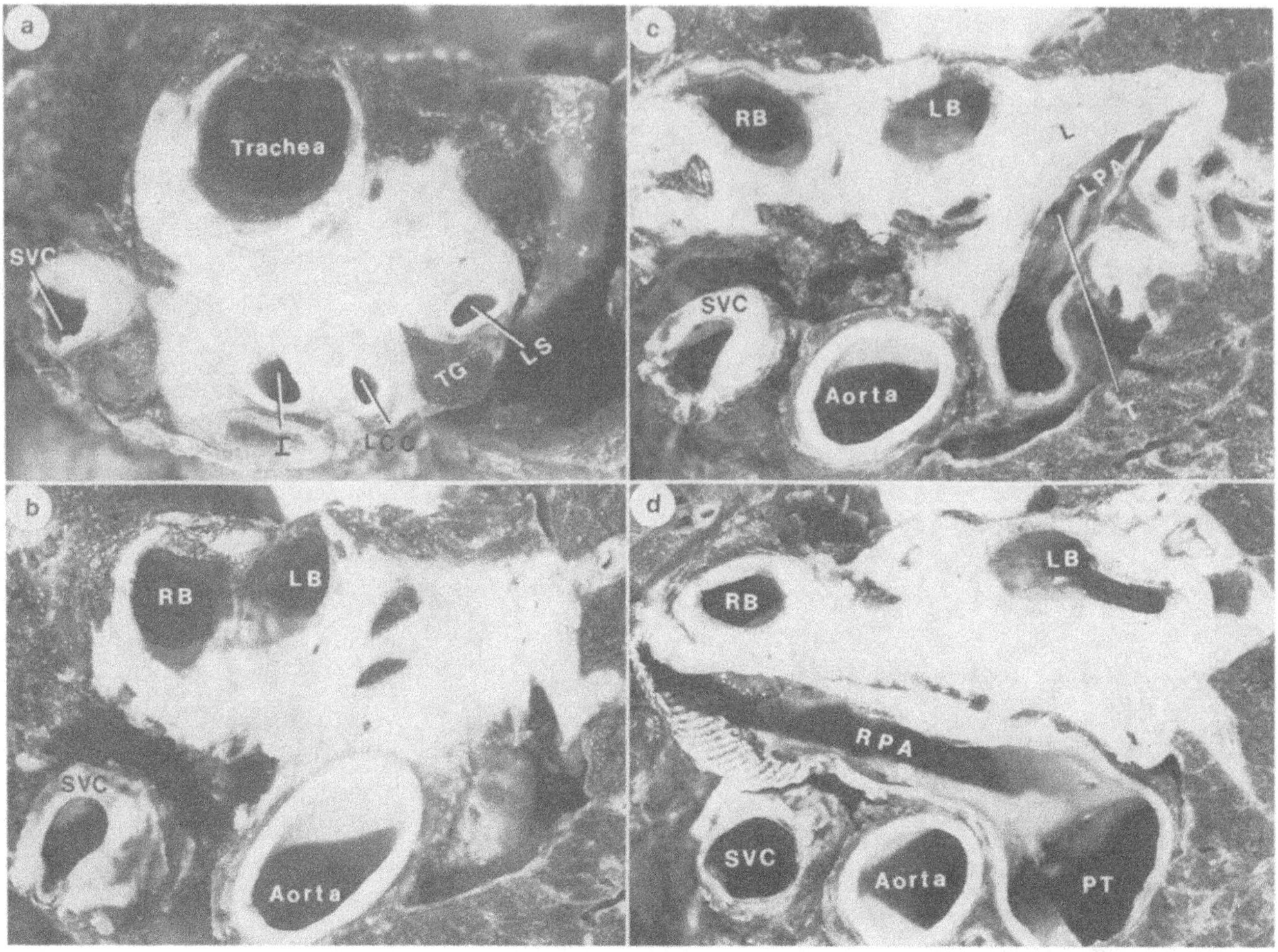

Figure 4. *Case 1. Transverse cuts through the mediastinum at successively more caudal levels.* ***a,*** *at the level of the innominate (I), left common carotid (LCC) and left subclavian (LS) arteries. Dense fibrous tissue (white) surrounds these structures and the trachea. The superior vena cava (SVC) is narrowed. TG = thymus gland.* ***b,*** *at level of the bifurcation of trachea into right (RB) and left bronchus (LB). The superior vena cava had been partially freed (at operation four days earlier) from the fibrous tissue.* ***c,*** *at level of left main pulmonary artery (LPA). The lumens of its major branches are totally compressed by the dense fibrous tissue and thrombus (T) is present in this artery.* ***d,*** *at level of right main pulmonary artery (RPA) and its grafted segment. Although the lumen of the proximal portion of this artery is patent, the branches to the middle and lower lobes remain markedly narrowed just beyond the graft. PT = pulmonary trunk.*

the narrowing was 22 mm Hg. Therapy with digoxin and furosemide was started.

Exertional dyspnea, orthopnea, dizziness and arthralgia associated with malaise and weight loss continued, however, and 28 months before death signs of superior vena caval obstruction appeared. A superior vena cavagram (Figure 6) disclosed severe narrowing at the level of the carina, and an 11 mm Hg gradient was measured between the cephalad portion of the superior vena cava and right atrium. A large pericardial effusion now was present. Results of histoplasma and coccidiodin complement fixation tests, and tests for antinuclear and rheumatoid factor were negative, but results of the tuberculin skin test were now strongly positive (42 mm). Pericardiocentesis yielded 500 ml of serosanguineous fluid with total protein 7 g/100 ml and mononuclear cells/ 10,000/mm^3; cultures of this fluid were negative for fungi and tuberculosis. Bronchoscopy yielded no abnormalities, but tomograms demonstrated an anterior mediastinal mass. Mediastinoscopy disclosed obliteration of the anterior mediastinal space by dense fibrous tissue. Consequently, 27 months before death, a saphenous vein was used to bypass the obstructed portion of superior vena cava. Biopsy specimens of the mediastinal mass revealed dense fibrous tissue with focal collections of mononuclear cells; of the parietal pericardium, diffuse chronic inflammation and fibrosis, and of mediastinal and scalene lymph nodes, reactive hyperplasia. Symptomatic improvement followed relief of the superior vena caval obstruction.

Pain in the right upper quadrant appeared intermittently beginning 12 months before death; one month before death, the patient had the abrupt onset of right upper quadrant pain and obstructive type jaundice. Laparotomy disclosed a dis-

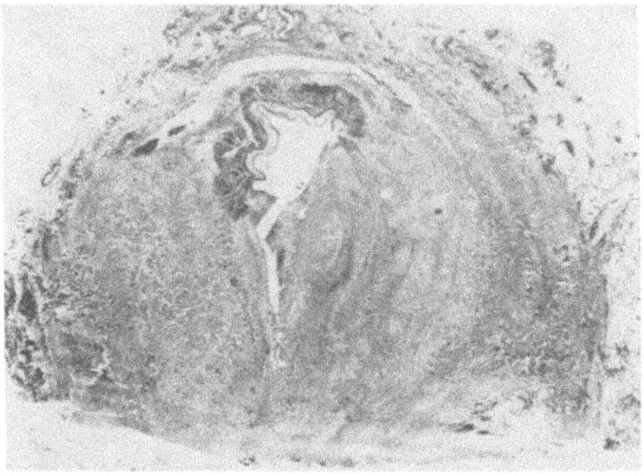

Figure 5. *Case 1. Histologic section of the left lower pulmonary vein. It is surrounded by dense fibrous tissue and its lumen is narrowed by extrinsic compression. Masson's trichrome stain; original magnification × 55.*

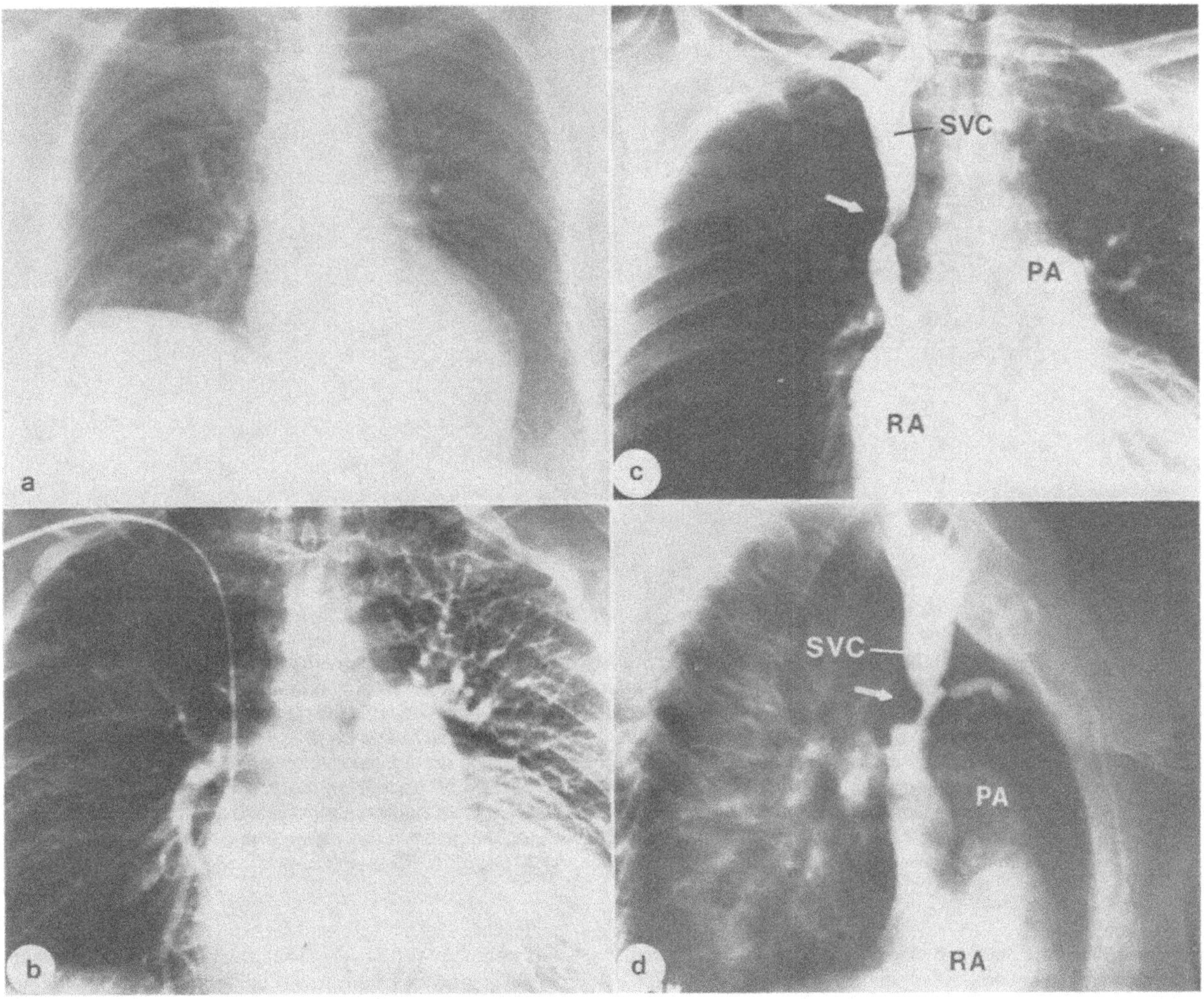

Figure 6. *Case 2.* ***a,*** *posteroanterior chest roentgenogram, and* ***b,*** *pulmonary angiogram 34 months before death. The cardiac silhouette is enlarged, and a large right pleural effusion is present. An arteriogram disclosed markedly diminished flow to the entire right lung with virtually no flow to the upper lobe. An area of discrete narrowing of the right pulmonary artery is present. A 23 mm Hg gradient was present across this area.* ***c*** *and* ***d,*** *superior vena cavagram 28 months before death. The lumen is severely narrowed at the level of the tracheal bifurcation (arrow). An 11 mm Hg gradient was measured across the narrowed segment.*

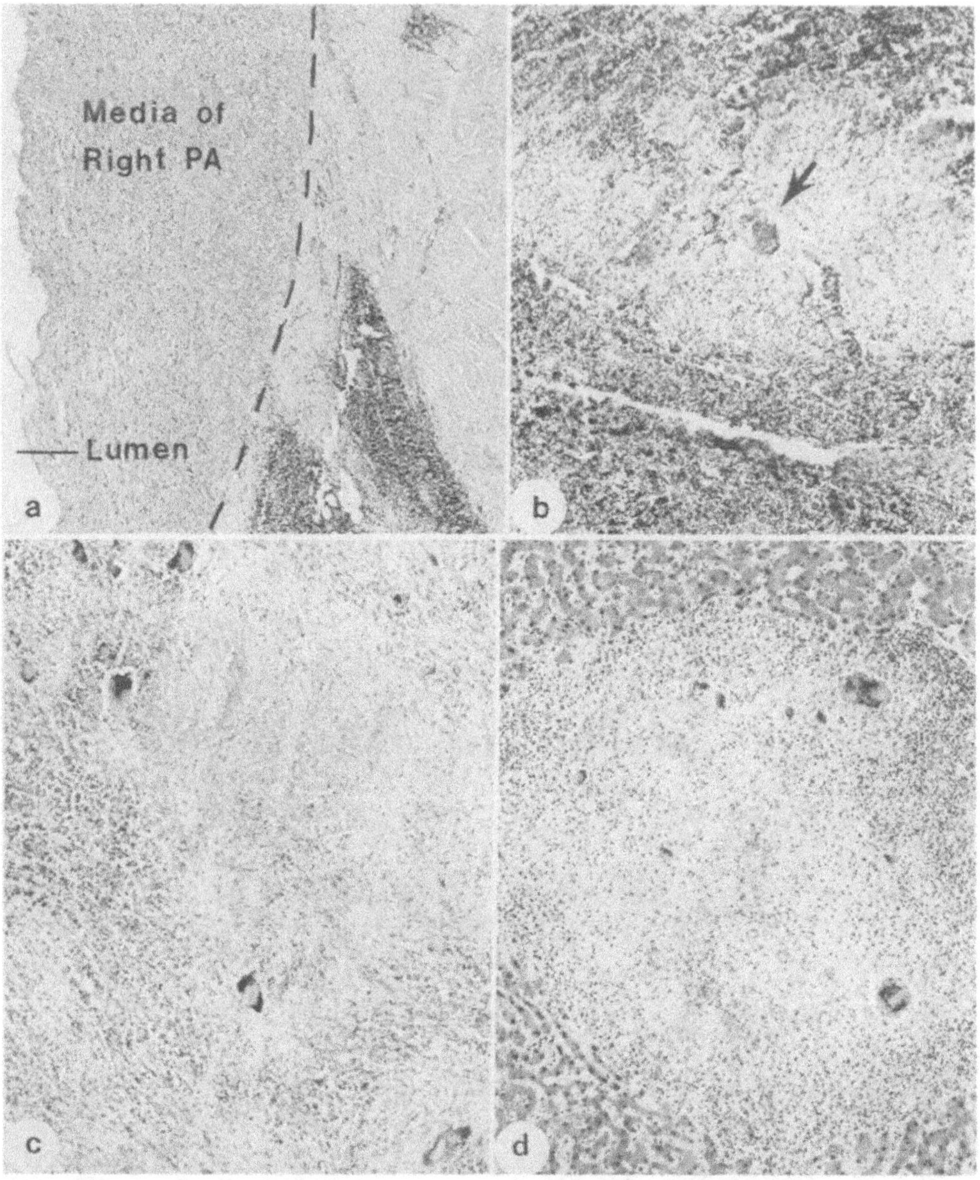

Figure 7. *Case 2.* ***a,*** *histologic section of the wall of the right pulmonary artery (PA) showing dense fibrous tissue with focal collections of mononuclear cells on its adventitial surface. The dense fibrous tissue encased the artery and caused marked narrowing of its lumen.* ***b,*** *histologic section of a mediastinal lymph node. A multinucleated giant cell (arrow) is present in an area of dense scar.* ***c,*** *histologic section of liver. A large caseating granuloma containing numerous giant cells is present.* ***d,*** *histologic section of a necrotic lymph node from the porta hepatis. Confluent granulomas with numerous giant cells and extensive central necrosis are present. Special stains revealed the presence of numerous acid-fast bacilli in these lymph nodes. Hematoxylin and eosin stains; original magnification × 54 (a), × 80 (b and c) and × 88 (d).*

tended gallbladder devoid of stones, and a hard fibrous mass surrounding and severely obstructing the common bile duct. Biopsy of the mass revealed only dense fibrous tissue with focal collections of chronic inflammatory cells. A cholecystojejunostomy was performed. Fifteen days postoperatively signs of thrombophlebitis in the lower extremities appeared, and heparin therapy was started. Two weeks later, the patient had the sudden onset of left-sided weakness followed by coma, and she died three days later.

At necropsy (WHC A74-343), the anterior and posterior mediastinal spaces were totally obliterated by dense fibrous tissue. The superior vena cava, ascending aorta, right and left main pulmonary arteries, major pulmonary veins and main stem bronchi were encased by fibrous tissue, and the lumens of the superior vena cava and right main pulmonary artery were severely narrowed by it. Although the lumen of the left main pulmonary artery was only slightly narrowed, the artery was totally inelastic due to the fibrous encasement. The pa-

TABLE I Observations in Previously Described Necropsy Patients with Pulmonary Hypertension Due to Fibrosing Mediastinitis (FM)

Source	Age (yr) and Sex	Cause of FM	ECG	PA Pressure (mm Hg) s/d (mean)	Obst. Main PA R	Obst. Main PA L	Obst. PV	PA Emboli	Narrowed Small PAs	IPF	Obst. SVC
Edwards, Burchell 1951 [18]	26,F	I	↓V	98/45	0	0	+	0	+	0	0
Davis, Andrus 1954 [19]	26,M	H	RVS	–	0	0	+	–	+	+	0
Bindelglass, Trubowitz 1958 [20]	25,M	I	RAD	–	0	0	+	0	+	0	0
Nelson et al. 1965 [21]	31,F	T	RVH	–	+	+	+	+	–	0	0
Clinicopathologic conference (JHHCPC 600747) 1966 [22]	42,F	H	RVS	82/45	0	0	+	0	+	+	0
Chesis, Dadey 1967 [23]	55, F	I	RAD P-pulm.	–	+	0	–	–	+	–	+
Nasser et al. 1967 [24]	21,F	I	RAD	50/22 (34)	0	0	+	–	+	0	0
Goodwin et al. 1972 [9]	27,F	H	RAD	–	+	0	+	+	+	0	+
Kittridge, Nash 1974 [25]	40,F	I	–	–	0	0	+	0	+	0	0

NOTE: H = histoplasmosis; I = idiopathic; IPF = idiopathic pulmonary fibrosis; L = left; Obst. = obstructed; PA = pulmonary artery; P-pulm. = P-pulmonale; PV = pulmonary vein; R = right; RAD = right axis deviation; RVH = right ventricular hypertrophy; RVS = right ventricular strain; SVC = superior vena cava; T = tuberculosis; V = voltage.

rietal pericardium was thickened and the pericardial space obliterated by numerous dense fibrous adhesions. The heart weighed 450 g; the walls of both ventricles were hypertrophied and the right-sided chambers were dilated. Histologic sections from mediastinum revealed dense hyalinized fibrous tissue with scattered foci of mononuclear cells (Figure 7). Several remnants of mediastinal lymph node contained granulomas with giant cells (Figure 7), but no acid-fast bacilli or fungi were found. Except for focal areas of intra-alveolar hemorrhage, the pulmonary parenchyma and intralung vessels were normal.

An extensive mass of dense fibrous tissue and enlarged lymph nodes was present in the porta hepatis, surrounding and compressing the bile duct. Histologically, it consisted of dense collagenous fibrous tissue, similar to that present in the mediastinum, surrounding regional lymph nodes which were virtually totally replaced by caseating granulomas containing numerous giant cells (Figure 7). Special stains disclosed acid-fast bacilli in the caseating granulomas. Caseating granulomas also were present in the liver (Figure 7), and in celiac and supraclavicular lymph nodes. Examination of histologic sections from several body organs, including the kidney, liver, heart, stomach, uterus, peripancreatic, periadrenal and perithyroidal fat, disclosed the presence of widespread segmental inflammation and fibrinoid necrosis of the walls of small- and medium-sized muscular arteries. Death resulted from a large subarachnoid hemorrhage.

COMMENTS

Although early reports [1,2] attributed it to syphilis, rheumatic fever or tuberculosis, fibrosing mediastinitis is now known to result most often from histoplasmosis [3–10]. Tuberculosis, however, remains a frequent cause [8,9,11,12]. The fibrosing mediastinitis in both our patients appears to have resulted from tuberculosis. In Case 1, the tuberculin skin test result was positive from childhood, the patient had an illness compatible with pulmonary tuberculosis two years before death and, although no acid-fast organisms were found at necropsy, she had received antituberculosis drugs during her last year. In Case 2, although the patient had polyarteritis nodosa, a condition which, on rare occasion, is associated with fibrosing mediastinitis [13], she also had untreated disseminated tuberculosis, which is the likely cause of her fibrosing mediastinitis.

Symptoms from fibrosing mediastinitis most often are due to obstruction of major systemic veins. Obstruction of the superior vena cava has been considered the hallmark of fibrosing mediastinitis [14–16]. Both our patients had obstructed superior vena cavae. The obstruction in Case 2 was operatively relieved 27 months before death [17].

Pulmonary hypertension from fibrosing mediastinitis is rare; it usually is due to obstruction of multiple major pulmonary veins and to secondary changes in the small intrapulmonary arteries. Among nine previously described necropsy patients (age range 21 to 42 years [average age 33 years]; seven women, three men) with fibrosing mediastinitis and pulmonary hypertension (Table I) [9,18–25], seven had obstruction of large pulmonary veins, the sole cause of the pulmonary hypertension in six. One other patient had pulmonary venous as well as pulmonary arterial obstruction. Each of these seven patients had severe secondary changes in the small intrapulmonary pulmonary arteries. Edwards and Burchell [18] in 1951 first described a patient with severe pulmonary arterial hypertension due to obstruction of three of four major pulmonary veins by fibrosing mediastinitis. In 1954, Davis and Andrus [19] described a similar patient whose initial clinical features strongly suggested mitral valve stenosis. Subsequently, additional patients with fibrosing mediastinitis were

TABLE II Causes of Pulmonary Hypertension in Patients with Fibrosing Mediastinitis

1. Obstruction of multiple large pulmonary veins
2. Obstruction of the right or both main pulmonary arteries
3. Associated pulmonary interstitial fibrosis with or without hypoxemia
4. Multiple occlusions of small intrapulmonary arteries by thromboembolic material
5. Combinations of these

described, and pulmonary hypertension due to pulmonary venous obstruction by fibrosing mediastinitis became well recognized [20].

Pulmonary hypertension in fibrosing mediastinitis may result from causes other than pulmonary venous obstruction (Table II). As illustrated by our two patients, obstruction of the main pulmonary arteries by fibrosing mediastinitis can cause pulmonary arterial hypertension in the absence of pulmonary venous hypertension. Both our patients had severe pulmonary arterial hypertension but normal pulmonary arterial wedge pressures. At necropsy, one (Case 1) had severe obstruction of both right and left main pulmonary arteries, partial obstruction of one major pulmonary vein and normal intrapulmonary arteries. A similar patient was described by Nelson et al. in 1965 [21]. In our Case 2, the right main pulmonary artery was severely narrowed, the left main pulmonary artery only mildly narrowed, none of the large pulmonary veins was obstructed and the intrapulmonary arteries of both lungs were normal.

Pulmonary hypertension has been shown, both clinically and experimentally to result from obstruction of only the right main pulmonary artery. Vogel and associates [26] ligated the right or left main pulmonary artery in 29 calves at sea level (17 calves) or at 5,280 feet above sea level (12 calves). At sea level, pulmonary hypertension developed in half the calves with right main pulmonary arterial ligation but in none with ligated left main pulmonary arteries. At the high altitude, however, ligation of the left main pulmonary artery also produced pulmonary hypertension. Cheris and Dadey [23] described a patient with fibrosing mediastinitis and pulmonary hypertension who had severe narrowing of only the right main pulmonary artery, and Cohn and associates [27] described a patient with isolated congenital stenosis of the right main pulmonary artery and severe pulmonary hypertension. Both patients had severe changes in the small intrapulmonary arteries. Why such changes were absent in the left lung in our Case 2 is unclear. It is clear, however, that fibrosing mediastinitis can cause pulmonary hypertension and cor pulmonale by obstructing only the right main pulmonary artery or both right and left main pulmonary arteries.

Another cause of pulmonary arterial hypertension in fibrosing mediastinitis is interstitial pulmonary fibrosis, which may be the consequence of fibrosing mediastinitis or due to the same condition which caused the fibrosing mediastinitis [28]. Two of the nine previously described necropsy patients with fibrosing mediastinitis and pulmonary hypertension also had considerable interstitial pulmonary fibrosis. How much the interstitial pulmonary fibrosis contributed to the pulmonary hypertension in them, however, is uncertain, because each also had obstruction of multiple large pulmonary veins.

Obstruction of multiple small intrapulmonary arteries by thromboembolic material also is a well known cause of pulmonary hypertension [29,30], and patients with fibrosing mediastinitis have an increased risk to thromboembolism. Superior vena caval constriction, the most frequent complication of fibrosing mediastinitis, is often accompanied by thrombosis of the residual lumen of the partially occluded vein. In 1903 Osler [31] described a patient with superior vena caval syndrome due to constriction of the superior vena cava by fibrosing mediastinitis, and the drawing of McCallum's autopsy findings show a thrombus in the residual lumen of the constricted vein. Among the nine previously described necropsy patients with fibrosing mediastinitis and pulmonary hypertension (Table I), two also had superior vena caval obstruction; at necropsy, two of the nine patients had thromboemboli in the lumens of multiple small intrapulmonary arteries.

Although patients with fibrosing mediastinitis with extensive changes in the small intrapulmonary arteries due to pulmonary venous obstruction or to thromboemboli and those with extensive interstitial pulmonary fibrosis are unlikely to benefit significantly from any form of therapy, patients with pulmonary hypertension due to obstruction of one or both main pulmonary arteries by fibrosing mediastinitis may be benefited by operative intervention unless the mediastinal fibrous tissue extends into the hilum of the lung as it did in our patient (Case 1).

REFERENCES

1. Knox LC: Chronic mediastinitis. Am J Med Sci 169: 807, 1925.
2. Keefer CS: Acute and chronic mediastinitis. A study of sixty cases. Arch Intern Med 62: 109, 1938.
3. Peabody JW Jr, Brown RB, Sullivan MB, et al.: Mediastinal granulomas. J Thorac Surg 35: 384, 1958.
4. Lull GF, Winn DF Jr: Chronic fibrous mediastinitis due to histoplasma capsulatum (histoplasmal mediastinitis). Report of three cases with different presenting symptoms. Radiology 73: 367, 1959.
5. Marshall RJ, Edmundowicz AC, Andrews CE: Chronic obstruction of the superior vena cava due to histoplasmosis.

A hemodynamic and angiographic correlation. Circulation 29: 604, 1964.

6. Clinicopathologic conference (JHH 664434). Bull Johns Hopkins Hosp 119: 288, 1966.
7. Hewlett TH, Steer A, Thomas DE: Progressive fibrosing mediastinitis. Ann Thorac Surg 2: 345, 1966.
8. Schowengerdt CG, Suyemoto R, Main FB: Granulomatous and fibrous mediastinitis: a review and analysis of 180 cases. J Thorac Cardiovasc Surg 57: 365, 1969.
9. Goodwin RA, Nickell JA, Des Prez RM: Mediastinal fibrosis complicating healed primary histoplasmosis and tuberculosis. Medicine (Baltimore) 51: 227, 1972.
10. Strimlan CV, Dines DE, Payne WS: Mediastinal granuloma. Mayo Clin Proc 50: 702, 1975.
11. Ferguson TB, Burford TH: Mediastinal granuloma. A 15-year experience. Ann Thorac Surg 1: 125, 1965.
12. McIntire FT, Sykes EM: Obstruction of the superior vena cava: a review of the literature and report of two personal cases. Ann Intern Med 30: 925, 1949.
13. Carton RW, Wong R: Multifocal fibrosclerosis manifested by vena caval obstruction and associated with vasculitis. Ann Intern Med 70: 81, 1969.
14. Erganian J, Wade LJ: Chronic fibrous mediastinitis with obstruction of the superior vena cava. J Thorac Surg 12: 275, 1943.
15. Hache L, Woolner LB, Bernatz PE: Idiopathic fibrous mediastinitis. Dis Chest 41: 9, 1962.
16. Miller RE, Sullivan FJ: Superior vena caval obstruction secondary to fibrosing mediastinitis. Ann Thorac Surg 15: 483, 1973.
17. Garcia J, Ramariz R, Bacos J, et al.: Technique of superior vena cava reconstruction in fibrosing mediastinitis. J Thorac Cardiovasc Surg 65: 547, 1973.
18. Edwards JE, Burchell HB: Multilobar pulmonary venous obstruction with pulmonary hypertension. "Protective" arterial lesions in the involved lobes. Arch Intern Med 87: 372, 1951.
19. Davis FW Jr, Andrus EC: Mitral stenosis in facsimile. N Engl J Med 251: 297, 1954.
20. Bindelglass IL, Trubowitz S: Pulmonary vein obstruction: an uncommon sequel to chronic fibrous mediastinitis. Ann Intern Med 48: 876, 1958.
21. Nelson WP, Lundberg GD, Dickerson RB: Pulmonary artery obstruction and cor pulmonale due to chronic fibrous mediastinitis. Am J Med 38: 279, 1965.
22. Clinicopathologic conference (JHH 600747). Bull Johns Hopkins Hosp 118: 73, 1966.
23. Cheris DN, Dadey JL: Fibrosing mediastinitis. An unusual cause for cor pulmonale. Am J Roentgenol Radium Ther Nucl Med 100: 328, 1967.
24. Nasser WK, Feigenbaum H, Fisch C: Clinical and hemodynamic diagnosis of pulmonary venous obstruction due to sclerosing mediastinitis. Am J Cardiol 20: 725, 1967.
25. Kittredge RD, Nash AD: The many facets of sclerosing fibrosis. Am J Roentgenol Radium Ther Nucl Med 122: 288, 1974.
26. Vogel JHK, McNamara DG, Hallman G, et al.: Effects of mild chronic hypoxia on the pulmonary circulation in calves with reactive pulmonary hypertension. Circ Res 21: 661, 1967.
27. Cohn LH, Sanders JH Jr, Collins JJ Jr: Surgical treatment of congenital unilateral pulmonary arterial stenosis with contralateral pulmonary hypertension. Am J Cardiol 38: 257, 1976.
28. Andrews EC: Five cases of an undescribed form of pulmonary interstitial fibrosis caused by obstruction of the pulmonary veins. Bull Johns Hopkins Hosp 100: 28, 1957.
29. Fowler NO, Black-Schaffer B, Scott RC, et al.: Idiopathic and thromboembolic pulmonary hypertension. Am J Med 40: 331, 1966.
30. Arnett EN, Battle WE, Russo JV, et al.: Intravenous injection of talc-containing drugs intended for oral use. A cause of pulmonary granulomatosis and pulmonary hypertension. Am J Med 60: 711, 1976.
31. Osler W: Obliteration of the superior vena cava. Bull Johns Hopkins Hosp 14: 169, 1903.

Anchoring Fibrils

A New Connective Tissue Structure in Fibrotic Lung Disease

Oichi Kawanami, MD, PhD, Victor J. Ferrans, MD, PhD, William C. Roberts, MD, Ronald G. Crystal, MD, and Jack D. Fulmer, MD

Electron microscopic studies of lung were made and compared in 17 patients with fibrotic lung disease (10 with idiopathic pulmonary fibrosis, 3 with collagen–vascular diseases, 3 with sarcoidosis, and 1 with chronic eosinophilic pneumonia) and in 5 control patients. In control patients, the alveolar epithelial cells were normal, and no hemidesmosomes were present between the plasma membranes and the basal laminae. In comparison, cuboidal alveolar epithelial cells were present in 15 of the patients with fibrotic lung disease; in 9 of these the alveolar epithelial cells were multilayered. In 7 of the latter 9 patients (5 with idiopathic pulmonary fibrosis and 2 with collagen–vascular diseases), the basal laminae of the alveolar epithelial cells were attached to the plasma membranes by hemidesmosomes and to the underlying interstitial connective tissue by "anchoring fibrils." These fibrils measured from 4000 to 6000 Å in length and from 200 to 600 Å in width. One or both ends of the anchoring fibrils inserted into the basal lamina, often forming arcs through which collagen fibrils and connective tissue microfibrils penetrated. Anchoring fibrils showed a complex pattern of transverse banding, which differed from that of collagen and appeared to be symmetric about the center of the fibril. These anchoring fibrils, which resemble those in normal skin and other tissues, were not found in lungs of control patients. In addition, there was a significant correlation between the severity of the pulmonary fibrosis and the presence of anchoring fibrils. These observations suggest that in severe fibrotic lung disease, anchoring fibrils reinforce the attachment of the basal lamina of multilayered alveolar epithelial cells to interstitial connective tissue. (Am J Pathol 92:389–410, 1978)

THE FIBROTIC LUNG DISORDERS are a heterogeneous group of diseases characterized morphologically by a derangement of fibrous tissue in the interstitium.[1,2] During the course of studies of the fine structure of lung tissue from patients with fibrotic lung disease, we have observed unusual connective tissue fibrils that appear to attach the basal lamina of alveolar epithelial cells to the underlying interstitial connective tissue. A description of the morphology and distribution of these fibrils, which correspond to the "anchoring fibrils" in the skin [3-16] and other tissues,[17-29] forms the basis of this communication.

From the Pathology Branch and the Pulmonary Branch, National Heart, Lung, and Blood Institute, National Institutes of Health, Bethesda, Maryland.

Accepted for publication April 5, 1978.

Address reprint requests to Oichi Kawanami, MD, PhD, Building 10, Room 7N208, National Heart, Lung, and Blood Institute, National Institutes of Health, Bethesda, MD 20014.

Materials and Methods

Fibrotic Lung Disease Group

Seventeen patients with fibrotic lung disease were studied (Table 1). Their mean age was 50 ± 3.7 years* (range, 23 to 69 years); 12 were men and 5 were women.

Ten patients were diagnosed as having idiopathic pulmonary fibrosis on the basis of the following criteria [1,2,30-32]: an interstitial pattern on chest roentgenogram; reduced total lung capacity or diffusion capacity, reduced compliance, exercise hypoxemia, and a normal forced expiratory volume in 1 sec/forced vital capacity (FEV_1%); no significant environmental exposure history, symptoms of hypersensitivity lung disease, history of chronic pulmonary infection, or evidence of left ventricular failure; no defined collagen–vascular disease; and a lung biopsy revealing interstitial and intra-alveolar inflammatory and immune effector cells and varying degrees of alveolar septal fibrosis, but without intra-alveolar fibrosis, granuloma, significant material identifiable by polarized light microscopy or evidence of bacteria, mycobacteria, or fungi.

Three patients were diagnosed as having fibrotic lung disease associated with collagen–vascular disease. Two of these patients (JV and CSW) had classic rheumatoid arthritis (American Rheumatism Association criteria) and the other (ON) had a mixed connective tissue syndrome.[33] The biopsy findings in these patients were indistinguishable from those in patients with idiopathic pulmonary fibrosis.

Three other patients (RPB, JAW, and DLM) were diagnosed as having sarcoidosis on the basis of the following criteria [34]: typical chest roentgenogram; clinical course typical of sarcoidosis; noncaseating granulomas on open lung biopsy; and negative cultures of the biopsy specimens for bacteria, mycobacteria, and fungi.

One patient (BC) was diagnosed as having chronic eosinophilic pneumonia [35] based on typical nonsegmental subpleural infiltrates on chest roentgenogram and lung biopsy showing intra-alveolar and interstitial eosinophils and scattered giant cells and plasma cells.

The mean duration of symptoms in the patients with fibrotic lung disease was 1.5 ± 0.2 years (Table 1). Ten of the patients were smokers and 7 were nonsmokers. Fourteen patients were receiving no therapy, 3 were taking prednisone, and 1 was taking chloroquine. The mean total lung capacity was 66.2 ± 4.3% predicted, vital capacity was 68.5 ± 5.4% predicted, and diffusing capacity was 53.4 ± 3.2% predicted, but forced expiratory volume in 1 sec/forced vital capacity was normal. The mean resting arterial oxygen tension (PaO_2) was 83.3 ± 3.0 mmHg, and the mean PaO_2 on exercise was 59.1 ± 3.6 mmHg. The severity of fibrosis in biopsy specimens was graded from minimal (+1) to severe (+4) as previously described.[31,32]

Control Group

Five patients were included in the control group. Their mean age was 27 ± 9.3 years (range, 14 to 64 years); 4 were men and 1 was a woman. Each of these patients had metastatic disease to the lung (osteogenic sarcoma in 4 patients and oat cell carcinoma in 1). Histologically normal lung tissue was obtained at the time of lobectomy or wedge biopsy for removal of metastatic nodules (Table 1).

Preparation of Tissues

For light microscopy, tissues were fixed with buffered formalin, embedded in paraffin, sectioned, and stained using the following methods: hematoxylin–eosin, Masson tri-

---

* All data are presented as mean ± SEM.

Table 1—Clinical Findings in 17 Patients With Pulmonary Fibrosis and 5 Control Patients

Patients	Age (yr)	Sex	Clinical diagnosis	Smoking history	Duration of symptom (yr)	Anti-inflammatory drug therapy	TLC (% predicted)	VC (% predicted)	D_{LCO} (% predicted)	PaO_2 (mmHg) Rest	PaO_2 (mmHg) Exercise
LY	65	♂	IPF	0	1.0	0	36	34	41	91.0	49.0
AM	48	♂	IPF	H	2.0	0	81	86	45	88.0	50.0
RM	69	♂	IPF	0	3.0	0	75	81	37	67.0	44.0
WD	43	♂	IPF	M	0.5	0	59	59	58	92.0	82.0
WK	68	♂	IPF	M	4.0	P, C	42	40	—	63.0	—
WES	66	♂	IPF	§	1.0	0	49	35	58	74.2	46.0
SFB	64	♀	IPF	0	0.5	0	57	69	58	79.3	52.0
WH	41	♂	IPF	L	2.0	0	46	50	52	79.2	49.0
EB	48	♂	IPF	H	1.5	0	86	83	48	80.5	56.8
MKL	46	♀	IPF	0	2.0	P	94	110	30	83.5	51.0
JV	57	♂	Rheumatoid arthritis	H	0.5	0	76	86	36	76.0	56.3
ON	27	♀	Mixed connective tissue disease	0	1.5	P	43	42	57	89.5	71.0
CSW	53	♀	Rheumatoid arthritis	L	0.5	0	84	94	67	98.5	78.8
RPB	39	♂	Sarcoidosis	0	1.5	0	70	70	70	84.2	81.0
JAW	24	♂	Sarcoidosis	0	1.0	0	77	69	68	—	—
DLM	23	♀	Sarcoidosis	H	1.0	0	77	80	71	111.0	—
BC	60	♂	Chronic eosinophilic pneumonia	L	0.2	0	74	77	58	75.2	60.3
Mean ± SEM	50.0 ± 3.7				1.5 ± 0.2		66.2 ± 4.3	68.5 ± 5.4	53.4 ± 3.2	83.3 ± 3.0	59.1 ± 3.6
Control patients											
LS	18	♂	Metastatic osteogenic sarcoma	—	0	0	60	43	97	—	—
MLS	20	♀	Metastatic osteogenic sarcoma	—	0	0	—	—	—	—	—
LL	19	♂	Metastatic osteogenic sarcoma	—	0	0	—	—	—	—	—
WKN	14	♂	Metastatic osteogenic sarcoma	—	0	0	—	—	—	—	—
BJC	64	♂	Metastatic oat cell carcinoma	H	0	0	108	98	46	—	—
Mean ± SEM	27.0 ± 9.3										

TLC = total lung capacity; VC = vital capacity, D_{LCO} = diffusing capacity, PaO_2 = arterial oxygen tension, IPF = idiopathic pulmonary fibrosis, 0 = none, H = heavy: > 25 pack-years, M = moderate: 10–25 pack-years, P = prednisone, C = chloroquine, — = information not available, § = cigar, L = light: < 10 pack-years.

chrome, Movat pentachrome, elastica–van Gieson, periodic acid–Schiff, Ziehl–Neelsen, and reticulin. For electron microscopy, tissues were fixed with 3% glutaraldehyde in 0.1 M phosphate buffer, pH 7.2, washed with several changes of 5% sucrose in 0.1 M phosphate buffer, pH 7.2, dehydrated in a graded series of ethanols and propylene oxide, and embedded in either Maraglas or Epon. Half-micron–thick sections were cut, stained with alkaline toluidine blue, and examined with a light microscope to select areas for ultrathin sectioning. Ultrathin sections were stained with an ethanolic solution of uranyl acetate and with Reynolds' lead citrate and examined with a JEOL 100B electron microscope.

Results

Morphologic Observations on Control Patients

In tissues from control patients, both Type I and Type II alveolar epithelial cells exhibited a normal morphology, and their basal surfaces were invested by a basal lamina that measured from 600 to 1000 Å in thickness and consisted of very finely fibrillar material of moderate electron density (Figures 1 through 4). In some areas (Figures 1 and 2), this material was in direct contact with the outer leaflet of the plasma membrane of the epithelial cell; in other areas the fibrillar material was separated from the plasma membrane by an electron-lucent space (lamina lucida) 200 to 300 Å in width. Adjacent alveolar epithelial cells were connected by desmosomes and tight junctions (Figure 3). Plasma membrane areas that were invested by basal lamina did not have any specialized junctional structures such as hemidesmosomes.

The interstitial space separating the basal lamina of alveolar epithelium from that of an adjacent capillary often was so narrow that the two basal laminae appeared to be confluent (Figure 4). In certain areas (Figure 1), a few collagen fibrils were present in small clusters in the space between the basal laminae of alveolar epithelium and capillary endothelium. These collagen fibrils measured from 500 to 900 Å in diameter, coursed parallel to the cell surfaces, and frequently were associated with connective tissue microfibrils. The latter measured from 120 to 180 Å in diameter and also formed small clusters. The arrangement and orientation of connective tissue microfibrils was highly irregular, and these structures often appeared enmeshed in basal lamina material (Figure 2). Alveolar septums contained a few elastic fibers, which were small and were composed, as are elastic fibers elsewhere,[36] of centrally located amorphous material (elastin) and peripherally located microfibrils. The latter were indistinguishable from connective tissue microfibrils not associated with elastin. Small amounts of proteoglycan material, composed of electron-dense, fine spicules and granules, were also present in areas of broadening of the alveolar septums.

Morphologic Observations on Patients With Fibrotic Lung Diseases

Fifteen of the 17 patients with fibrotic lung diseases did not have the normal pattern of Type I and Type II alveolar epithelial cells but, rather, had alveolar epithelial cells that were cuboidal. These cells were associated with alveolar septums that were thickened by connective tissue composed of collagen fibrils, elastic fibers, connective tissue microfibrils, proteoglycan material, and accumulations of material resembling that in basal laminae.

The cuboidal alveolar epithelial cells showed a multilayered arrangement (Figures 5 and 6) in 9 of the 17 patients. Study of serial half-micron–thick sections indicated that this multilayering was not the result of artifacts produced by tangential planes of sectioning. Cuboidal alveolar epithelial cells were characterized by plump, cuboidal, or even columnar shapes; oval, elongated or indented nuclei; short, irregularly shaped microvilli along the luminal surfaces; few or no lamellar bodies of the type in normal Type II alveolar epithelial cells; moderate amounts of smooth-surfaced endoplasmic reticulum; well-developed rough-surfaced endoplasmic reticulum and Golgi complexes; and small to moderate numbers of mitochondria. These cells had highly irregular lateral surfaces, with large, clear spaces between adjacent cells. Intercellular junctions consisted of desmosomes and tight junctions. Cytoplasmic processes of various sizes (Figure 7) extended from the basal portions of cuboidal alveolar epithelial cells into the underlying interstitium. Most of these processes were invested by basal laminae. In some areas, however, the basal laminae showed discontinuities through which these processes protruded. The basal laminae often were greatly thickened (Figures 7 and 8), sometimes up to 4000 Å in width. The basal lamina typically appeared composed of a lamina lucida and a lamina densa. The lamina lucida was an electron-lucent layer adjacent to the plasma membrane of the epithelial cell and measured up to 600 Å in width. The remainder of the thickness of the basal lamina consisted of the lamina densa, which was composed of a finely fibrillar or filamentous material of moderate electron density.

Hemidesmosomes (Figures 9 and 10) were found along the basal portions of the cuboidal alveolar epithelial cells in 7 (5 of the 10 patients with idiopathic pulmonary fibrosis and 2 of the 3 patients with connective tissue diseases) of the 9 patients in whom such cells were multilayered. Hemidesmosomes were characterized by the following components: a) a condensation of electron-dense material (attachment plaque) associated with 100-Å filaments along the inner (cytoplasmic) surface of the plasma membrane, b) a subbasal dense plaque adjacent to the outer (extracellular) surface of the plasma membrane, and c) fine filaments that connected one side of the subbasal dense plaque to the plasma membrane and the other side of this plaque to the basal lamina. The basal lamina usually appeared denser at the sites of these connections than it did elsewhere. In 2 of the 7 patients, the hemidesmosomes appeared to be incompletely formed and lacked a subbasal dense plaque (Figure 11).

Small extracellular fibrils with the features described below were encountered (Figures 7 through 10 and 12 through 15) in each of the 7 patients with pulmonary fibrosis in whom hemidesmosomes were present in cuboidal alveolar epithelial cells. These fibrils will be referred to in this communication as "anchoring fibrils" because of their morphologic similarity to the so-called anchoring fibrils that occur in other tissues.[3-29] Anchoring fibrils were associated with the basal laminae of cuboidal alveolar epithelial cells but not with those of normal Type I or Type II alveolar epithelial cells. However, in the 7 patients in whom such structures were present, anchoring fibrils and hemidesmosomes were associated with unilayered as well as multilayered cuboidal alveolar epithelial cells.

Comparison of the clinical and pathologic features of the 5 patients with idiopathic pulmonary fibrosis who had anchoring fibrils and those of the 5 patients with idiopathic pulmonary fibrosis who did not have anchoring fibrils revealed significant differences with respect to the degree of severity of the fibrosis, which was greater ($P = 0.002$) in the patients with anchoring fibrils. The latter patients also had longer duration of symptoms, smaller total lung capacities, vital capacities, diffusion capacities, and more marked exercise hypoxemia than did the patients who did not have anchoring fibrils. However, because the patient groups were small, these values were not significantly different at the $P < 0.05$ level.

Anchoring fibrils measured up to 6000 Å in length and up to 600 Å in width and showed a complex pattern of transverse banding. They often were arc-shaped (Figures 12 through 15) rather than straight, and their ends were broader than their middle portions (Figures 12 and 15). One or both ends of the fibrils frequently appeared to be separated into two slightly divergent terminal portions. Each of the two ends of the arc formed by an anchoring fibril appeared to attach to the basal lamina of an alveolar epithelial cell (Figures 13 through 15), especially in regions where the basal lamina was focally condensed and showed increased electron density (Figures 7 and 12). Some anchoring fibrils inserted into accumulations of material that resembled that of basal lamina; however, such accumulations were located deep in the interstitium without showing continuity with the basal lamina proper (Figure 8). Anchoring fibrils frequently attached in the vicinity of hemidesmosomes (Figures 9 and 10) but were not in direct contact with these structures. Some anchoring fibrils (Figures 9 and 10) appeared attached to the basal lamina at only one of their ends and, due to the plane of sectioning, the site of attachment of the other end could not be determined. Some of these anchoring fibrils appeared oriented perpendicular to the basal portions of the epithelial cells. The ends of the anchoring fibrils were composed of extremely fine filaments, which spread out and became enmeshed into the filamentous material of the basal lamina. In addition, a filamentous substructure was evident along the entire length of some anchoring fibrils. A few collagen fibrils (Figures 7, 13, and 15) and connective tissue microfibrils (Figure 14) were present in the spaces between the basal lamina and the arcs formed by the anchoring fibrils, thus binding the epithelial cells to the underlying stroma.

The banding pattern of anchoring fibrils was clearly different from that of collagen fibrils. Some anchoring fibrils (Figures 13 through 15) showed bilateral symmetry of their banding pattern, which appeared similar to that of anchoring fibrils in mouse uterus [26] and human cervix.[27] As in those other tissues, the anchoring fibrils in lung showed some variations in their pattern of banding. The smallest anchoring fibrils, which measured only approximately 200 Å in diameter, showed less distinct banding patterns and often were difficult to distinguish from connective tissue microfibrils.

Discussion

Anchoring fibrils were first described in 1960 by Brody,[3] who observed them in normal human skin and called them "reticular filaments." These fibrils filled out the spaces between adjacent cell processes extending from the stratum basale into the dermis. Palade and Farquhar [5] introduced the term "anchoring fibrils" in their report describing such fibrils in the skin of amphibians and in the skin, lingual mucosa, and gastric fundic mocusa of the rat. Palade and Farquhar [5] concluded that the anchoring fibrils secured the minute outfoldings of the basement membrane along the dermal–epidermal junction. Other studies (Table 2) have confirmed the presence of anchoring fibrils in normal human skin,[6-10] in skin of patients with dermatitis herpetiformis,[15] and in a cylindroma.[16] In dermatitis herpetiformis, the anchoring fibrils in the skin have been shown to bind IgA.[15] Of special interest is the absence of anchoring fibrils from the skin of patients with epidermolysis bullosa dystrophica–recessive.[11] It has been postulated that the defect in this disease resides in the dermis and is associated with impaired formation of anchoring fibrils.[11] It also has been

Table 2—Pulmonary Biopsy Findings in 17 Patients With Pulmonary Fibrosis and 5 Control Patients

Patients	Biopsy sites	Degree of fibrosis	Cuboidal metaplasia	Epithelial multi-layering	Epithelial hemides-mosomes	Epithelial basal lamina thickening	Anchoring fibrils
LY	Lingula	+4	+	+	+	+	+
AM	Lingula	+3	+	0	0	+	0
RM	Lingula	+4	+	+	+	+	+
WD	Lingula	+1	0	0	0	0	0
WK	Lingula	+4	+	+	+	+	+
WES	RUL	+4	+	+	+	+	+
	Lingula	+2					
	RLL	+4					
SFB	Lingula	+3	+	+	0	+	0
WH	LUL	+3	+	0	0	+	0
	LLL	+3					
EB	LUL	+1	+	0	0	0	0
MKL	RLL	+4	+	+	+*	+	+
JV	Lingula	+4	+	+	0	0	0
ON	LUL	+4	+	+	+	+	+
CSW	Lingula	+2	+	+	+*	+	+
RPB	Lingula	+1	+	0	0	0	0
	LLL	+1					
JAW	Lingula	+3	+	0	0	0	0
DLM	RUL	+2	0	0	0	0	0
BC	Lingula	+2	+	0	0	0	0
	RLL	+2					
Control patients							
LS	LLL	0	0	0	0	0	0
MLS	RUL	0	0	0	0	0	0
LL	LLL	0	0	0	0	0	0
WKN	RUL	0	0	0	0	0	0
	RLL	0					
BJC	Lingula	0	0	0	0	0	0

Degree of fibrosis graded from 0 to +4 as described by Fulmer et al [31]; + = present, 0 = absent, RUL = right upper lobe, RLL = right lower lobe, LUL = left upper lobe, LLL = left lower lobe, * = incompletely formed hemidesmosomes (see text).

suggested, on the basis of dermis–epidermis recombination experiments,[8,9] that anchoring fibrils of the skin are a dermal derivative since the presence of viable dermis is necessary for their formation. Anchoring fibrils also have been found in human and rat oral mucosa,[17-20] amphibian notochord,[12,13] human and rat gingiva,[21-24] human cervical mucosa,[25-27] mouse uterus,[28] and human vaginal mucosa [29] and along Schwann cells in unmyelinated nerve fibers in human skin.[6] Thus, it would appear that anchoring fibrils constitute a distinct family of connective tissue fibrils that are consistently associated with the basal laminae of epithelial cells in various organs.

To our knowledge, anchoring fibrils have not been previously described in normal or abnormal lung tissue. It is possible that they have been missed because they are clearly recognizable only at relatively high magnifications. We did not find such fibrils in lungs from our control patients; however, we cannot exclude the possibility that they occur in small numbers in normal lung.

Structure of Anchoring Fibrils

The morphologic features of anchoring fibrils in the tissues listed in Table 3 are generally similar, except for the strikingly different pattern of banding of the fibrils in amphibian tissues and for the symmetry or asymmetry of the banding of the fibrils in other tissues (Table 3). There is general agreement that the banding pattern in each tissue shows a certain amount of variation. Termination of one of the ends of each fibril in the basal lamina is the most prevalent pattern of arrangement observed in skin.[8-11] Nevertheless, reports of other tissues [5-7,9-11,19,25,27] have described the attachment of both ends of the anchoring fibrils to the basal lamina, forming loops through which collagen fibrils and microfibrils are inserted in a weaving pattern. Such an arrangement also was found in the present study, suggesting that anchoring fibrils form a network that serves to attach the basal laminae of epithelial cells to the subjacent connective tissue. Hemidesmosomes appear to play a similar role in reinforcing the attachment of epithelial cells to their basal laminae. It should be noted that bundles of nonbanded anchoring filaments have been described in embryonic feathers [37] and in skin of various aquatic chordates.[38,39] The relationship of such bundles of filaments to the banded anchoring fibrils is not known.

The chemical nature of banded anchoring fibrils is not known. It has been suggested [28] that they are a dimeric form of aggregates of collagen or tropocollagen, particularly since antiparallel packing of the protein molecules with opposing ends in register is a feature common to such aggregates,[40-42] but the banding pattern of anchoring fibrils does not correspond to that of the aggregates of any of the known types of collagen. Anchoring fibrils in skin have been reported to be destroyed by bacterial collagenase.[10] Nevertheless, considerable caution is necessary in interpreting this observation because of the presence of impurities in the collagenase preparation.[10]

Significance of Anchoring Fibrils in Lung of Patients With Fibrotic Lung Disease

On review of our observations, it became evident that the following requisites seem to be necessary for the development of anchoring fibrils in

Table 3—Reports of Occurrence of Anchoring Fibrils in Various Tissues

Authors and reference	Species	Tissue	Condition	Cell type	Anchoring fibrils		
					Length (Å)	Diameter (Å)	Symmetry of banding
Brody[3]	Human	Skin	Normal	Basal cell	—	—	—
Farquhar and Palade[4]	Rana, Bufo, Xenopus, Amblystoma	Skin	Normal	Basal cell	—	—	—
Palade and Farquhar[5]	Rana, Bufo, Xenopus, Amblystoma	Skin	Normal	Basal cell	4000	200–750	0
	Rat	Skin	Normal	Basal cell	—	—	—
		Lingual and gastric fundic mucosa	Normal	Basal epithelial cell	—	—	—
Swanson and Helwig[6]	Human	Skin	Normal	Basal cell Schwann cell	—	200–600	—
Kobayasi[7]	Human	Skin	Normal	Basal cell	—	—	—
Briggaman et al[8-11]	Human	Skin	Normal	Basal cell	—	—	0
Bruns[12]	Rana	Skin	Normal	Basal cell	7500	300–1000	+
		Notochord	Normal	Notochord cell			
Bruns and Gross[13]	Rana	Notochord	Normal	Notochord cell	—	—	+
Caputo and Peluchetti[14]	Human	Skin	Normal	Basal cell	—	—	—
Yaoita and Katz[15]	Human	Skin	Dermatitis herpetiformis	Basal cell	—	—	—
Hashimoto and Lever[16]	Human	Skin	Cylindroma	Tumor cell	—	—	—

Stern[17]	Human Rat	Oral mucosa	Normal	Basal epithelial cell	—	100	—
Frithiof[18]	Human	Oral mucosa	Normal Hyperplasia Carcinoma	Basal cell	—	—	—
Susi et al [19]	Human	Oral mucosa	Normal	Basal epithelial cell	2500	200–400	—
Shimono and Clementi [20]	Rat	Oral mucosa	Normal	Basal epithelial cell	—	—	—
Schroeder and Theilade[21]	Human	Gingiva	Normal	Basal epithelial cell	—	—	—
Nikai et al [22]	Human	Gingiva	Chronic desquamative gingivitis	Basal epithelial cell	—	—	—
Sugimoto et al [23]	Human	Gingiva	Hyperplasia Periodontitis	Basal epithelial cell	5000	150–480	—
Takarada et al[24]	Human	Gingiva	Hyperplasia Periodontitis	Basal epithelial cell	—	1100	+
Younes et al [25]	Human	Cervix	Normal	Epithelial cell	—	150–200	—
Hackemann et al [26]	Human	Cervix	Normal	Basal cell	—	—	—
Laguens [27]	Human	Cervix	Normal	Epithelial cell	2000–5000	—	+
Rowlatt [28]	Mouse	Uterus	Normal	Epithelial cell	4000	—	+
Rupec and Hoffmeister [29]	Human	Vagina	Normal	Mucosal cell	—	—	—
Kawanami et al (present study)	Human	Lung	Severe pulmonary fibrosis	Metaplastic alveolar epithelial cell	4000–6000	200–600	+

— = information not available, 0 = absent, + = present.

lung tissue: a) severe degree of pulmonary fibrosis; b) cuboidal metaplasia and multilayering of the alveolar epithelial cells; c) cytoplasmic processes extending from the cuboidal cells into the underlying connective tissue, and d) presence of hemidesmosomes along the basal portions of the cuboidal alveolar epithelial cells. Thus, it may be concluded that anchoring fibrils develop in lung, not simply as a component of fibrous connective tissue, but as part of a more complex phenomenon associated with cuboidal metaplasia of the alveolar epithelial cells. It remains to be determined how these changes in cell shape and morphology relate to the need for the development of structures, such as hemidesmosomes and anchoring fibrils, that are capable of reinforcing the attachment of epithelial cells to thickened, fibrotic alveolar walls. The question of the induction of these changes in pulmonary fibrosis is particularly intriguing because such changes may be preceded by a phase of damage and desquamation of alveolar epithelium and are associated with disordering of connective tissue in pulmonary interstitium.[1,31,32]

References

1. Crystal RG, Fulmer JD, Roberts WC, Moss ML, Line BR, Reynolds HY: Idiopathic pulmonary fibrosis: Clinical, histologic, radiographic, physiologic, scintigraphic, cytologic, and biochemical aspects. Ann Intern Med 85:769–788, 1976
2. Reynolds HY, Fulmer JD, Kazmierowski JA, Roberts WC, Frank MM, Crystal RG: Analysis of cellular and protein content of broncho-alveolar lavage fluid from patients with idiopathic pulmonary fibrosis and chronic hypersensitivity pneumonitis. J Clin Invest 59:165–175, 1977
3. Brody I: The ultrastructure of the tonofibrils in the keratinization process of normal human epidermis. J Ultrastruct Res 4:264–297, 1960
4. Farquhar MG, Palade GE: Cell junctions in amphibian skin. J Cell Biol 26:263–291, 1965
5. Palade GE, Farquhar MG: A special fibril of the dermis. J Cell Biol 27:215–224, 1965
6. Swanson JL, Helwig EB: Special fibrils of human dermis. J Invest Dermatol 50:195–199, 1968
7. Kobayasi T: Electron microscopy of the elastic fibers and the dermal membrane in normal human skin. Acta Derm Venereol (Stockh) 48:303–312, 1968
8. Briggaman RA, Wheeler CE: Epidermal-dermal interactions in adult human skin: Role of dermis in epidermal maintenance. J Invest Dermatol 51:454–465, 1968
9. Briggaman RA, Dalldorf FG, Wheeler CE Jr: Formation and origin of basal lamina and anchoring fibrils in adult human skin. J Cell Biol 51:384–395, 1971
10. Briggaman RA, Wheeler CE Jr: The epidermal-dermal junction. J Invest Dermatol 65:71–84, 1975
11. Briggaman RA, Wheeler CE Jr: Epidermolysis bullosa dystrophica-recessive: A possible role of anchoring fibrils in the pathogenesis. J Invest Dermatol 65:203–211, 1975
12. Bruns RR: A symmetrical, extracellular fibril. J Cell Biol 42:418–430, 1969
13. Bruns RR, Gross J: Studies on the tadpole tail. I. Structure and organization of the notochord and its covering layers in Rana catesbeiana. Am J Anat 128:193–224, 1970
14. Caputo R, Peluchetti D: The junctions of normal human epidermis: A freeze-

fracture study. J Ultrastruct Res 61:44–61, 1977
15. Yaoita H, Katz SI: Immunoelectronmicroscopic localization of IgA in skin of patients with dermatitis herpetiformis. J Invest Dermatol 67:502–506, 1976
16. Hashimoto K, Lever WF: Histogenesis of skin appendage tumors. Arch Dermatol 100:356–369, 1969
17. Stern IB: Electron microscopic observations of oral epithelium. I. Basal cells and the basement membrane. Periodontics 3:224–238, 1965
18. Frithiof L: Ultrastructure of the basement membrane in normal and hyperplastic human oral epithelium compared with that in preinvasive and invasive carcinoma. Acta Pathol Microbiol Scand (Suppl 200):1–63, 1969
19. Susi FR, Belt WD, Kelly JW: Fine structure of fibrillar complexes associated with the basement membrane in human oral mucosa. J Cell Biol 34:686–690, 1967
20. Shimono M, Clementi F: Intercellular junctions of oral epithelium. I. Studies with freeze-fracture and tracing methods of normal rat keratinized oral epithelium. J Ultrastruct Res 56:121–136, 1976
21. Schroeder HE, Theilade J: Electron microscopy of normal human gingival epithelium. J Periodont Res 1:95–119, 1966
22. Nikai H, Rose GG, Cattoni M: Electron microscopic study of chronic desquamative gingivitis. J Periodont Res 6(Suppl):7–30, 1971
23. Sugimoto A, Rose GG, Takarada H, Cattoni M: Ultrastructural changes of basal lamina and anchoring fibrils of gingiva in vitro. J Periodont Res 8:127–142, 1973
24. Takarada H, Cattoni M, Sugimoto A, Rose GG: Ultrastructural studies of human gingiva. IV. Anchoring fibrils and perforations of the basal lamina in chronic periodontitis. J Periodont 45:809–814, 1974
25. Younes MS, Steele HD, Robertson EM, Bencosme SA: Correlative light and electron microscope study of the basement membrane of the human ectocervix. Am J Obstet Gynecol 92:163–171, 1965
26. Hackemann M, Grubb C, Hill KR: The ultrastructure of normal squamous epithelium of the human cervix uteri. J Ultrastruct Res 22:443–457, 1968
27. Laguens R: Subepithelial fibrils associated with the basement membrane of human cervical epithelium. J Ultrastruct Res 41:202–208, 1972
28. Rowlatt C: Subepithelial fibrils associated with the basal lamina under simple epithelia in mouse uterus: Possible tropocollagen aggregates. J Ultrastruct Res 26:44–51, 1969
29. Rupec M, Hoffmeister H: Zur Ultrastruktur de Halbdesmosomen. Dermatologica 138:453–458, 1969
30. Fulmer JD, Roberts WC, von Gal ER, Crystal RG: Small airways in idiopathic pulmonary fibrosis: Comparison of morphologic and physiologic observations. J Clin Invest 60:595–610, 1977
31. Fulmer JD, von Gal ER, Roberts WC, Crystal RG: Morphologic-physiologic correlates of the severity of fibrosis in idiopathic pulmonary fibrosis. (Submitted)
32. Fulmer JD, Bienkowski RS, Cowan MJ, Bruel SD, Bradley KM, Ferrans VJ, Roberts WC, Crystal RG: Collagen concentration and rates of synthesis in idiopathic pulmonary fibrosis. (Submitted)
33. Rodman GF, McEwen C, Wallace SL: Primer on the rheumatic diseases. JAMA 224:662–812, 1973
34. Siltzbach LE: Sarcoidosis: Clinical features and management. Med Clin North Am 51:483–502, 1967
35. Carrington CB, Addington WW, Goff AM, Madoff IM, Marks A, Schwaber JR, Gaensler EA: Chronic eosinophilic pneumonia. N Engl J Med 280:787–798, 1969
36. Ross R: The elastic fiber: A review. J Histochem Cytochem 21:199–208, 1973
37. Kallman F, Evans J, Wessels NK: Anchor filament bundles in embryonic feather germs and skin. J Cell Biol 32:236–240, 1967
38. Nakao T: Some observations on the fine structure of the epidermal-dermal junction

in the skin of the frog tadpole, Rana rugosa. Am J Anat 140:533–550, 1974
39. Fox H: Anchoring fibrils of the basal lamina and basement lamella in the skin of aquatic chordates. J Microscopie Biol Cell 26:43–46, 1976
40. Chapman JA, Armitage PM: An analysis of fibrous long spacing forms of collagen. Connect Tissue Res 1:31–37, 1972
41. Doyle BB, Hulmes DJS, Miller A, Parry DAD, Piez KA, Woodhead-Galloway J: Axially projected collagen structures. Proc R Soc Lond (Biol) 187:37–46, 1974
42. Weinstock M: Centrosymmetrical cross-band structures in the matrix of rat incisor predentin and dentin. J Ultrastruct Res 61:218–229, 1977

Acknowledgments

The authors wish to express their appreciation for the skilled assistance of Mrs. Octavia Dejoie (electron microscopy), Mrs. Ester Wilhoite (photography), and Mrs. Dorothy Veigle (secretarial and editorial work).

Figures 1 through 4 and 6 through 15 are electron micrographs of sections stained with alcoholic uranyl acetate and lead citrate. Figure 5 is a light micrograph. Figures 1 through 4 are from control patient BJC. Figures 5 through 15 are from patients with idiopathic pulmonary fibrosis; Figures 5, 6, and 8 through 12 are from patient LY; Figure 7 is from patient WFK; and Figures 13 through 15 are from patient MKL.

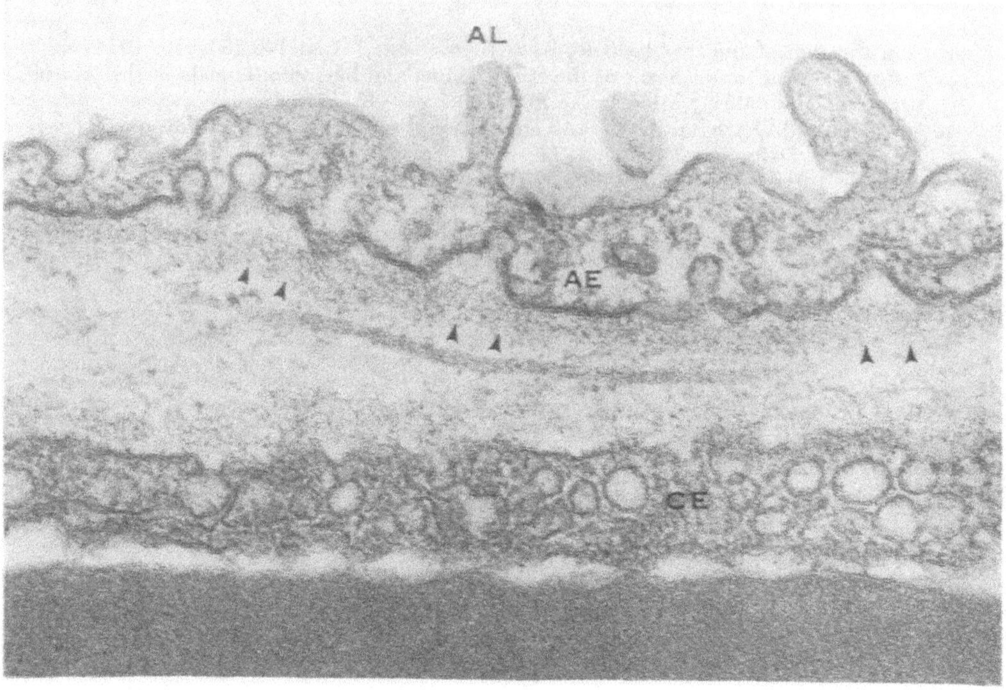

1

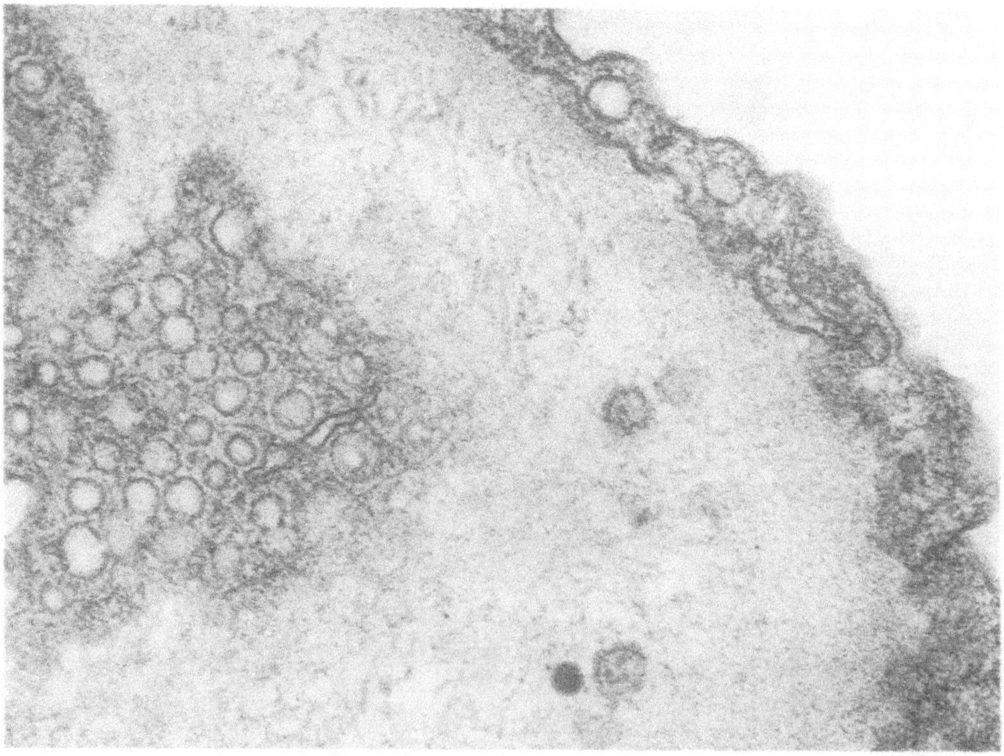

2

Figure 1—Air-blood barrier in control lung. Alveolar lumen (*AL*) is bordered by cytoplasm of Type 1 alveolar epithelial cell (*AE*). Basal lamina (*arrowheads*) of this cell is separated from basal lamina of capillary endothelial cell (*CE*) by narrow interstitial space in which collagen fibrils and strands of material presumed to be proteoglycans are present. (× 67,500) **Figure 2**—Air-blood barrier in control lung. Type I alveolar epithelial cell (*right*) is separated from capillary endothelial cell (*left*) by interstitial space that contains connective tissue microfibrils (*upper center*) and fine strands of proteoglycan material (*lower center*). (× 60,000)

3

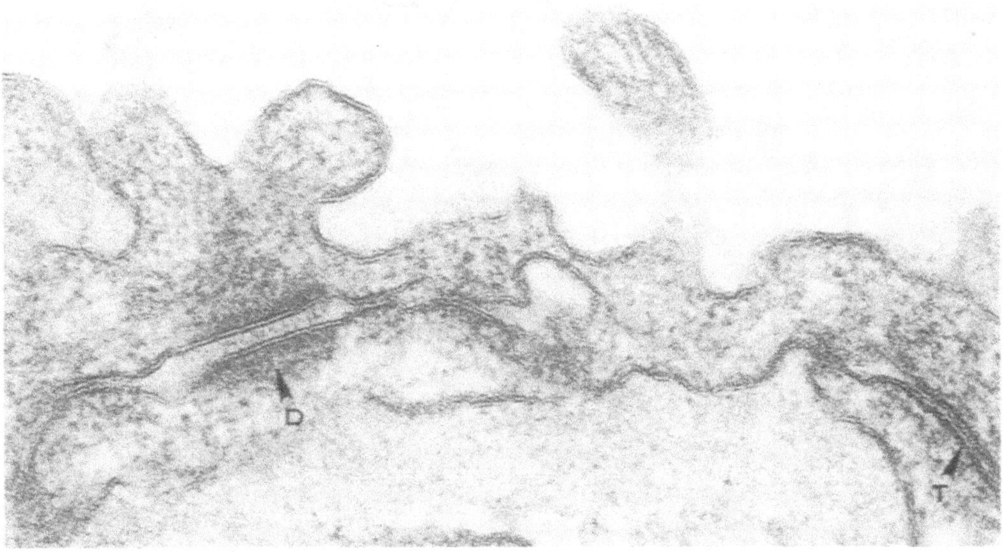

4

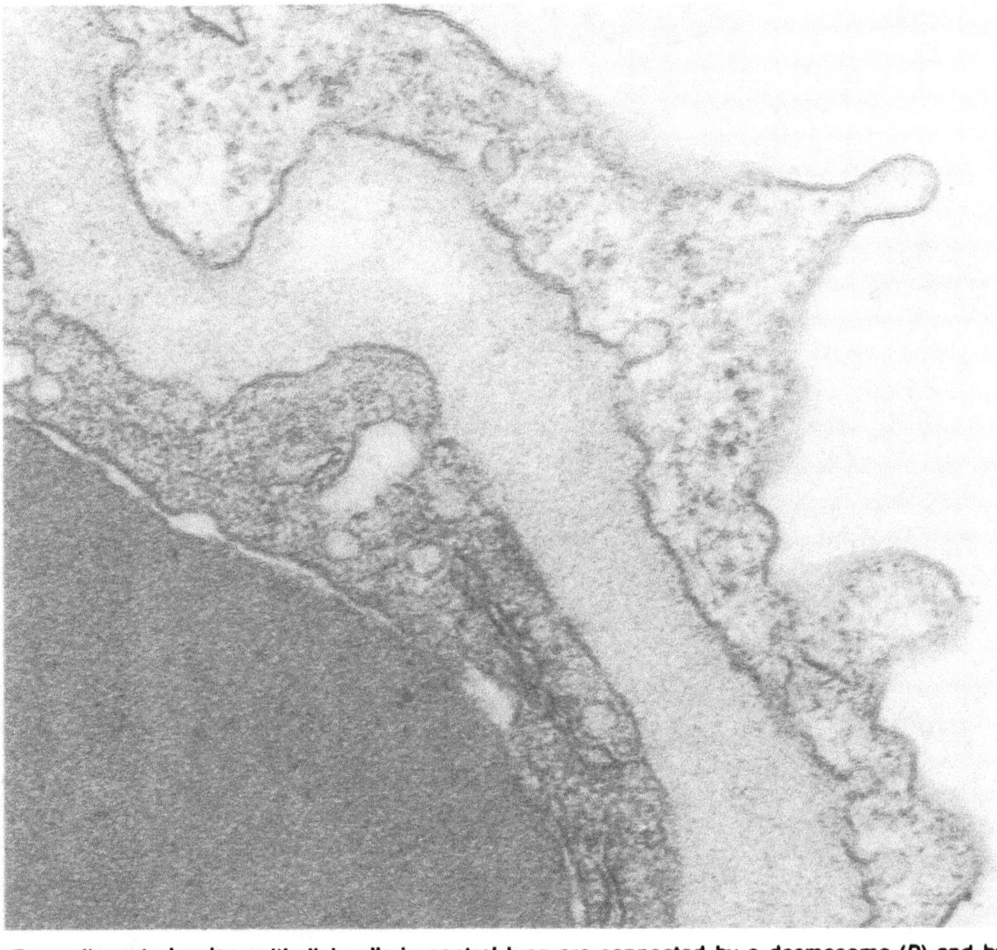

Figure 3—Two adjacent alveolar epithelial cells in control lung are connected by a desmosome (*D*) and by a tight junction (*T*). (× 110,000) **Figure 4**—Area of confluence of the basal laminae of an alveolar epithelial cell (*upper center* and *right*) and a capillary endothelial cell (*lower left*) in control lung. Note absence of other connective tissue components in this area. (× 75,000)

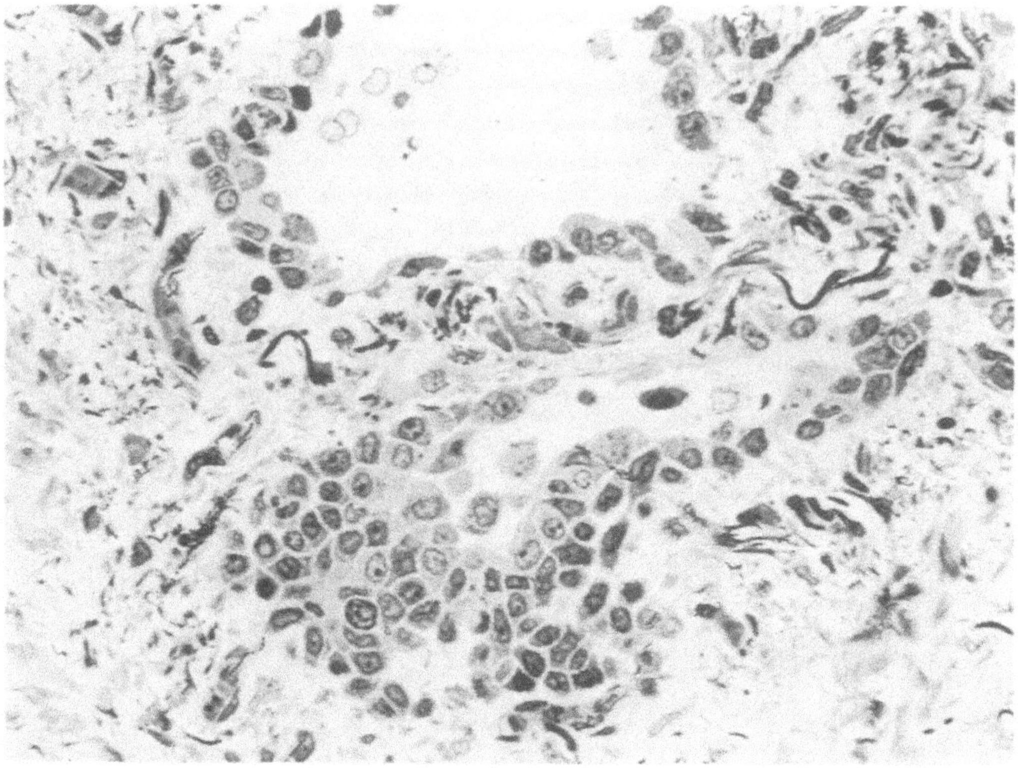

5

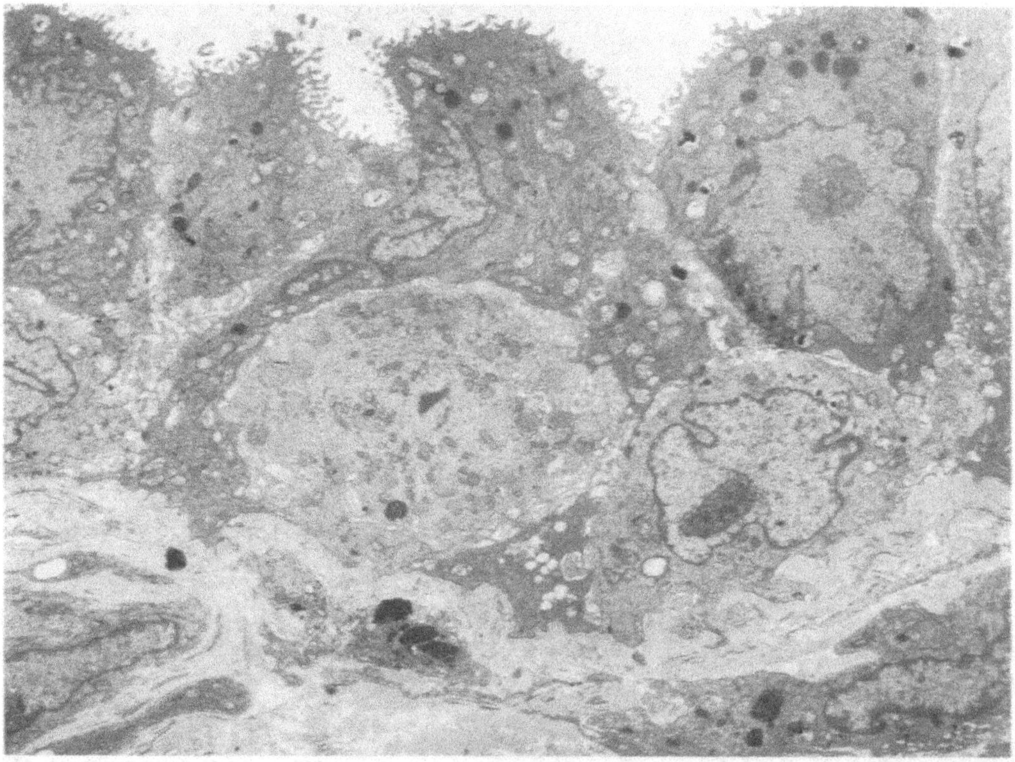

6

Figure 5—Light micrograph of alveoli that are lined by multilayered, cuboidal cells and are surrounded by dense fibrous tissue. Plastic-embedded tissue. (Alkaline toluidine blue stain, × 400) **Figure 6**—Low magnification view of alveolus lined by cuboidal, multilayered alveolar epithelial cells. Small, irregular microvilli are present along the luminal surfaces of these cells. Their cytoplasm contains dense bodies, mitochondria, and smooth- and rough-surfaced endoplasmic reticulum. The plasma membranes in the basal portions of the cells display highly irregular protrusions that are invested by basal lamina and extend into the underlying connective tissue. (× 5000)

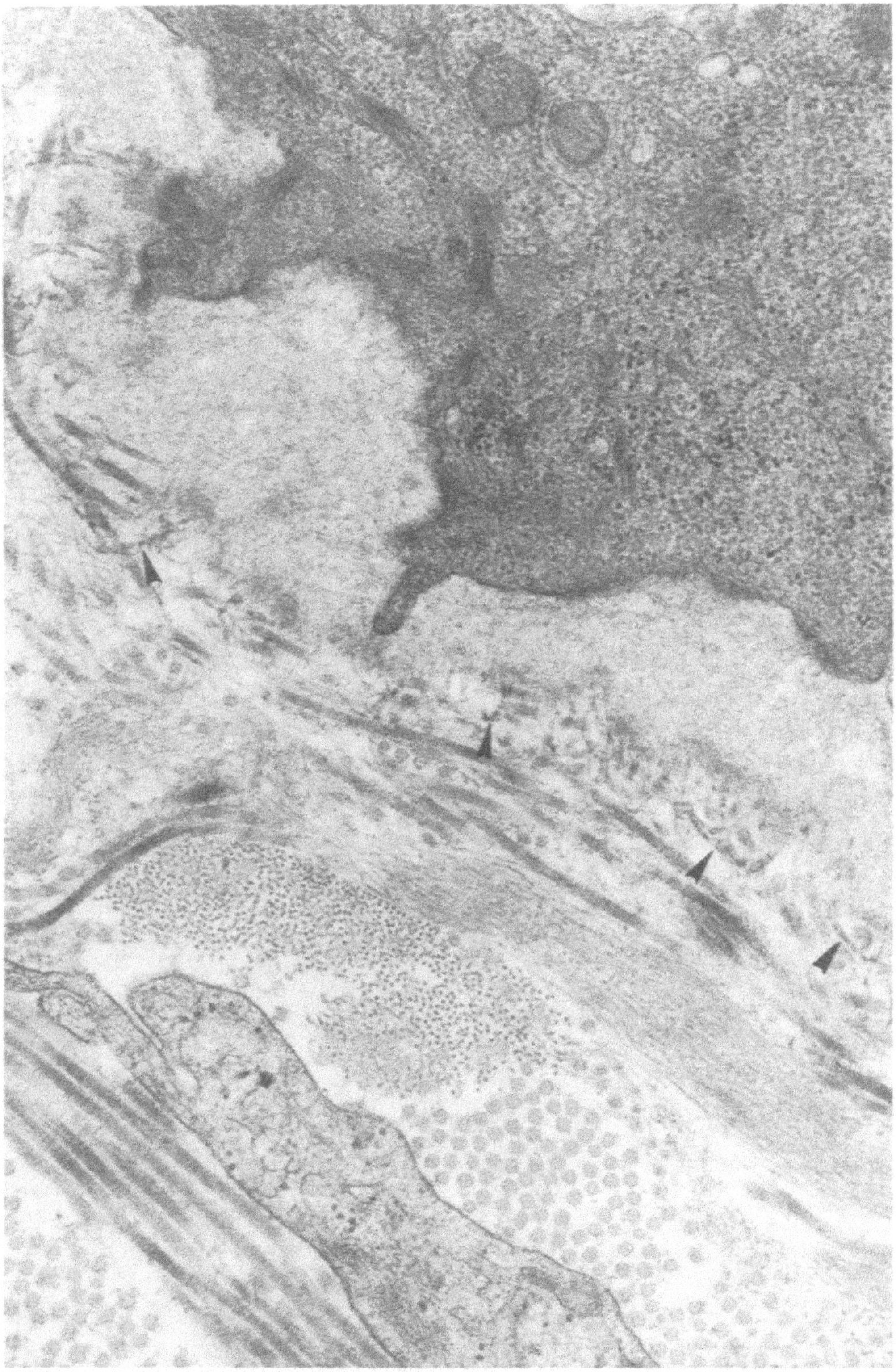

Figure 7—View of basal portion of cytoplasm of metaplastic alveolar epithelial cell and subjacent connective tissue. The cell contains mitochondria, glycogen granules, and bundles of cytoplasmic filaments. Cytoplasmic processes extended into the basal lamina, which is greatly thickened. Numerous arc-shaped anchoring fibrils (*arrowheads*) are located adjacent to the outer border of the basal lamina. This border is denser than the remainder of the basal lamina. Collagen fibrils and connective tissue microfibrils are woven through the loops formed by the anchoring fibrils. Part of a fibroblast (*bottom*) is surrounded by bundles of collagen fibrils and connective tissue microfibrils. (× 40,500)

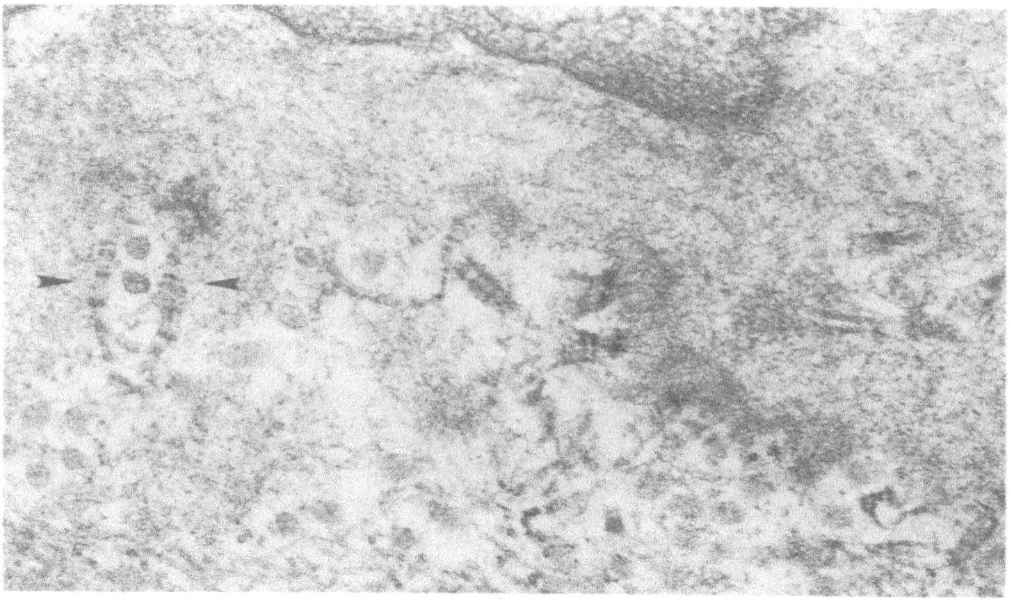

8

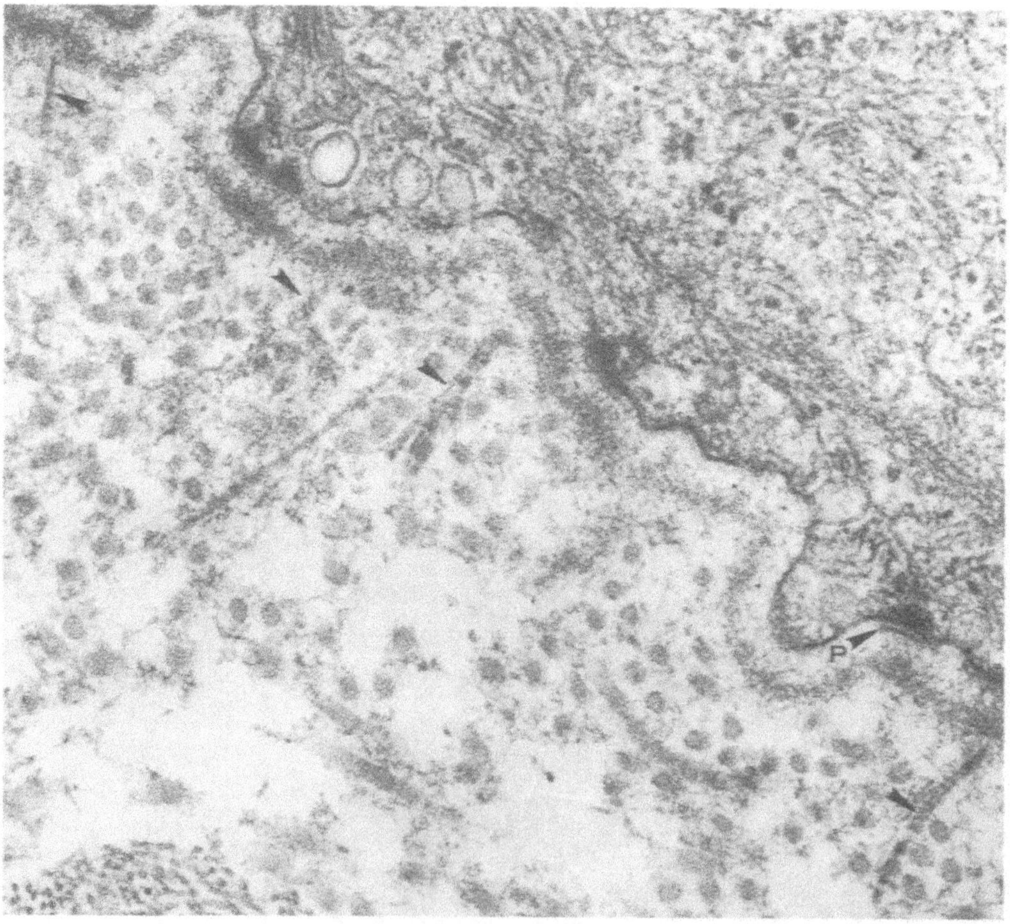

9

Figure 8—Several anchoring fibrils show a filamentous substructure and terminate in thickened basal lamina that surrounds cuboidal alveolar epithelial cell (*top*). One anchoring fibril (*arrowheads*) forms an arc through which two collagen fibrils are inserted. The banding pattern of this fibril is symmetric about the center of the arc. Note basal-lamina-like material (*center*) which appears separate from the basal lamina proper. (× 71,000) **Figure 9**—View of hemidesmosomes and of anchoring fibrils (*arrowheads*), which appear oriented perpendicular to the basal lamina, on the basal surface of cuboidal alveolar epithelial cell. Cytoplasmic filaments are abundant in this cell. Note well-developed subbasal plaque (*P*) in hemidesmosomes and fine filaments which extend from this plaque to the lamina densa region of the basal lamina. The banding of these anchoring fibrils does not appear symmetric. (×75,000)

Figure 10—Two hemidesmosomes have prominent condensations of electron-dense material against the inner surface of the plasma membrane, subbasal plaques adjacent to the outer surface of the plasma membrane, and fine filaments connecting the subbasal plaque to the basal lamina. The latter is thickened and reduplicated. Two anchoring fibrils (*single arrowheads*) insert into the basal lamina adjacent to hemidesmosomes. Other structures (*double arrowheads*) also may represent obliquely sectioned anchoring fibrils. (× 62,500)

Figure 11—Focal condensations of electron-dense material against the inner surface of the plasma membrane in the basal region of a cuboidal alveolar epithelial cell are associated with fine filaments that extend from the outer surface of the plasma membrane to the lamina densa region of the basal lamina. Such structural complexes are regarded as representing an early stage in the formation of hemidesmosomes. Spreading filaments at the end of an anchoring fibril (*arrowheads*) insert into basal lamina. (× 76,800)

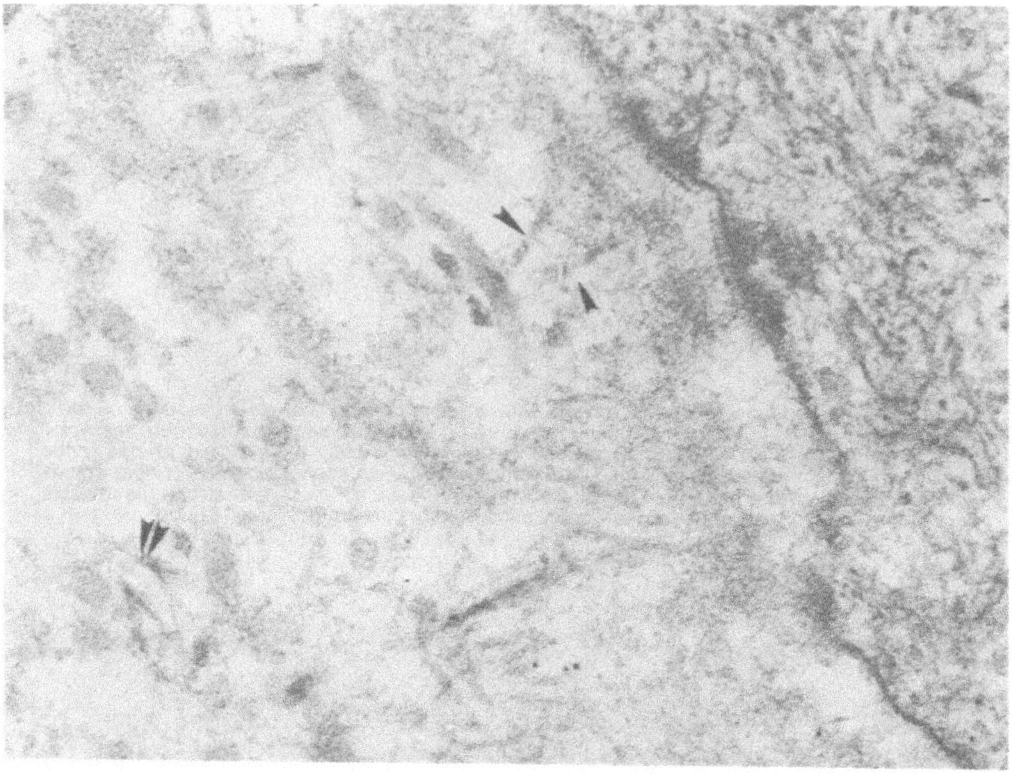

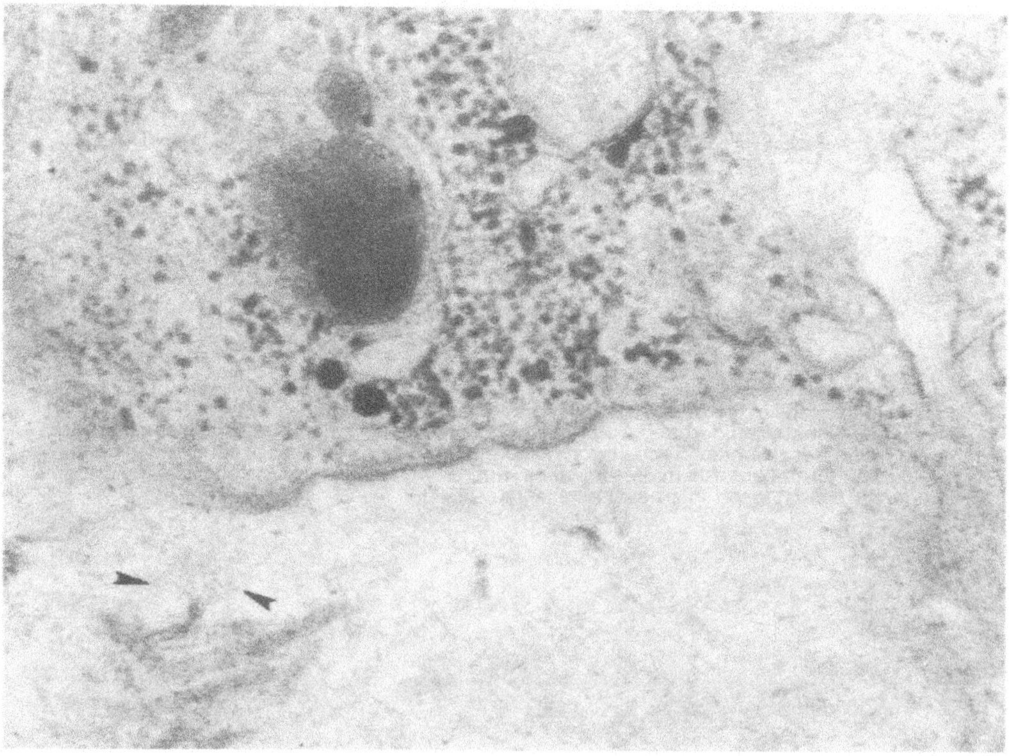

12 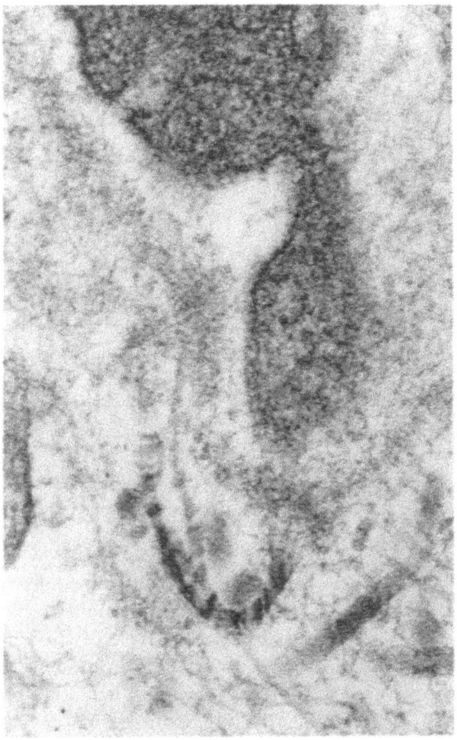

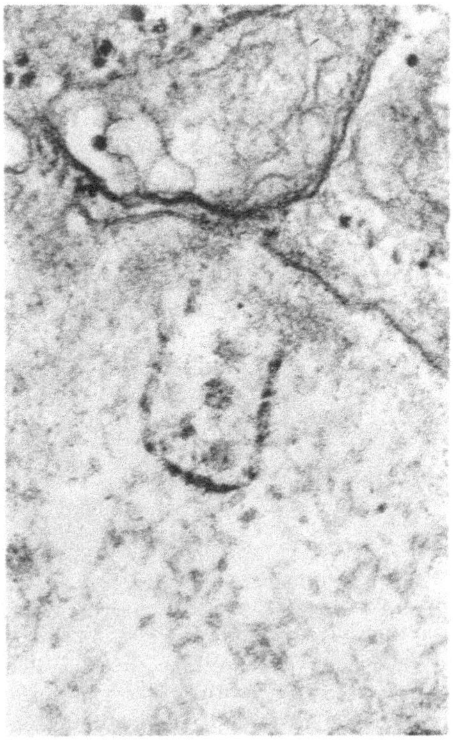 13

14 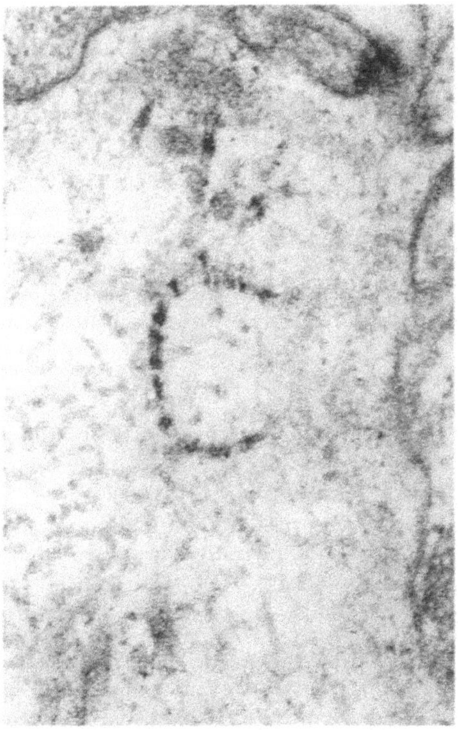

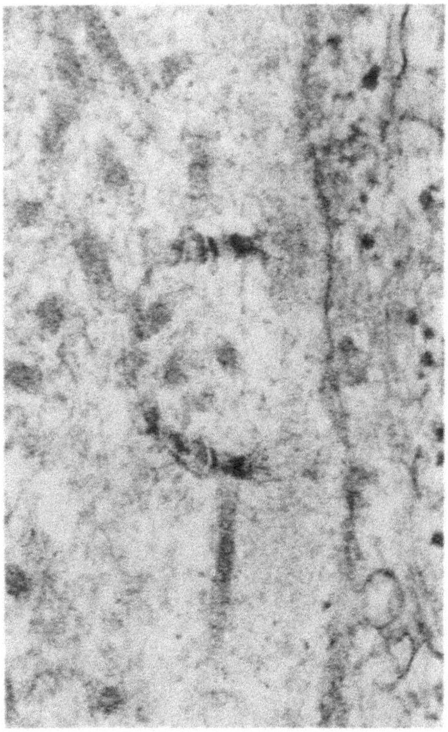 15

Figures 12 through 15—High magnification views of anchoring fibrils. **Figure 12**—Protruding cytoplasmic processes of cuboidal alveolar epithelial cell are invested by basal lamina which is composed of fine fibrillar elements and is connected to fine strands of glycosaminoglycan and to connective tissue microfibrils. Both ends of an arc-shaped anchoring fibril insert into the basal lamina. Two collagen fibrils and one banded fibril (possibly another anchoring fibril) are seen inside the arc formed by the anchoring fibril. (× 95,000) **Figure 13**—Both ends of an arc-shaped anchoring fibril terminate on condensed basal lamina along the plasma membrane of cuboidal alveolar epithelial cell. Banding pattern appears symmetric but is not as well defined as in Figures 14 and 15. Some collagen fibrils are present in the arc. (× 100,000) **Figure 14**—Arc-shaped anchoring fibril shows distinctive symmetric bands, particularly in its central portion. A few connective tissue microfibrils are enclosed within the arc. (× 100,000) **Figure 15**—Symmetric banding of large, arc-shaped anchoring fibril is especially clear at both ends, where the fibril inserts into the basal lamina. (× 100,000)

Gallium-67 Citrate Scanning in the Staging of Idiopathic Pulmonary Fibrosis: Correlation with Physiologic and Morphologic Features and Bronchoalveolar Lavage[1-3]

BRUCE R. LINE, JACK D. FULMER, HERBERT Y. REYNOLDS, WILLIAM C. ROBERTS, A. ERIC JONES, EUGENE K. HARRIS, and RONALD G. CRYSTAL

SUMMARY

Idiopathic pulmonary fibrosis is a fatal disorder characterized by interstitial fibrosis and parenchymal inflammation. Current concepts of this disease suggest that the inflammation precedes and probably induces the fibrotic state. To evaluate the extent and relative activity of the inflammatory process, we scanned patients with idiopathic pulmonary fibrosis using gallium-67, a radionuclide known to concentrate in regions of inflammation. To quantify the amount of isotope in the lung parenchyma, the ^{67}Ga-index was developed, a parameter derived from estimates of the size of regional pulmonary uptake, the uptake intensity, and its texture. Evaluation of ^{67}Ga scans in 30 patients with idiopathic pulmonary fibrosis and 19 control subjects demonstrated that the ^{67}Ga-index in the group with idiopathic pulmonary fibrosis was significantly higher ($P < 0.001$) than that in the control group. When compared with lung biopsy morphologic studies in 22 patients with idiopathic pulmonary fibrosis, the ^{67}Ga-index correlated with the degree of interstitial cellularity ($P < 0.05$) and the degree of alveolar cellularity ($P < 0.005$). When compared with cellular analysis of bronchoalveolar lavage fluid in 17 patients with idiopathic pulmonary fibrosis, the ^{67}Ga-index correlated with the differential percentage of neutrophils ($P < 0.05$), but not lymphocytes, eosinophils, or macrophages.

These studies indicate that ^{67}Ga accumulates in the lungs of patients with idiopathic pulmonary fibrosis and is probably associated with the active inflammatory state. The associations of the ^{67}Ga-index with morphologic features and bronchoalveolar lavage analysis suggest that quantitative evaluation of these scans may be useful in staging the activity of idiopathic pulmonary fibrosis and following responses to therapy.

Introduction

Idiopathic pulmonary fibrosis (IPF) is a fatal disorder characterized clinically by exertional breathlessness, radiographically by an interstitial infiltrative pattern, and physiologically by decreased lung volumes, decreased diffusing capacity of the lung for CO (D_{LCO}), and hypoxemia that worsens with exercise (1–11). The disease usually presents in middle age and follows a progressive downhill course during an average of 4 years (10, 12).

Lung biopsies of patients with IPF reveal

(*Received in original form January 5, 1978 and in revised form April 7, 1978*)

[1] From the Laboratory of Applied Studies, Division of Computer Research and Technology; the Pulmonary Branch and the Laboratory of Pathology, National Heart, Lung, and Blood Institute; the Laboratory of Clinical Investigation, National Institute of Allergy and Infectious Diseases; and the Department of Nuclear Medicine, Clinical Center, National Institutes of Health, Bethesda, MD 20014.

[2] Presented in part at the Annual Meeting of the American Thoracic Society, Scientific Session 14D, May 19, May 1976.

[3] Requests for reprints should be addressed to Pulmonary Branch, Room 6N260, Bldg. 10, National Institutes of Health, Bethesda, MD 20014.

varying degrees of inflammation and fibrosis (10, 13–15). The inflammatory component is characterized by interstitial and intra-alveolar infiltrates composed mainly of mononuclear cells, with smaller numbers of neutrophils and eosinophils. The fibrotic component is limited to the interstitium and is characterized by a derangement of collagen fibers (16, 17).

Although many of the physiologic manifestations of IPF result from interstitial fibrosis, current concepts suggest that the inflammatory component ("alveolitis") plays a central role in the pathogenesis and clinical course of this disorder (10). First, it is likely that the alveolitis precedes and contributes to the development of fibrosis (18, 19). Second, whereas the fibrotic component is probably irreversible once established, the inflammatory process may be amenable to therapy (13). Consequently, to evaluate and treat patients with IPF, it is necessary to stage the extent of parenchymal inflammation, preferably on a repetitive basis. This, however, is not an easy task because (*1*) the inflammation is limited to the lung tissues and does not manifest itself systemically; (*2*) no physiologic methods have been shown to reflect the degree of inflammation in these patients; (*3*) a lung biopsy, the definitive procedure for staging the alveolitis of IPF, is rarely performed more than once; and (*4*) the amount of inflammation in any region probably changes through the course of the disease or with therapy.

Thus, a method that was noninvasive and that would estimate the degree of parenchymal inflammation in all parts of the lung would be useful to stage IPF and to follow the effectiveness of therapy directed against the alveolitis of the disease.

One approach that fulfills these requirements is to use a radioactive tracer that concentrates in areas of active inflammation. Gallium-67 is such a radionuclide; it is known to concentrate in inflammatory foci found in a variety of infectious and granulomatous disorders; it is easily imaged; and it is used noninvasively (20–31).

To evaluate the usefulness of ^{67}Ga scans as an index of the alveolitis associated with IPF, we scanned 30 patients with this disease, quantified their pulmonary uptake of ^{67}Ga, and correlated this uptake with physiologic, morphologic, and bronchoscopic lavage assessments of their parenchymal inflammation.

Materials and Methods

Study population. Thirty patients with IPF were chosen randomly from a group of more than 200 patients with interstitial lung disease referred to the Pulmonary Branch, National Heart, Lung and Blood Institute during an 18-month period. The criteria used to make the diagnosis of IPF included (8–11) (*1*) clinical criteria: no significant exposure to environmental agents, no symptoms of extrinsic allergic alveolitis, no history of chronic pulmonary infection or left ventricular failure; (*2*) radiographic criteria: evidence of interstitial lung disease; (*3*) physiologic criteria: decreased total lung capacity (TLC) and/or DLco, normal ratio of forced expiratory volume in 1 sec (FEV_1) to forced vital capacity (FVC), static deflation volume-pressure curve shifted downward and to the right, and an exercise-induced decrease in the arterial Po_2; and (*4*) morphologic criteria: varying degrees of interstitial fibrosis with interstitial and intra-alveolar inflammatory cells consisting primarily of lymphocytes, macrophages, and monocytes, but including neutrophils and eosinophils; no granuloma, vasculitis, intra-alveolar fibrosis, or inorganic material identified by polarized light microscopy; and negative cultures for bacteria, mycobacteria and fungi.

The 30 patients with IPF included 18 men and 12 women with a mean ± SE age of 47.6 ± 2.6 years (table 1). The average duration of symptoms at the time of study was 3.5 years, but two thirds of the patients had had the disease for 2 years or less. Seven patients were current cigarette smokers, 11 patients had stopped smoking at least 6 months before the study, and the remaining 12 patients had never smoked. One half of the patients were untreated at the time of ^{67}Ga scanning, and one-half were taking prednisone (mean dose, 29.0 ± 4.6 mg daily; range, 10 to 60 mg daily). All patients had normal blood hemoglobin and total leukocyte counts. The mean values for vital capacity (VC) (53.2 ± 3.2 per cent predicted), TLC (56.8 ± 2.7 per cent predicted, DLco (45.6 ± 3.6 per cent predicted), and FEV_1/FVC (108.0 ± 2.4 per cent predicted) were typical for patients with IPF in mid-course of their disease (10). Five patients had a defined collagen-vascular disorder, including systemic lupus erythematosus (Patients KM and EK), rheumatoid arthritis (Patient VJ), and a mixed connective tissue syndrome (Patients ON and AM). Two of these patients (Patients KM and AM) had a decreased FEV_1/FVC, which, although unusual for IPF in mid-course, is seen in association with collagen-vascular disorders (33). Within the limits of fiberoptic bronchoscopy, both of these patients had normal airways.

A control group of patients free of fibrotic lung disease was selected from a review of 1,550 patients scanned with ^{67}Ga during the 18-month period of IPF group study. Patients were considered for the control group only if a chest roentgenogram and pulmonary function studies were obtained within 1 month of the ^{67}Ga scan. Nineteen patients met the following criteria used for control group selec-

TABLE 1

CLINICAL, PHYSIOLOGIC, SCINTIGRAPHIC, MORPHOLOGIC, AND BRONCHOALVEOLAR LAVAGE DATA FROM 30 PATIENTS WITH IDIOPATHIC PULMONARY FIBROSIS

	Clinical Data					Physiologic Data*				Scintigraphic Data	Morphologic Data			Bronchoalveolar Lavage Data						
Patient	Age (*years*)	Sex	Duration of Symptoms (*years*)	Smoking History	Drug Therapy	Vital Capacity (*% pred.*)	Total Lung Capacity (*% pred.*)	Diffusing Capacity (*% pred.*)	FEV_1/FVC, % (*% pred.*)	67Ga-Index†	Fibrosis Rank	Interstitial Cellularity Rank	Alveolar Cellularity Rank	Fluid Recovered (%)	Total Cells Recovered ($\times 10^6$)	Viable Cells (%)	Neutrophils (%)	Lymphocytes (%)	Eosinophils (%)	Macrophages (%)
NC	27	M	2.0	L	P	28	44	74	112	100	4	3	2	–	–	–	–	–	–	–
BT	47	F	0.5	M	O	48	50	96	112	125	4	3	2	–	–	–	–	–	–	–
AD	67	M	0.5	HX	P	59	61	49	122	70	4	2	2	70	8.2	94	18	12	1	39
JCS	61	M	2.0	HX	O	55	82	57	109	120	4	4	2	30	23.0	96	16	9	1	74
SC	43	M	10.0	H	P	78	78	11	102	165	–	–	–	32	15.9	93	24	7	5	64
PR	31	F	0.5	M	P	60	67	47	102	105	2	3	3	30	36.0	70	4	13	6	77
KM	29	F	10.0	N	O	60	70	43	65	55	–	–	–	–	–	–	–	–	–	–
EB	48	M	1.5	H	O	83	86	48	96	25	1	1	1	38	8.2	92	6	7	0	87
AH	26	F	2.0	LX	O	75	72	66	97	35	2	2	2	65	7.6	96	5	15	0	80
WH	41	M	2.0	LX	P	50	46	52	113	155'.	3	2	3	42	16.0	98	50	8	2	40
AR	75	M	2.5	H	O	56	57	36	118	180	–	–	–	15	1.3	89	36	13	5	46
JKS	46	M	2.0	MX	P	65	68	30	123	30	4	4	2	–	–	–	–	–	–	–
LF	54	F	8.0	N	P	82	88	27	108	55	–	–	–	–	–	–	–	–	–	–
WES	66	M	1.0	CX	O	35	49	58	104	190	4	3	2	6	9.6	91	14	20	10	56
VJ	27	F	0.5	N	P	50	50	71	114	2	1	1	1	–	–	–	–	–	–	–
RC	66	M	0.5	N	O	71	64	42	109	45	3	3	3	30	3.1	90	19	2	8	71
EK	46	F	2.0	L	P	58	57	75	105	30	3	2	1	30	8.0	82	11	6	6	77
RF	61	M	0.5	CX	P	63	52	23	115	56	4	3	3	30	5.2	60	20	7	1	72
RS	52	M	2.0	N	P	33	33	25	120	70	4	3	3	–	–	–	–	–	–	–
OH	27	F	1.0	N	P	45	43	57	125	55	4	3	2	50	12.0	88	9	18	4	69
EV	51	F	10.0	MX	P	40	40	20	91	70	–	–	–	28	8.7	90	9	6	1	84
ET	56	M	5.0	N	O	62	53	44	105	65	4	2	–	45	14.6	93	10	15	3	72
WD	42	M	0.5	N	O	59	59	58	114	60	1	1	2	20	10.0	88	18	6	0	76
BM	54	M	5.0	HX	O	58	57	36	98	75	–	–	–	–	–	–	–	–	–	–
AM	37	F	14.0	N	P	56	55	41	80	35	–	–	–	28	4.7	60	2	7	2	89
BS	53	M	2.0	HX	O	32	38	22	119	150	4	2	2	–	–	–	–	–	–	–
JS	58	M	7.0	M	O	15	50	46	123	25	4	1	1	–	–	–	–	–	–	–
RH	28	F	0.5	M	P	28	39	37	104	20	–	–	–	–	–	–	–	–	–	–
FR	41	F	1.1	N	O	26	33	–**	126	145	4	4	3	–	–	–	–	–	–	–
WL	67	M	10.0	HX	O	65	62	31	109	50	4	2	2	–	–	–	–	–	–	–
Mean ± SD	47.6 ± 14.2		3.5 ± 3.8			53.2 ± 17.3	56.8 ± 14.9	45.6 ± 19.2	108.0 ± 13.4	78.3 ± 52.1	3.3 ± 1.1	2.5 ± 1.0	2.1 ± 0.7	34.6 ± 16.2	11.3 ± 8.3	86.5 ± 11.2	17.7 ± 14.4	10.0 ± 4.9	3.2 ± 0.3	68.1 ± 15.8

Definitions of abbreviations: FEV_1 = 1-sec forced expiratory volume; FVC = forced vital capacity; L = light cigarette smoker (< 10 pack-years); M = medium cigarette smoker (10–25 pack-years); H = heavy cigarette smoker; X = ex-smoker for more than 6 months; CX = ex-cigar smoker; N = nonsmoker; P = taking prednisone; O = not taking anti-inflammatory medication at time of study.

*The methods used for these studies are detailed by Fulmer and associates (32).

†Mean values of 3 readers.

**Not done because the patient was too ill to perform this test at the time of scan; more recent studies have been compatible with idiopathic pulmonary fibrosis.

TABLE 2

CLINICAL, PHYSIOLOGIC, AND SCINTIGRAPHIC DATA IN 19 CONTROL SUBJECTS

	Clinical Data				Physiologic Data					Scintigraphic Data
Patient	Age (*years*)	Sex	Smoking History	Major Diagnosis	Vital Capacity (*% pred.*)	Total Lung Capacity (*% pred.*)	Diffusing Capacity (*% pred.*)	FEV_1/FVC, % (*% pred.*)	Physiologic Diagnosis	(^{67}*Ga-index*)
ME	65	F	H	Aortic valve disease	95	112	110	109	Normal	3
BN	68	F	H	Squamous cell carcinoma of the mouth	108	122	88	104	Normal	13
AM	44	M	N	Lymphoma	142	142	116	95	Normal	0
HP	49	F	M	Lymphosarcoma	59	124	75	38	Emphysema	28
LL	53	F	H	Normal	105	125	115	102	Normal	32
AK	43	F	M	Squamous cell carcinoma of the mouth	92	123	110	96	Normal	3
VM	38	M	N	Normal	98	110	82	96	Normal	27
AG	49	M	N	Lymphoma	96	99	54	101	Decreased diffusing capacity of unknown origin	12
RS	28	M	N	Hilar adenopathy	111	119	97	98	Normal	17
BK	71	F	H	Squamous cell carcinoma of the vulva	107	116	52	91	Emphysema	15
BH	45	F	H	Squamous cell carcinoma of the larynx	90	104	92	95	Normal	45
HB	68	M	H	Squamous cell carcinoma of the mouth	106	100	52	95	Early emphysema	15
RW	30	M	N	Melanoma	87	104	75	86	Emphysema	35
FL	60	M	H	Melanoma	94	130	72	70	Emphysema	10
MS	57	F	N	Amyloidosis	75	120	80	114	Chest wall disease	13
CM*	64	M	H	Adenocarcinoma of the lung	57	91	36	84	Emphysema	5
CL	67	F	N	Rheumatic heart disease	87	150	133	100	Normal	43
VG	51	F	H	Fever of unknown origin	86	111	90	97	Normal	43
HM	64	M	H	Squamous cell carcinoma of the mouth	82	124	77	95	Emphysema	0
Mean ± SD	53.4 ± 13.0				93.5 ± 19.1	117.2 ± 14.8	84.5 ± 25.3	92.9 ± 16.1		18.9 ± 14.8

Definitions of abbreviations: FEV_1 = forced expiratory volume in 1 sec; FVC = forced vital capacity; H = heavy cigarette smoker (> 25 pack-years); M = medium cigarette smoker (10 to 25 pack-years); N = nonsmoker.

*Patient CM was studied 7 years after right middle and right lower lobe resection for adenocarcinoma.

tion: no history or radiographic evidence of interstitial disease, no primary or metastatic tumors in the lung, and no recent (within 2 years) chest irradiation or chemotherapy (table 2). Of the 9 men and 10 women in the control group (mean age, 53.4 ± 3.0 years), 10 were free of lung disease by pulmonary function studies, 7 had physiologic studies consistent with emphysema, one had an isolated decrease in D_{LCO} of unknown origin, and one had a restrictive pattern secondary to chest wall disease. Ten patients were heavy cigarette smokers (> 25 pack-years), 2 had moderate smoking histories (10 to 25 pack-years), and 7 did not smoke. All chest ^{67}Ga scans in the control group were similar to those found in normal subjects.

Isotope and scanning technique. Gallium-67 is an amphoteric, cyclotron-produced radionuclide with a physical half-life of 78 hours (34). Each patient was injected intravenously with 50 μCi of [^{67}Ga] citrate (New England Nuclear Corp, Billerica, MA) per kg of body weight. Forty-eight hours later, after bowel cleansing, anterior and posterior scans from the neck to the pelvis were recorded with an Ohio-Nuclear (Solon, Ohio) 5-inch dual-probe rectilinear scanner using 5:1 image reduction.

Scan evaluation. All scans were reviewed independently by 3 members of the Clinical Center Nuclear Medicine staff without knowledge of the clinical histories. The final ^{67}Ga-index for each patient was the average value of these 3 estimates. Only the posterior ^{67}Ga scans were evaluated, because they were less sensitive to image variations due to patient size, sex, and body habitus than the anterior scans. To quantify the pulmonary ^{67}Ga uptake, each region of increased ^{67}Ga accumulation was characterized by recording its image area intensity and textural features on a diagram of the posterior pulmonary segments. The following criteria were used to estimate the value of each feature (figure 1): (*1*) area of ^{67}Ga uptake. So that patients of different size could be compared, each region of ^{67}Ga uptake on the posterior scan was taken to represent a portion (0 to 100 per cent) of the total lung image. This feature provided the height and width of the volume of involved lung relative to the total lung surface. In the example shown in figure 1, the uptake in the right lung involved 20 per cent of the total posterior lung fields, whereas the 2 areas of uptake in the left lung involved 10 per cent and 5 per cent, respectively.

(*2*) Intensity of ^{67}Ga uptake was used to estimate the combined effect of the concentration of tracer and the depth of involved lung, neither of which was measurable directly from the image. To minimize the effects of background or nonspecific uptake, contrast variations between images of different studies, and different imaging film characteristics, the intensity of ^{67}Ga concentration in different regions of lung was graded on a scale of 0 to 4 using internal, nonpulmonary features of each scan. Background uptake (intensity 0) was chosen to be equivalent to a

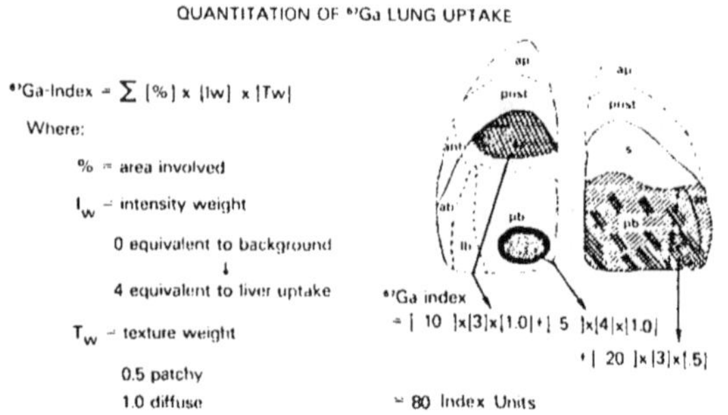

Fig. 1. Quantification of gallium-67 lung uptake. The ^{67}Ga-index is a summation of values, one for each region of the posterior lung image showing increased ^{67}Ga uptake. Each value is computed from a product of the regional per cent of total lung area (%), the regional intensity (I_w), and the regional texture (T_w). In the example, the increased uptake in the left superior segment involves 10 per cent of the lung area, has a moderate intensity (I_w = 3), a diffuse uptake (T_w = 1.0), and accounts for 30 ^{67}Ga-index units. Two additional regions in the basal lung zones are included in the final summation of 80 index units.

region of the scan below the level of the kidneys, because normal lung and normal empty bowel show similar levels of nonspecific uptake (35). Variations in body morphologic features do not affect this estimate, because the nonspecific background associated with muscle and adipose tissue is relatively low (35). Intensity 4 was used to represent any region with an intensity equal to or greater than the uptake of the liver. The remaining intensity values were spaced equally between the scale endpoints of 0 and plus-4. In the example in figure 1, the left upper region had an intensity of 3, the left lower region had an intensity of 4, the right lower region had an intensity of 3, and the remainder of the lung had an intensity of 0 (background).

(*3*) The texture of ^{67}Ga uptake in each area was also used to quantify ^{67}Ga uptake, because the pattern of regional tracer accumulation was not always uniform. The textural patterns were classified as patchy (nonhomogeneous regions) or diffuse (areas of homogeneous tracer distribution with ill-defined margins). Patchy areas were given a weight of 0.5, and diffuse regions were given a weight of 1.0. In the example in figure 1, the areas of ^{67}Ga uptake in the left lung were diffuse, and the region in the right lung was patchy.

The ^{67}Ga-lung index was computed from area, intensity, and textural features, as shown in figure 1. The product of the area percentage (per cent), the intensity weight (Iw), and the texture weight (Tw) was determined for each region of increased ^{67}Ga uptake (intensity > 0); the products from each area of uptake were then summed to obtain the ^{67}Ga-index. In the example in figure 1, the region in the left upper zone was estimated to occupy 10 per cent of the lung surface, to have an Iw of 3 relative to the span set by the background and liver intensities, and to have a diffuse texture (Tw = 1.0). The product of these values was equivalent to 30 ^{67}Ga-index units. Similarly, products were computed for the diffuse region in the left base and the patchy region in the right lower lung. Finally, a total lung ^{67}Ga-index of 80 units was obtained by summing the values computed for each area.

Tests of the validity of the ^{67}Ga-index. To validate the ^{67}Ga-index as a quantitative measure of ^{67}Ga uptake, all scans were examined by 3 readers independently, and the mean ± SD was calculated for each subject. The SD of the 3 readers was approximately 10 for mean values < 50, 15 for mean values between 50 and 70, and ≥25 for mean indices > 75. To examine the significance of differences in ^{67}Ga-indices between patients with IPF (as a group) and control subjects (as a group), nonparametric tests were used. Methods such as the t test or analysis of variance could not be used because they require either a constant variance or a known, precise relationship between the variance and the mean. The nonparametric Wilcoxon rank-sum test showed that the values of each reader for the IPF patients were significantly higher than the same reader's values for the control subjects ($P < 0.001$), thus validating the ability of the ^{67}Ga-index to discriminate between patients with IPF and control subjects. To evaluate whether any reader was consistently higher or lower than his colleagues, each triplet of ^{67}Ga-index values (one value from each reader) for a given subject was ordered by magnitude, and the individual values were ranked 1, 2, or 3. The mean ranks for the 3 readers were then compared using Friedman's Chi-square test. One reader consistently evaluated the control scans with a slightly higher ^{67}Ga-index than his colleagues, although over-all, the average index for the 3 readers was always less than 50 for the control group. The average of control ^{67}Ga-indices reported by this reader was 25, compared to 15 for the other 2. The readers showed no consistent biases, relative to each other, with respect to the scans from the patients with IPF.

Evaluation of lung biopsies. Of the group of 30 patients with IPF, 9 had had lung biopsies within 3 months of the ^{67}Ga scan, and 13 had had biopsies within 3 months to 1 year of the scan (table 1). Six of the remaining 8 patients had had biopsies more than 1 year before the scan; for this reason, their morphologic data were not used for statistical comparisons. Two patients did not undergo lung biopsy for clinical reasons. For statistical comparisons with the results of ^{67}Ga scanning, all biopsies were evaluated in a single-blind fashion to grade the degrees of fibrosis, interstitial cellularity, and alveolar cellularity on a scale of 1 to 4 (32).

Bronchoalveolar lavage. Seventeen of the 30 patients with IPF underwent fiberoptic bronchoscopy (Olympus BF-B2, New Hyde Park, NY) within 1 week after the ^{67}Ga scan (table 1). Within the limits of the procedure, all of these patients showed normal airways. The tip of the bronchoscope was wedged into a subsegmental airway of the lingula, where 100 ml of sterile saline were infused in divided portions and immediately aspirated. The lavage fluid was centrifuged on completion of the procedure, and the cell pellet was analyzed for the total number, viability, and differential count of the recovered cells. Details of both this procedure and of the lavage fluid analysis are reported elsewhere (9, 36).

Statistical methods. Five statistical methods were used for data analysis: Pearson correlation (37), Spearman correlation (37), the 2-tailed "Student's" t test (37), the Wilcoxon rank-sum test (38), and the Friedman's Chi-square (39) test. To facilitate discussion of the analysis, data were grouped as follows: "clinical data" included age, sex, duration of symptoms, smoking history, and drug therapy; "physiologic data" included VC, TLC, DLCO, and FEV_1/

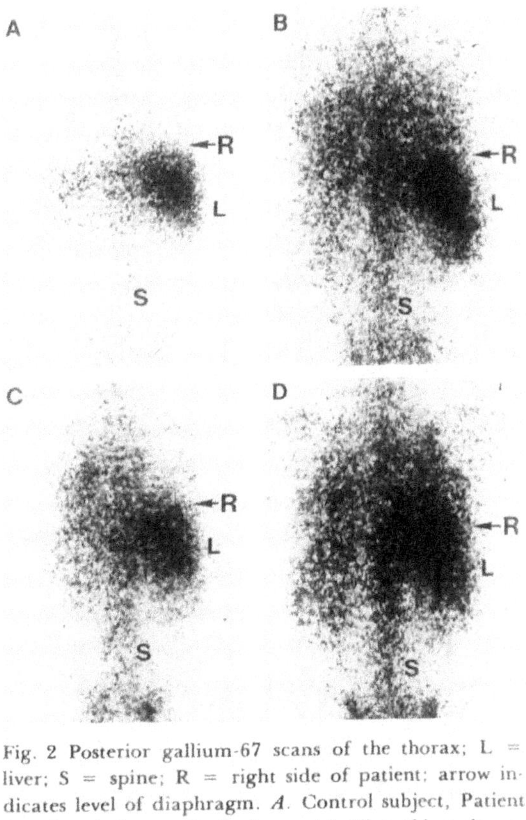

Fig. 2 Posterior gallium-67 scans of the thorax; L = liver; S = spine; R = right side of patient: arrow indicates level of diaphragm. *A.* Control subject, Patient MS; ^{67}Ga-index = 13. Patients with idiopathic pulmonary fibrosis (*B, C, D,*). *B.* Patient WH; ^{67}Ga-index = 155. *C.* Patient EV; ^{67}Ga-index = 70. *D.* Patient WES; ^{67}Ga-index = 190. The typical pattern seen in the patients with IPF was a diffuse bibasilar distribution, sometimes asymmetric, involving one lung to a greater extent than the other.

FVC; "morphologic data" included fibrosis rank, interstitial cellularity rank, and alveolar cellularity rank; and "bronchoalveolar lavage data" included volume of fluid recovered, total cells recovered, cells/volume recovered, per cent viable cells, and differential cell count.

The form of the data dictated the choice of statistical methods used in comparisons between the ^{67}Ga-indices and the clinical, physiologic, morphologic, and bronchoalveolar lavage data. When comparisons were made with continuous data, the Pearson correlation procedure was used. When the data were ranked, Spearman's correlation procedure was used. When the data were separable into 2 groups, the 2-tailed "Student's" t test was used. Nonparametric methods (Wilcoxon rank-sum, Friedman's Chi-square) were used to evaluate the variation of ^{67}Ga-index scoring between independent readers.

Results

Gallium-67 scanning. Forty-eight hours after the intravenous administration of [^{67}Ga]citrate, control subjects showed little ^{67}Ga uptake in the chest (figure 2A), except for a low-level (intensity = 1), diffuse uptake in the lower lung zones. This accumulation might partially represent the contribution of rib uptake, which has been found to contain several times the nonspecific activity of normal lung (35). One hundred per cent (19 of 19) of the control patients had a ^{67}Ga-index of less than 50; over-all, the mean ^{67}Ga-index in the control group was 18.9 ± 3.4 index units (table 2, figure 3).

In comparison, 70 per cent (21 of 30) of patients with IPF showed significant accumulations of ^{67}Ga in the lung (table 1, figure 2 B–D). The remaining 30 per cent had little ^{67}Ga uptake in the chest (table 1, figure 3). In general, the ^{67}Ga scans with indices >50 showed uptake most frequently in the lower lung fields, but often involving one lung to a greater extent than the other. Most regions of increased tracer accumulation had diffuse texture patterns (80 per cent of the scans with indices >50), whereas patchy areas accounted for 20 per cent of the regions.

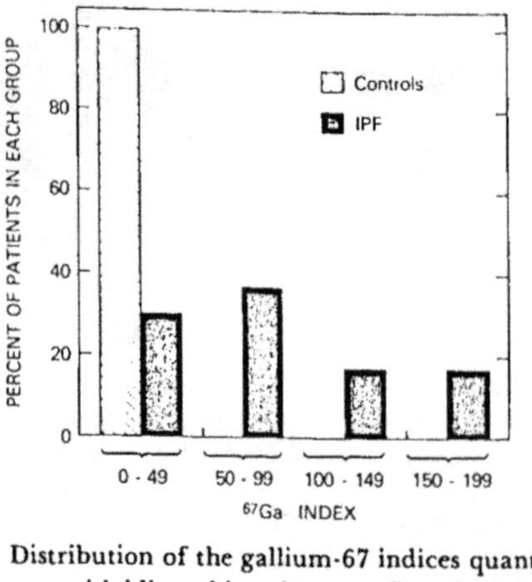

Fig. 3. Distribution of the gallium-67 indices quantified in the group with idiopathic pulmonary fibrosis (IPF) and the control group. One hundred per cent (19 of 19) of control subjects had values within the range of indices less than 50 index units; 70 per cent (21 of 30) of patients with IPF had index values greater than 50 units.

Comparisons of ^{67}Ga-index with clinical, physiologic, morphologic, and bronchoalveolar lavage data in IPF. There were no significant associations between the ^{67}Ga-index and patient age, sex, duration of symptoms, smoking history (pack-years), current smoking status, or drug therapy (table 3). Likewise, there were no significant relationships between the ^{67}Ga-index and VC, TLC, D_{LCO} or FEV_1/FVC.

The typical open-lung biopsy demonstrated moderate to severe interstitial fibrosis (average rank, 3.3 ± 0.2), moderate interstitial cellularity (rank, 2.5 ± 0.2), and moderate alveolar cellularity (rank, 2.1 ± 0.2) (table 1). There were significant associations between the ^{67}Ga-index and both the interstitial cellularity rank ($P = 0.038$) and the alveolar cellularity rank ($P = 0.004$) (table 3). The fibrosis rank on the open-lung biopsies tended to increase with the level of ^{67}Ga uptake, but the correlation was not significant at the 95 per cent confidence level.

Both the concentration of cells in the lavage fluid (number of cells per ml recovered) and the percentage of neutrophils among the recovered cells showed significant associations with the ^{67}Ga-index (table 3). There was also a negative association between the ^{67}Ga-index and the relative number of macrophages present, but this was probably related to the increase in the percentage of neutrophils.

Discussion

Most patients with IPF accumulated detectable concentrations of ^{67}Ga in their lung parenchyma 48 hours after intravenous injection of the tracer. In contrast, control patients did not show significant pulmonary ^{67}Ga uptake. The significant correlations between the ^{67}Ga-index and the alveolar and interstitial cellularity rank and the percentage of neutrophils recovered in lavage fluid suggested that the accumulation of ^{67}Ga in the lungs of these patients reflected the degree of their parenchymal inflammation.

TABLE 3

COMPARISON OF GALLIUM-67 LUNG INDICES WITH CLINICAL, PHYSIOLOGIC, MORPHOLOGIC, AND BRONCHOALVEOLAR LAVAGE DATA IN 30 PATIENTS WITH IDIOPATHIC PULMONARY FIBROSIS

^{67}Ga Lung Index Compared with	N	^{67}Ga-Index Mean*	Rho	P
Clinical data				
Age†, years	30	78.8	0.291	0.118
Sex*				
Male	18	90.6		0.130
Female	12	61.0		
Duration of symptoms†	30		0.110	0.564
Smoking history†, pack-years	30		0.260	0.164
Smoking status*				
Current smoker	5	72.0		0.756
Non- or ex-smoker	25	80.1		
Drug therapy*				
None	15	86.8		0.408
Prednisone	15	70.7		
Physiologic data†				
Vital capacity	30		−0.198	0.291
Total lung capacity	30		−0.155	0.414
Diffusing capacity	29		−0.064	0.741
FEV_1/FVC, %	30		0.176	0.352
Morphologic data**				
Fibrosis rank	22		0.392	0.071
Interstitial cellularity rank	22		0.445	0.033
Alveolar cellularity rank	22		0.584	0.004
Bronchoalveolar Lavage data†				
Fluid recovered, %	17		−0.442	0.076
Total cells recovered	17		0.256	0.322
Cells/volume recovered	17		0.549	0.022
Per cent viable cells	17		0.291	0.257
Differential cell count, %				
Neutrophils	17		0.485	0.049
Lymphocytes	17		0.337	0.186
Eosinophils	17		0.441	0.077
Macrophages	17		−0.659	0.004

Data are from table 1.
*Comparisons made between mean values of the ^{67}Ga-index using the 2-tailed "Student's" t test.
†Comparisons made using Pearson correlation procedure.
**Comparisons made using Spearman correlation procedure.

As a rule, interpretations of ^{67}Ga scans of the thorax use qualitative terms to describe the intensity and the distribution of tracer uptake (40) and therefore are difficult to use for patient comparisons or to follow disease progression. To correlate the pulmonary uptake of ^{67}Ga in IPF with quantitative measurements of lung structure and function, the ^{67}Ga-index was developed. This index is designed to minimize the effects of body morphologic features, imaging technique, and interpretation subjectivity on the quantification of pulmonary uptake of ^{67}Ga. The index provides a semiquantitative measure of the volume of lung tissue containing a uniform unit-intensity ^{67}Ga uptake from estimates of the area (per cent area), depth (intensity), and homogeneity (texture) of the involved lung. Statistical evaluation of the ^{67}Ga-index validated its ability to discriminate between the IPF group and the control group and showed no bias between readers producing ^{67}Ga-index values in patients with IPF.

A ^{67}Ga-index of 50 was used to represent a reasonable boundary between the normal and abnormal ^{67}Ga lung scan. The validity of this empiric threshold is suggested by the observations that: (*1*) 70 per cent of patients with IPF had ^{67}Ga-indices greater than 50, whereas 100 per cent of control subjects had indices less than 50; (*2*) the statistical analysis of the ^{67}Ga-indices of control subjects and patients with IPF indicated that the index distinguished between the 2 groups ($P < 0.001$); and (3) the mean value of the ^{67}Ga-index for each reader was always greater than 50 in the IPF patients and was always less than 50 in the control subjects.

There were no significant associations between the ^{67}Ga-index and the clinical data (table 3). For example, the degree of ^{67}Ga pulmonary uptake did not correlate with patient age or sex, findings that are consistent with results in other patient populations (34, 41). Because the number of cells in the bronchoalveolar lavage fluid from smokers is greater than the number recovered from nonsmokers (9, 36), it is important to note that neither the control subjects nor the patients with IPF showed a significant ^{67}Ga-index correlation with smoking history (number of pack-years) or smoking status (current or non-smoker).

Although patients receiving corticosteroids had lower mean ^{67}Ga-index values than untreated patients, the presence or absence of steroid therapy at the time of scan did not significantly affect the degree of ^{67}Ga uptake as measured by the ^{67}Ga-index. It should be noted, however, that there was a wide variation among dosages at the time of scan and that the same patients were not evaluated before and after therapy. Thus, these data are insufficient to determine whether corticosteroid therapy significantly decreases parenchymal inflammation in IPF.

The quantitative assessment of ^{67}Ga uptake in patients with IPF did not correlate with any of the physiologic measurements. This is reasonable, because the magnitudes of lung volumes, diffusing capacity, and forced expiratory flows are probably related to prior lung damage (10, 11) and do not necessarily reflect the current inflammatory process.

In comparison, there were significant associations between the ^{67}Ga-index and the degree of both the interstitial and the alveolar cellularity found in the lung biopsies. Because increased biopsy cellularity is characteristic of active inflammatory disease (10, 13, 15, 18, 19), these findings support the use of the ^{67}Ga-lung index in staging the active inflammatory process. In conjunction with this, the ^{67}Ga-index was not related to the degree of fibrosis seen on lung biopsy. This is consistent with the experience of others who have used ^{67}Ga scanning to differentiate normally healed surgical scars from those that conceal inflammation or abscess (42, 43).

The finding that the ^{67}Ga-index correlates with the percentage of neutrophils present in lavage fluid provides further evidence that ^{67}Ga uptake in IPF is related to the degree of parenchymal inflammation. The correlation of the ^{67}Ga-index with the number of cells recovered per ml of lavage fluid is probably related to the presence of neutrophils, because analyses of normal lavage fluid show the same number of cells found in patients with IPF, but relatively few, if any, neutrophils (9, 36).

Although the mechanisms of pulmonary ^{67}Ga uptake in patients with IPF are not clear (44–48), taken together, the biopsy and bronchoalveolar correlative data suggest that patients with low ^{67}Ga-indices are those with relatively little alveolitis, whereas those with high ^{67}Ga-indices have significant degrees of parenchymal inflammation. These findings are in agreement with the concept that the uptake of ^{67}Ga in inflammatory lesions is, in part, dependent on the presence of a leukocytic mass capable of binding the radioisotope (25, 47). Thus, visualization of the alveolitis of IPF by ^{67}Ga scans probably results from isotope-laden cells in parenchyma in which there is active inflammation. It is also reasonable that normal lung tissue is not seen in ^{67}Ga scans, because it has a very low concentration of inflammatory cells.

Idiopathic pulmonary fibrosis is but one of a wide variety of inflammatory, granulomatous, and neoplastic disease states of the lung that demonstrate ^{67}Ga uptake. Patients with primary and metastatic tumors, infections, abscesses, tuberculosis, sarcoidosis, and pneumoconioses all can have positive pulmonary ^{67}Ga scans (20–31, 49). Thus, we consider the ^{67}Ga scan to be useful as an indicator of the regional parenchymal alveolitis of IPF, but not as a diagnostic test for the disease.

In comparison to the lung biopsy, the ^{67}Ga scan is noninvasive. Because it involves radiation exposures comparable to radiographic studies (23), it can be repeated to assess longitudinally the degree of inflammation in the parenchyma as a whole. ^{67}Ga scanning should prove useful in gauging the progression of IPF and the efficacy of therapeutic protocols in the management of this disease.

Acknowledgment

The writers wish to thank Charles Lewallen for scan interpretation and Nancy Goldberg for aid in the statistical analysis. We are grateful for the expert technical assistance provided by Joseph F. Wilson and Bonnie A. Mack. We are also grateful to Edwyna von Gal, who coordinated all of the clinical studies.

References

1. Hamman, L., and Rich, A. R.: Acute diffuse interstitial fibrosis of the lungs, Bull Johns Hopkins Hosp, 1944, *74*, 177.
2. Austrian, R., McClement, J. H., Renzetti, A. D., Jr., Donald, K. W., Riley, R. L., and Cournand, A.: Clinical and physiologic features of some types of pulmonary diseases with impairment of alveolar-capillary diffusion: The syndrome of "alveolar-capillary block," Am J Med, 1951, *11*, 667.
3. Ruben, E. H., and Lubliner, R.: The Hamman-Rich syndrome: Review of the literature and analysis of 15 cases, Medicine (Baltimore), 1957, *36*, 397.
4. Herbert, F. A., Nahmias, B. B., Gaensler, E. A., and MacMahen, H. E.: Pathophysiology of interstitial pulmonary fibrosis: Report of 19 cases and follow-up with corticosteroids, Arch Intern Med, 1962, *110*, 628.
5. Livingstone, J. L., Lewis, J. G., Reid, L., and Jefferson, K. E.: Diffuse interstitial pulmonary fibrosis: Clinical, radiological, and pathological study based on 45 patients, Q J Med, 1964, *33*, 71.
6. Marks, A.: Diffuse interstitial pulmonary fibrosis, Med Clin North Am, 1967, *51*, 439.
7. DeRemee, R. A., Harrison, E. G., Jr., and Anderson, H. A.: The concept of classical interstitial pneumonitis-fibrosis (CIP-F) as a clinicopathologic syndrome, Chest, 1972, *61*, 213.
8. Kravis, T. C., Ahmed, A., Brown, T. E., Fulmer, J. D., and Crystal, R. G.: Pathogenic mechanisms in pulmonary fibrosis: Collagen-induced migration inhibition factor production and cytotoxicity mediated by lymphocytes, J Clin Invest, 1976, *58*, 1223.
9. Reynolds, H. Y., Fulmer, J. D., Kazmierowski, J. A., Roberts, W. C., Frank, M. M., and Crystal, R. G.: Analysis of cellular and protein content of bronchoalveolar-lavage fluid from patients with idiopathic pulmonary fibrosis and chronic hypersensitivity pneumonitis, J Clin Invest, 1977, *59*, 165.
10. Crystal, R. G., Fulmer, J. D., Roberts, W. C., Moss, M. L., Line, B. R., and Reynolds, H. Y.: Idiopathic pulmonary fibrosis: Clinical, histologic, radiographic, physiologic, scintigraphic, cytologic, and biochemical aspects, Ann Intern Med, 1976, *85*, 769.
11. Fulmer, J. D., and Crystal, R. G.: The biochemical basis of pulmonary function, in *The Biochemical Basis of Pulmonary Function*, R. G. Crystal, ed., Marcel Dekker, Inc., New York, 1976, pp. 419–466.
12. Stack, B. H. R., Choo-Kang, Y. F. J., and Heard, B. E.: The prognosis of cryptogenic fibrosing alveolitis, Thorax, 1972, *27*, 535
13. Scadding, J. G., and Hinson, K. F. W.: Diffuse fibrosing alveolitis (diffuse interstitial fibrosis of the lungs): Correlation of history at biopsy with prognosis, Thorax, 1967, *22*, 291.
14. Liebow, A. A.: New concepts and entities in pulmonary disease, in *The Lung*, A. A. Liebow and D. E. Smith, ed., Williams and Wilkins, Baltimore, 1968, pp. 332–365.
15. Scadding, J. G.: Diffuse alveolar fibrosis, Thorax, 1974, *29*, 271.
16. Cassen, S. M., Divertie, M. B., and Brown, A. L., Jr.: Fine structure morphometry on biopsy specimens of human lung, Chest, 1974, *65*, 275.
17. Brody, A. R., and Craighead, J. E.: Interstitial associations of cells lining airspaces in human pulmonary fibrosis, Virchow's Arch [Pathol Anat], 1976, *372*, 39.
18. Spencer, H.: Interstitial pneumonia, Annu Rev Med, 1967, *18*, 423.
19. Spencer, H.: Chronic interstitial pneumonia, in *The Lung*, A. A. Liebow and D. E. Smith, ed., Williams and Wilkins, Baltimore, 1968, pp. 134–150.
20. Ito, Y., Okuyama, S., Awano, T., Takahashi, K., Sato, T., and Kanno, I.: Diagnostic evaluation of 67-Ga scanning of lung cancer and other diseases, Radiology, 1971, *101*, 355.
21. Lavender, P. J., Lowe, J., Barker, J. R., Burn, J. I., and Chaudri, M. A.: Gallium 67 citrate scanning in neoplastic and inflammatory lesions, Br J Radiol, 1971, *44*, 361.
22. Higasi, T., Nakayama, Y., Murata, A., Nakamura, K., Sugiyama, M., Kawaguchi, T., and Suzuki, S.: Clinical evaluation of ^{67}Ga-citrate scanning, J Nucl Med, 1972, *13*, 196.
23. Langhammer, H., Glaubitt, G., Grebe, S. F., Hampe, J. F., Haubold, U., Hor, G., Kaul, A., Koeppe, P., Koppenhange, J., Roedler, H. D., and van der Schoot, J. B.: ^{67}Ga for tumor scanning, J Nucl Med, 1972, *13*, 25.
24. van der Schoot, J. B., Groen, A. S., and de Jong, J.: Gallium-67 scintigraphy in lung diseases, Thorax, 1972, *27*, 543.
25. Burleson, R. L., Johnson, M. C., and Head, H.: Scintigraphic demonstration of experimental abscesses with intravenous ^{67}Ga citrate and ^{67}Ga labeled blood leukocytes, Ann Surg, 1973, *178*, 446.
26. Heshiki, A., Schatz, S. L., McKusick, K. A., Bowersox, D. W., Soin, J. S., and Wagner, H. N.: Gallium-67 citrate scanning in patients with pulmonary sarcoidosis, J Roentgenol, 1974, *122*, 744.
27. Kinoshita, F., Ushio, T., Maekawa, A., Ariwa, R., and Kubo, A.: Scintiscanning of pulmonary diseases with ^{67}Ga-citrate, J Nucl Med, 1974, *15*, 227.
28. Siemsen, J. K., Sargent, E. N., Grebe, S. F., Winsor, D. W., Wentz, D., and Jacobson, G.: Pulmonary concentration of ^{67}Ga in pneumoconiosis, Radiology, 1974, *120*, 815.
29. Silva, J., and Harvey, W. C.: Detection of infections with gallium-67 and scintigraphic imaging

J Infect Dis, 1974, *130*, 125.
30. Niden, A. H., Mishkin, F. S., and Khurana, M. M. L.: ^{67}Gallium citrate lung scans in interstitial lung disease, Chest 1976, *69*, (Supplement, p. 266).
31. Siemsen, J. K., Grebe, S. F., Sargent, E. N., and Wentz, D.: Gallium-67 scintigraphy of pulmonary diseases as a complement to radiography, Radiology, 1976, *118*, 371.
32. Fulmer, J. D., Roberts, W. C., von Gal, E. R., and Crystal, R. G.: Small airways in idiopathic pulmonary fibrosis: Comparison of morphologic and physiologic observations, J Clin Invest, 1977, *60*, 595.
33. Gold, W. M., and Jennings, D. B.: Pulmonary function in patients with systemic lupus erythematosus, Am Rev Respir Dis, 1966, *93*, 556.
34. Kinsman, S.: Radiological Health Handbook, ed. 8, U.S. Dept. Health, Education, and Welfare, Washington, D.C., 1960, p. 256.
35. Nelson, B., Hayes, R. L., Edwards, C. L., Kniseley, R. M., and Andrews, G. A.: Distribution of gallium in human tissues after intravenous administration, J Nucl Med, 1972, *13*, 92.
36. Reynolds, H. Y., and Newball, H. N.: Analysis of proteins and respiratory cells obtained from human lungs by bronchial lavage, J Lab Clin Med, 1974, *84*, 559.
37. Snedecor, G. W., and Cochran, W. G.: Statistical Methods, ed. 6, Iowa State University Press, Ames, Iowa, 1967, pp. 54–194.
38. Noether, G. E.: Elements of Nonparametric Statistics, John Wiley and Sons, New York, 1967, pp. 31–35.
39. Brownlee, K. A.: Statistical Theory and Methodology in Science and Engineering, John Wiley and Sons, New York, 1965, pp. 260–262.
40. Larson, S. M., Milder, M. S., and Johnston, G. S.: Interpretation of the 67-Ga photoscan, J Nucl Med, 1973, *14*, 208.
41. Watson, E. E., Cloutier, R. J., and Gibbs, W. D.: Whole-body retention of ^{67}Ga-citrate; J Nucl Med, 1973, *14*, 840.
42. Harvey, C. H., Podoloff, D. A., and Kopp, D. T.: ^{67}Gallium in 68 consecutive infection searches, J Nucl Med, 1975, *16*, 2.
43. Teates, C. D., and Hunter, J. G.: Gallium scanning as a screening test for inflammatory lesions, Radiology, 1975, *116*, 383.
44. Gunasekera, S. W., King, L. J., and Lavender, P. J.: The behaviour of tracer gallium-67 towards serum proteins, Clin Chim Acta, 1972, *39*, 401.
45. Clausen, J., Edeling, C., and Fogh, J.: Binding to human serum proteins and tumor components, Cancer Res, 1974, *34*, 1931.
46. Swartzendruber, D. C., Nelson, B., and Hayes, R.: Gallium-67 localization in lysosomal-like granules of leukemic and non-leukemic murine tissues, J Natl Cancer Inst, 1971, *46*, 941.
47. Mertz, T., McKusick, K., and Wagner, H. N.: Mechanism of ^{67}Ga association with lymphocytes, Cancer Res, 1974, *34*, 2495.
48. Gelrud, L. G., Arseneau, J. C., Milder, M. S., Kramer, R. J., Swann, S. J., Canellos, G. P., and Johnston, G. S.: The kinetics of gallium-67 incorporation into inflammatory lesions: Experimental and clinical studies, J Lab Clin Med, 1974, *83*, 489.
49. Dige-Peterson, H., Heckscher, R., and Hertz, M.: 67-Ga-scintigraphy in non-malignant lung diseases, Scand J Respir Dis, 1972, *53*, 314.

Cells, Collagen and Idiopathic Pulmonary Fibrosis *

Ronald G. Crystal, Jack D. Fulmer, Bruce J. Baum, John Bernardo, Kathryn H. Bradley, Sally D. Bruel, Norton A. Elson, Gerald A. Fells, Victor J. Ferrans, James E. Gadek, Gary W. Hunninghake, Oichi Kawanami, Jeffrey A. Kelman, Bruce R. Line, John A. McDonald, Byron D. McLees, William C. Roberts, David M. Rosenberg, Paul Tolstoshev, Edwyna Von Gal and Steven E. Weinberger

Pulmonary Branch and Pathology Branch, National Heart, Lung, and Blood Institute, and Department of Nuclear Medicine, Clincial Center, National Institutes of Health, Bethesda, Maryland, USA

Abstract. Idiopathic pulmonary fibrosis (IPF) is a usually fatal disorder of lung with clearly defined clinical, roentgenographic, physiologic, morphologic, scintigraphic and bronchoalveolar lavage features. Current concepts of the pathogenesis of this disorder suggest a central role for a chronic alveolitis in causing changes in parenchymal cell populations and derangements in interstitial collagen. Of the many inflammatory and immune effector cells comprising the alveolitis of IPF, it is likely that the neutrophil is the most important mediator of parenchymal damage. To follow the status of lung neutrophils in patients with this disease, two methods have been utilized. Both gallium-67 scanning and bronchoalveolar lavage quantitate the extent of the alveolitis and can be used to stage and follow these patients. The treatment of IPF remains controversial, but it is likely that corticosteroids reduce the alveolitis and prolong the lifespan of these patients.

Key words: Lung - Cells - Collagen - Idiopathic pulmonary fibrosis - Alveolitis

---

Introduction

The interstitial lung diseases are chronic, diffuse, non-infectious, non-neoplastic disorders primarily affecting alveoli. In mid-course, these disorders are generally characterized roentgenographically by a nodular or reticular pattern, physiologically by decreased lung volumes and diffusing capacity, and morphologically by alveoli with altered cellular populations and deranged interstitial collagen. Because the deranged interstitial col-

* Presented at the 43rd Annual Meeting, American College of Chest Physicians, Las Vegas, Nevada, November 1977

lagen gives the alveolar septae a thickened, scarlike appearance when visualized by light microscopy, the term "interstitial fibrosis" is commonly used to describe this finding.

There are approximately 130 defined interstitial diseases, but the etiology can be identified in only about 30% of affected individuals [6]. The remaining 70% are categorized into specifically defined diseases, of which the most prevalent are idiopathic pulmonary fibrosis (IPF), chronic interstitial lung disease associated with the collagen-vascular disorders, and sarcoidosis. As an example of the current concepts of pathogenesis of the interstitial disorders, we will use IPF to demonstrate how alterations in alveolar cell populations can result in structural and functional abnormalities of gas-exchanging units.

Idiopathic Pulmonary Fibrosis

Because the etiology of IPF is unknown, and because lung biopsies from these patients do not have relatively unique morphologic features (e.g., granulomata), the diagnosis of IPF has often been considered "nonspecific" by pulmonary clinicians. However, as more information has accrued concerning these patients, it is apparent that IPF is a specific, independent disease entity, with clearly defined clinical, roentgenographic, physiologic, morphologic, scintigraphic and bronchoalveolar lavage features, including [4]:

1. Clinical. A history of breathlessness, particularly with exercise; no history suggesting a known etiology; no history or clinical evidence suggesting left ventricular failure or a defined collagen-vascular disease; no evidence of bronchitis; no history suggestive of hypersensitivity pneumonitis; and no exposure to inhalants or drugs known to cause interstitial lung disease;
2. Roentgenographic. A diffuse interstitial pattern on chest film; and no adenopathy;
3. Physiologic. Reduced total lung capacity or diffusing capacity; normal forced expiratory volume in 1 s/forced vital capacity; mild resting hypoxemia which worsens with exercise; and a deflation volume-pressure curve shifted downward and to the right;
4. Morphologic. Varying degrees of interstitial fibrosis; interstitial and intra-alveolar alveolitis[1] consisting predominantly of macrophages and lymphocytes but also including neutrophils and eosinophils; peribronchial inflammation and fibrosis; and no vasculitis, granulomata or significant refractile bodies by polarized light microscopy;
5. Scintigraphic. Diffuse uptake of gallium-67 in the lung parenchyma but not in lymph nodes; and
6. Bronchoalveolar lavage. Fluid recovered consisting of an increased proportion of polymorphonuclear leukocytes, normal lymphocyte subpopulations, and elevated levels of IgG.

[1] In reference to the interstitial lung disorders, "alveolitis" refers to the inflammatory and immune effector cells that accumulate within the interstitium and alveolar air spaces.

As the name implies, the process which incites the development of IPF is unknown, and all attempts to identify a responsible exogenous agent, such as a virus, have been unrewarding. Whatever the inciting process, the concept has arisen that genetic and host-acquired factors likely modulate susceptibility to IPF as well as the rate at which the disorder follows its characteristic pathogenic path.

In cases of early IPF that are biopsied, it is apparent that there is little, if any, fibrosis, but that the alveolar structures have two other distinguishing features (Fig. 1). First, there is a characteristic alveolitis, in which effector cells of the inflammatory and immune system accumulate within the alveolar interstitium and in the air spaces. Second, there are alterations in parenchymal cells, including changes in the proportions of epithelial, endothelial and interstitial cells that comprise the alveolus.

Although it is possible that some of the alveolitis and alterations in parenchymal cell populations are reversible, sequential biopsies have demonstrated that by the time IPF is in mid-course, the early changes have led to a progressive derangement of interstitial collagen (i.e., fibrosis) that is most likely irreversible once present (Fig. 2).

As this process continues, there are progressive alterations in the alveolar cellular and non-cellular structures such that the alveoli no longer can act as gas-exchanging units. As more and more alveoli follow this pathogenetic route, alveolar structures are no longer recognizable and are replaced by cystic spaces (Fig. 3). This late-stage IPF is termed "end-stage lung" and soon progresses to a state where the lung can no longer fulfill its function in gas exchange, and the patient dies.

It is clear from this discussion that three prominent features in the pathogenesis of IPF are: (1) a chronic alveolitis, (2) changes in parenchymal cell populations, and (3) a derangement in interstitial collagen (Fig. 4). Although it is useful to conceptualize each feature separately, it is important to understand that they are interdependent processes in which the cellular events within the alveolar structures lead to a progressive interstitial fibrosis and eventual destruction of the lung as a gas-exchanging organ. To understand how this may occur on a cellular level, it is first necessary to define the structure of the normal alveolus and how this structure is maintained.

The Normal Alveolus. The alveolus of the normal adult lung is comprised of four major parenchymal cells (epithelial type I, epithelial type II, capillary endothelial, interstitial mesenchymal) and two effector cell populations derived from the inflammatory and immune systems (alveolar macrophages, lymphocytes) [30]. The structural support for these cells is provided by the non-cellular connective tissue constituents of the alveolar interstitium, including collagen, elastic fibers, and proteoglycans [15, 17, 19]. Of these, collagen is the most abundant, comprising 15-20% of the alveolar dry weight and 60-70% of interstitial connective tissue. The other connective tissue components are critical to normal interstitial function, but as far as is known, they do not play an important role in the pathogenesis of IPF.

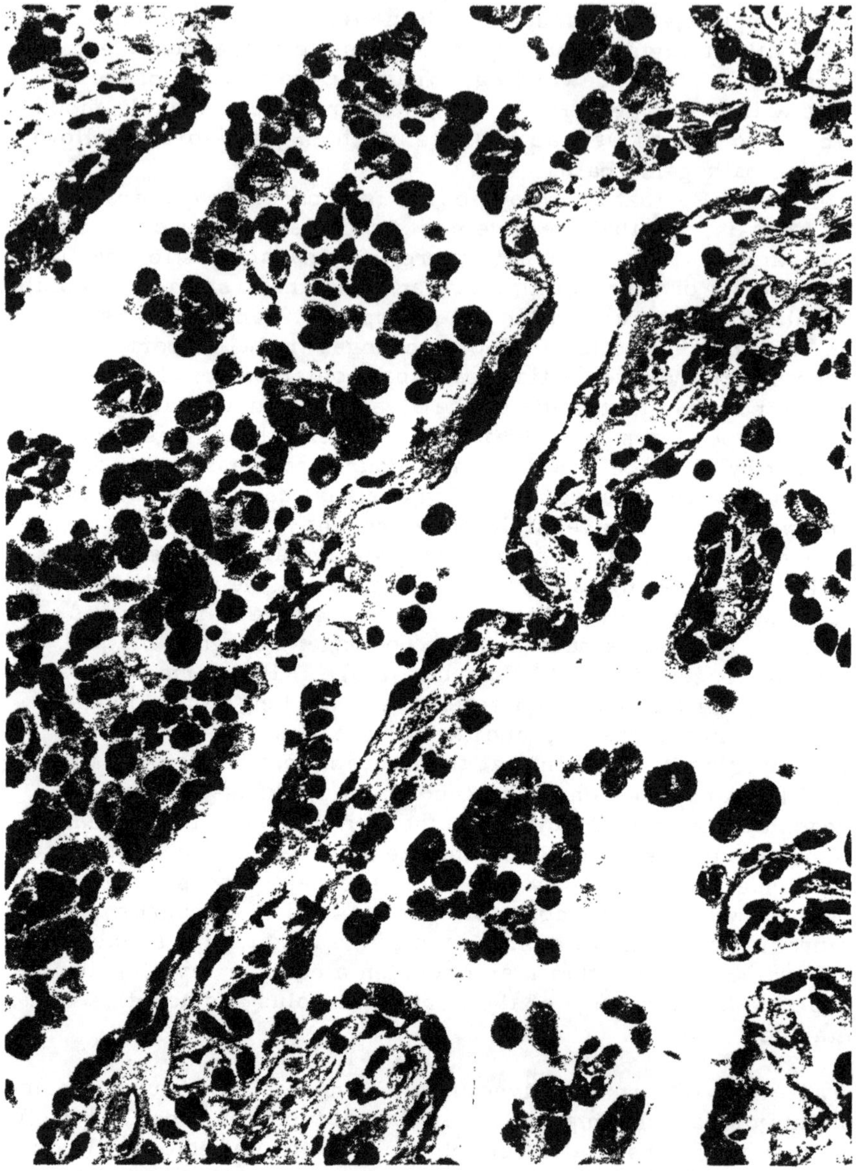

Fig. 1. Alveoli in lung biopsy specimen from patient with early IPF show minimal thickening but contain numerous inflammatory cells, including macrophages, polymorphonuclear leukocytes and lymphocytes. Hematoxylin and eosin stain, X 400.

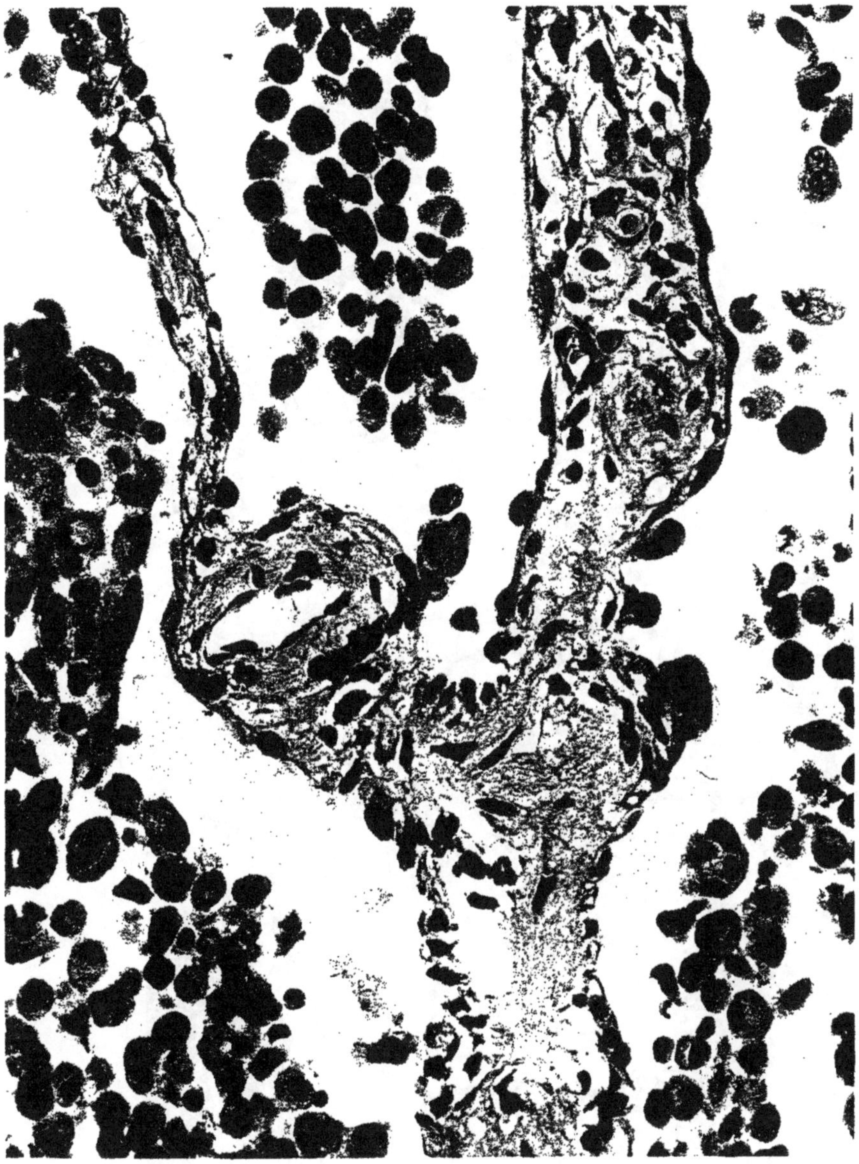

Fig. 2. Lung biopsy from patient with mid-course IPF showing inflammatory cells associated with marked thickening of the alveolar walls by fibrous connective tissue. Hematoxylin and eosin stain, X 400.

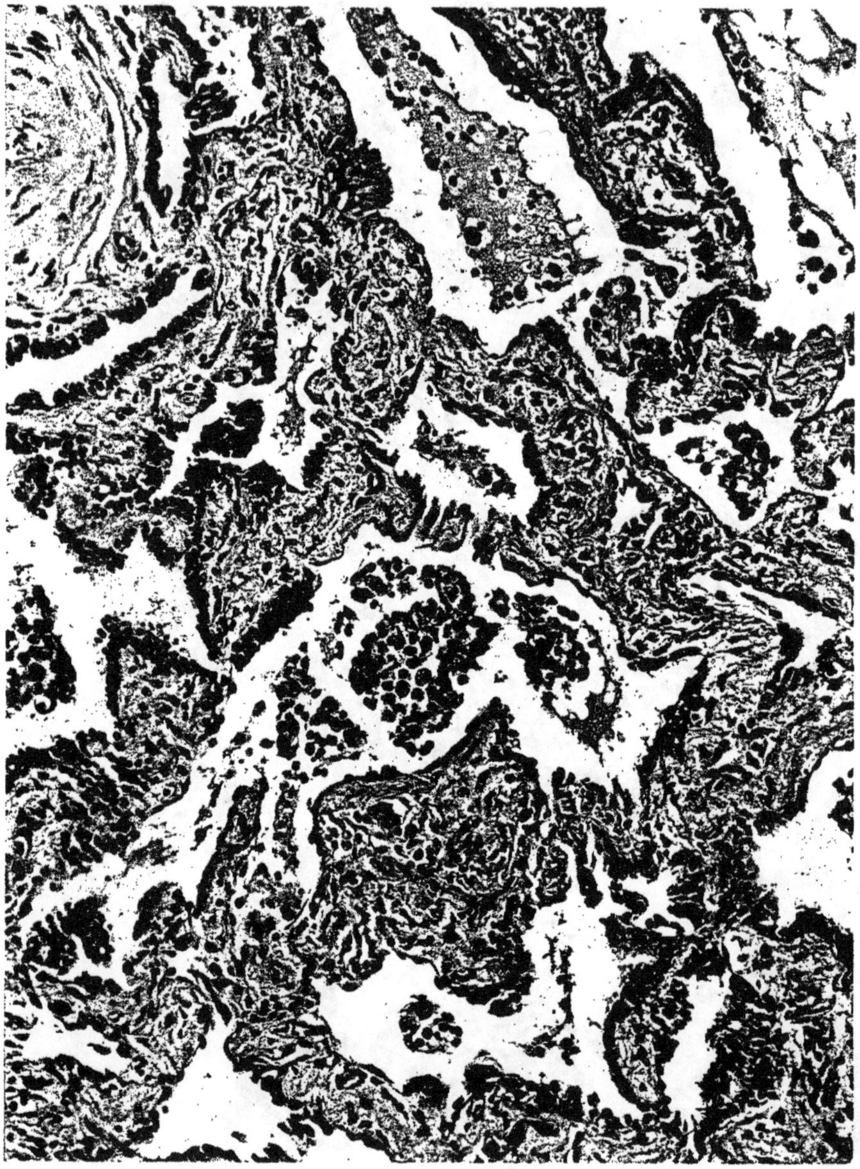

Fig. 3. Severely fibrotic, thickened and distorted alveolar walls in late IPF; cystic spaces that contain exudated material and numerous macrophages are evident. The epithelial cells vary in appearance; in some areas they are cuboidal and even multilayered. Hematoxylin and eosin stain, X 180.

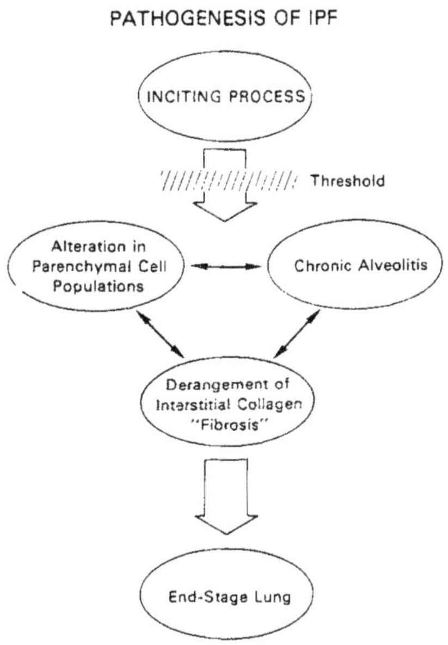

Fig. 4. Current concept of the pathogenesis of idiopathic pulmonary fibrosis (IPF). Although the inciting process has not been identified, it is likely that there exists a general threshold of alveolar injury above which characteristic pathogenic processes occur that result in IPF. See text for details.

The normal alveolar interstitium contains at least three types of collagen, each of which has a characteristic amino acid sequence [3, 15, 17]. Type I collagen (60-65% of the total) forms 500-1,000 μm banded fibers that usually run parallel to basement membrane. Most studies suggest that type I collagen is the most highly organized, least compliant form of interstitial collagen, and it plays a critical role in maintaining normal alveolar structure and function. Type III collagen (30-35% of the total) appears as 150-350 μm randomly dispersed fibrils that probably contribute to alveolar structure and function via their influence on the way in which type collagen forms fibers. The remaining collagen (< 5%) is that present in the basement membrane found beneath the alveolar epithelial and endothelial cells. The structure of alveolar basement membrane is not known, but from analogy to other basement membranes, it probably is composed of noncollagen glycoproteins together with collagens that are distinct from type I and type III. There is growing evidence that basement membrane collagens may differ depending on the cell responsible for synthesis, suggesting that the alveolar interstitium may include at least two types of basement membrane collagen (i.e., endothelial and epithelial). Alveolar basement membrane probably does not influence mechanical properties significantly, but it likely plays a critical role in directing the growth patterns of epithelial and endothelial cells following parenchymal injury.

Although it was originally thought that only mesenchymal, fibroblast-like cells could synthesize collagen, it is now known that a variety of differentiated cells are capable of this process [14, 15, 17]. Studies of individual cell types maintained in tissue culture suggest that most of the cells within the normal alveolar unit play an important role in production of the interstitial collagens (Table 1).

Table 1. Maintenance of interstitial collagen in normal lung and idiopathic

Cell type	Normal lung	
	Relative numbers	Role in the maintenance of interstitial collagen
Parenchymal cells		
Type I epithelial	8% of total parenchymal cells[a]	Probably synthesizes type I and III; ? synthesizes basement membrane
Type II epithelial	14% of total parenchymal cells	No known role
Capillary endothelial	39% of total parenchymal cells	Basement membrane synthesis[b]
Mesenchymal		
Fibroblast-like	39% of total parenchymal cells	Synthesizes types I and III collagen in a ratio of 10:1; secretes a collagenase that attacks collagens I and III at equal rates
Smooth muscle	Very rare	———
Inflammatory and immune effector cells		
Macrophage	80-90% of total effector cells	Produces collagenase which attacks types I and III collagen at an equal rate
Lymphocyte	10-20% of total effector cells; 70% T, 25%B	In collaboration with macrophages, probably suppresses collagen synthesis by fibroblasts [39]
Neutrophils	Very rare	———
Mast cells	Very rare	———
Eosinophils	Very rare	———

[a]Estimates are from rat lung [38].

[b]By analogy to endothelial cells derived from arteries and veins of sources other than lung [22].

pulmonary fibrosis

Idiophatic pulmonary fibrosis	
Relative numbers	Role in the derangement of interstitial collagen
Marked loss	Shifts in epithelial cell types probably affect the relative amounts and locations of interstitial collagen, but specific effects are unknown
Replacement of type I cells by a type II - like cell	
Decreased	Unknown
Increased	Predominant collagen-synthesizing cell of the IPF parenchyma; increased numbers probably play a critical role in the alterations of collagen found in IPF; unknown if differentiated state normal or altered in IPF
Increased	Synthesizes types I and III collagen and basement membrane[c]; likely alters relative collagen composition
Increased	IPF macrophages spontaneously secrete neutrophil chemotactic factor [11]
Increased	Proportions of T- and B - cells normal [24]; subpopulation produces MIF[d] in response to collagen [29]; may influence macrophages to secrete more collagenase[e];? loss of normal suppression of collagen synthesis
Increased	Collagenase attacks type I collagen selectively [20]; other neutral proteases destroy fibronectin [33]
Increased	Unknown
Increased	Unknown

[c]By analogy to smooth muscle cells derived from sources other than lung [32].

[d]MIF = Macrophage migration inhibiton factor.

[e]By analogy to studies of guinea pig cells in which activated lymphocytes induce peritoneal macrophages to secrete collagenase [37].

The synthesis of collagen, however, is only one side of the complex process involved in the maintenance of collagen in the normal lung. In the adult lung parenchyma, collagen is continually being synthesized, yet the amount of parenchymal collagen does not change [1, 2]. To provide this constancy, the normal parenchyma must have mechanisms to degrade collagen at the same rate at which it is produced. However, collagen is an unusual macromolecule in that only one class of enzymes, termed collagenases, is capable of degrading it under the physiologic conditions of the extracellular milieu. Thus, to maintain the normal alveolar interstitium, the cells of the alveolus must not only synthesize collagen, but they must also provide collagenase(s) to degrade it [18, 20, 21]. Although the production of collagenase is usually associated with cells of the inflammatory system (e.g., macrophages, neutrophils), tissue culture studies have demonstrated that parenchymal cells (e.g., mesenchymal cells) can also secrete a collagenase capable of attacking the major interstitial collagens [20, 40] (Table 1).

Cells, Collagen and IPF

The original light microscopic descriptions of IPF suggested that the "fibrosis" was simply an accumulation of interstitial collagen mediated by "activated" fibroblasts responding to "injury" [13, 36]. However, as more information has accrued using ultrastructural and biochemical techniques, it has become apparent that the "fibrosis" of IPF is much more complex and includes the following [5, 7, 26, 35]: (1) although the collagen is evenly distributed throughout the normal interstitium, in IPF there are localized accumulations such that some septa are markedly widened, whereas others are not (Fig. 2); (2) while the type I fibers of the normal interstitium (Fig. 5) are contained in sharply defined, relatively thin bundles running parallel to basement membrane, some fiber bundles in IPF are thickened, twisted, frayed and randomly oriented (Fig. 6); (3) on the average, the IPF interstitium contains relatively more type I and less type III collagen; and (4) basement membranes in the IPF lung are thickened, but in some areas they are thinned and occasionally disrupted, particularly on the epithelial surface.

This information, together with the knowledge that maintenance of interstitial collagen in the normal lung requires the balance of synthetic and degradative processes by a variety of cells, suggests that the "fibrosis" of IPF is not simply secondary to increased synthesis by "activated" fibroblasts. Rather the deranged collagen of the IPF interstitium must result from a number of processes involving multiple cell types in which the coordinated control of collagen synthesis and degradation is lost.

The key to understanding the pathogenesis of the fibrosis of IPF is the concept that this balance of collagen synthesis and degradation is upset through changes in the cells present in the alveolar structures. Most importantly, IPF is associated with significant alterations in all of the alveolar parenchymal cells (epithelial, endothelial and mesenchymal) as well as profound changes in the inflammatory and immune effector cells that are present within the alveolar structures.

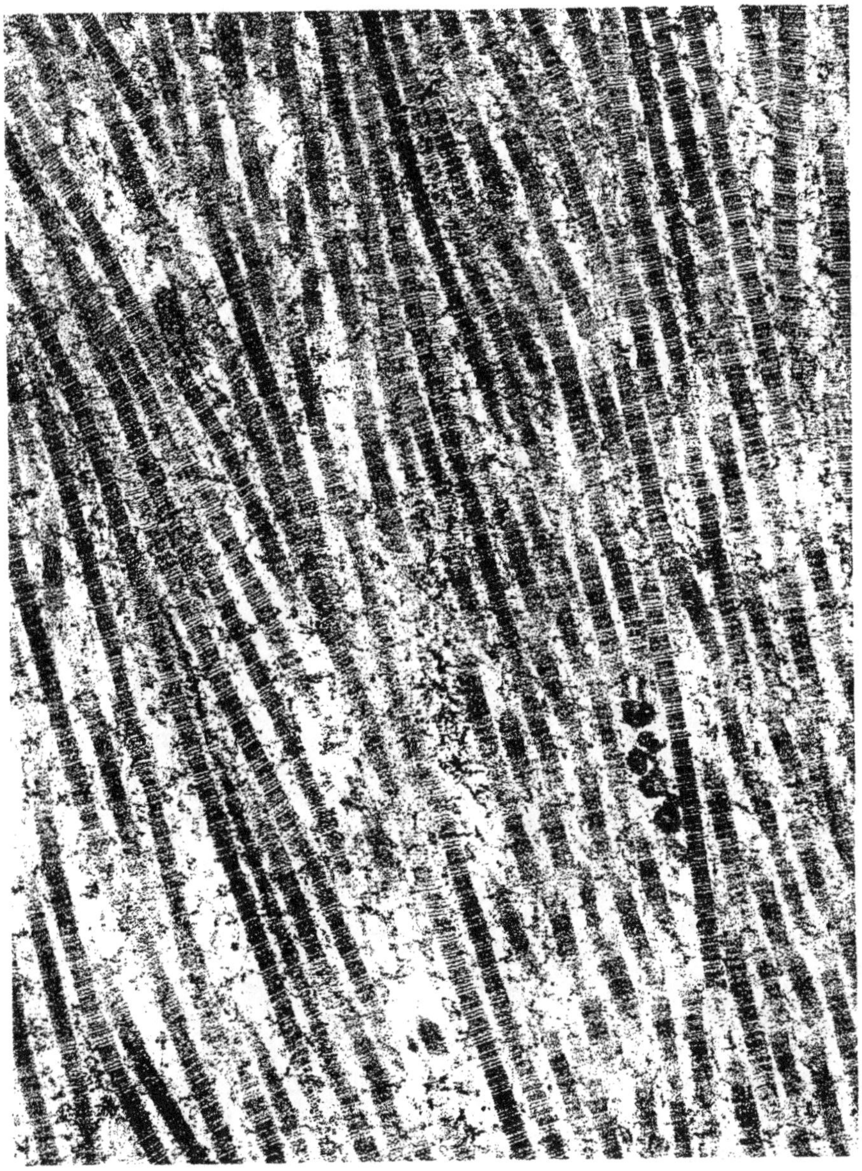

Fig. 5. Well-oriented interstitial collagen fibrils (presumed to be type I collagen) with typical periodic banding are associated with fine strands of material that probably represents proteoglycans. Pulmonary tissue removed from control patient (20-year-old woman) at the time of biopsy of metastatic (osteogenic sarcoma) pulmonary nodule. X 50, 000.

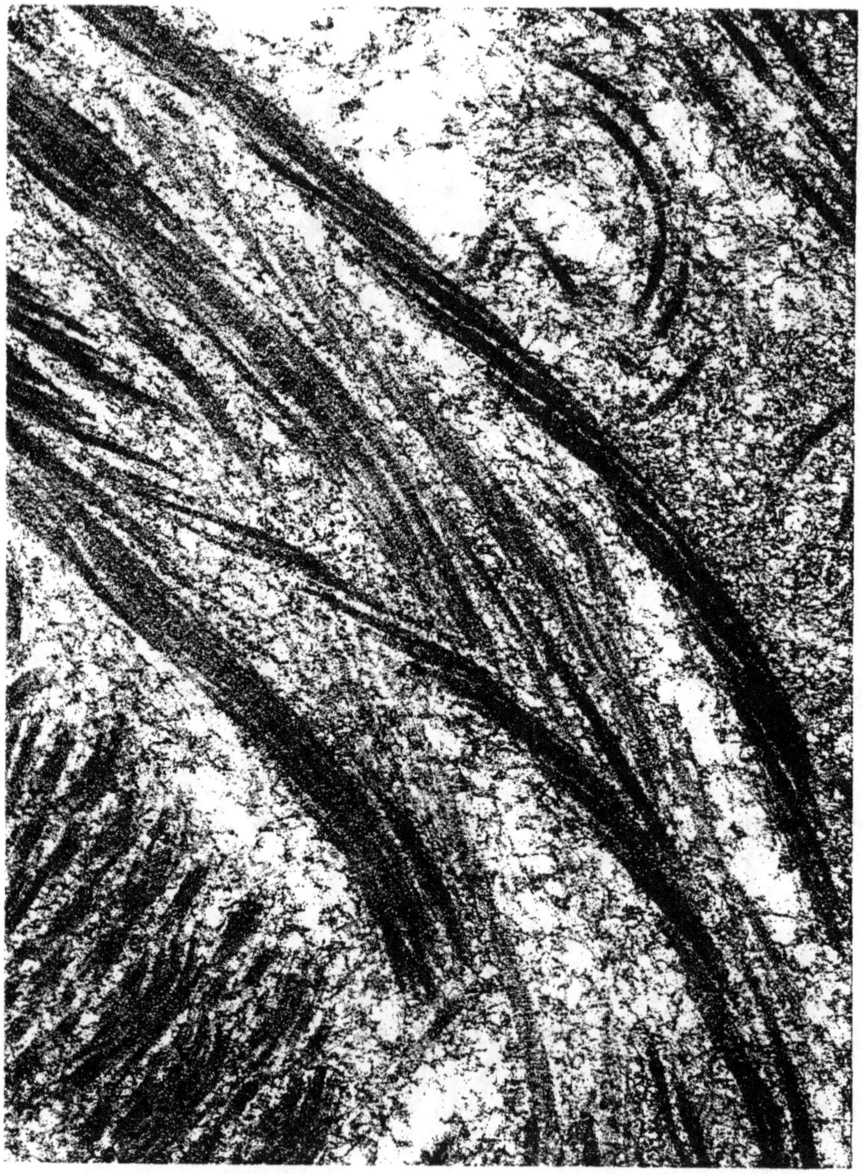

Fig. 6. Twisted, frayed, spiraling bundles of collagen (compare with normal collagen shown at same magnification in Fig. 5) are diversely oriented and are surrounded by abundant strands of material presumed to be proteoglycans. Tissue from same IPF patient as in light micrograph of Fig. 2. X 50, 000.

Status of the Parenchymal Cell Populations in IPF. Although quantitative morphometric studies have not been carried out in lung biopsy specimens from patients with this disease, the general consensus is that the alveolar parenchymal cell populations in IPF in mid-course are modified in several ways, including [4]: (1) a marked decrease in the numbers of type I epithelial cells and a concomitant increase in the numbers of an epithelial cell that has many of the features of the fully differentiated type II epithelial cell (Figs. 7, 8); (2) a probable decrease in the total number of capillary endothelial cells; (3) an apparent increase in the total numbers of mesenchymal cells, including more fibroblast-like cells similar to those of the normal interstitium as well as the addition of clusters of smooth muscle cells (Figs. 7, 9); and (4) a striking derangement in the topologic associations between alveolar parenchymal cells and between these cells and the interstitial connective tissue matrix (Figs. 2, 3, 7, 9, 10).

In terms of the maintenance of collagen within the alveolar interstitium, such changes have multiple consequences (Table 1). Since the type I epithelial cell [8] and the endothelial cell [22] both synthesize collagen, the loss of these cells must have an effect on collagen homeostasis within the interstitium. In addition, since fibroblast-like mesenchymal cells synthesize collagen, the increased number of these cells is likely responsible for the localized accumulation of collagen in some alveolar septa [14, 16]. Although smooth muscle cells have not been cultured from the alveolar interstitium of patients with IPF, they have been isolated from other human sources, and they clearly synthesize types I and III collagen as well as basement membrane [32]. It is probable, therefore, that the clusters of smooth muscle cells within the IPF interstitium are responsible for at least some of the derangements of collagen found in this disorder.

The striking topologic derangement of the alveolar parenchymal cells in IPF is manifest in several ways [4, 26]: (1) cells are found in different locations, particularly the mesenchymal cells which are randomly distributed throughout the IPF interstitium; (2) cells are found piling up on one another (Fig. 3), most characteristically seen in the type II-like epithelial cells which replace the lost type I epithelial cells; (3) epithelial cell-basement membrane interactions are disturbed in IPF, as manifest by the partial separation of some epithelial cells from their basement membrane and by the presence of hemi-desmisomes attaching some epithelial cells to the underlying basement membrane (Fig. 10). In addition, anchoring fibrils attach the basement membrane to the underlying connective tissue (Fig. 10) [26]. One potential consequence of these topologic abnormalities is that parenchymal cells capable of collagen synthesis are found in the wrong locations and are oriented in the wrong directions. Although unproven, it is probable that this results in the deposition of collagen in improper locations and orientations, which are some of the characteristic findings in IPF.

The Chronic Alveolitis of IPF. The current concepts of pathogenesis of the fibrosis of IPF suggest two important roles for the effector cells of the inflammatory and immune systems that comprise the chronic alveolitis of the disease. First, a number of cells can alter collagen directly by secreting a collagenase and thus upsetting the relative balance between collagen synthesis and destruction within the interstitium. Second, the inflammatory and immune effector cells of the chronic alveolitis can

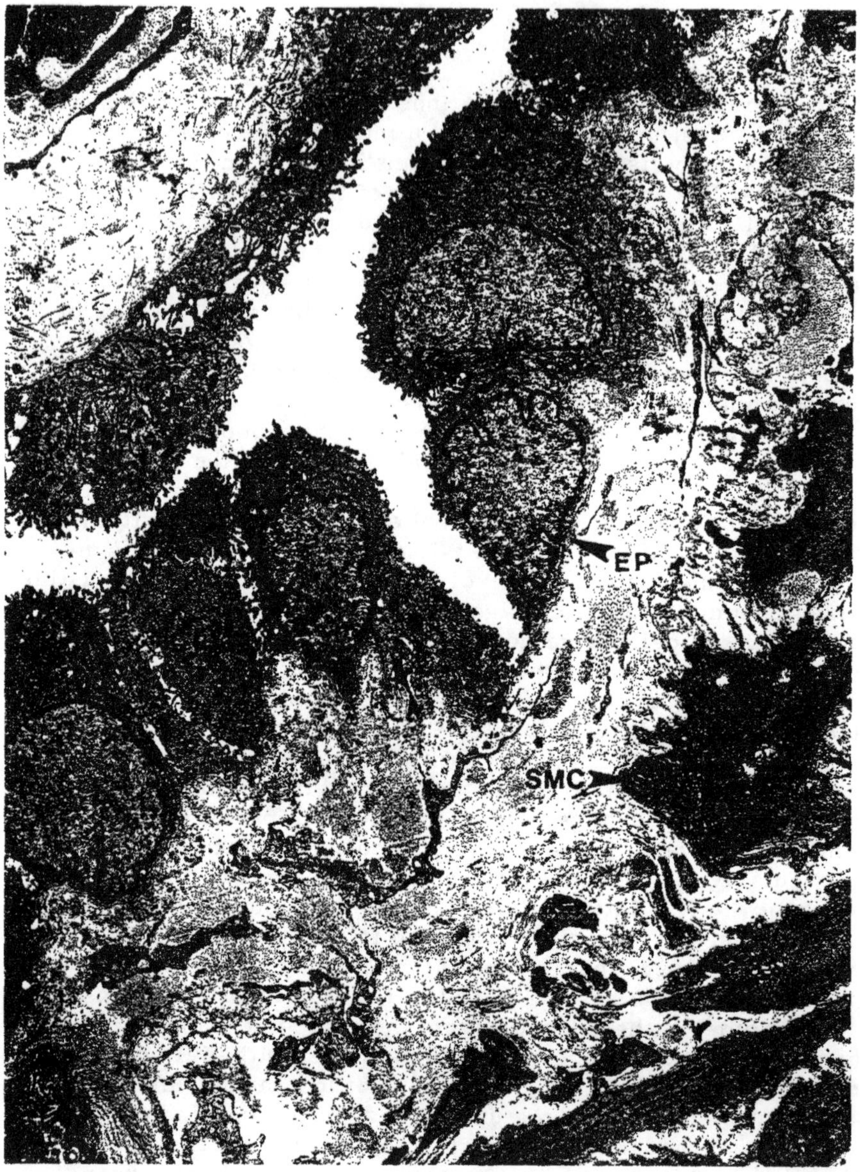

Fig. 7. Electron micrograph of alveolus in IPF. The alveolus is lined by cuboidal epithelial cells (EP), the luminal surfaces of which have numerous small cytoplasmic processes. Subjacent to the epithelium is a wide layer of dense, disordered fibrous connective tissue and a cluster of smooth muscle cells (SMC). X 5,480.

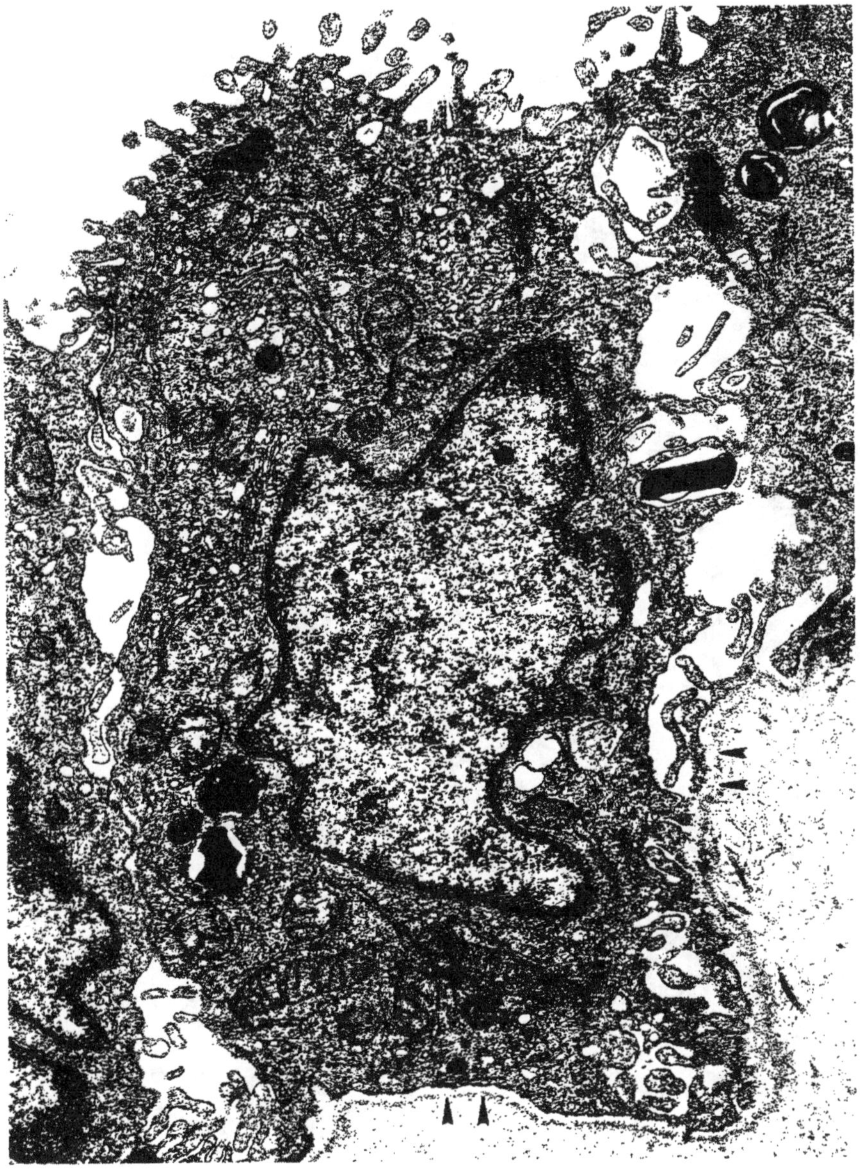

Fig. 8. View of cuboidal epithelial cells similar to those shown at low magnification in Fig. 7. The luminal surface is characterized by numerous short microvilli; the nucleus is idented, and the basement membrane (arrowheads) is prominent. The cytoplasm contains a well-developed Golgi complex, mitochondria, a few cisterns of rough-surfaced endoplasmic reticulum, and sparse numbers of lamellar bodies resembling those in normal type II alveolar epithelial cells. In contrast to normal alveolar epithelial cells, the cell in the center is loosely attached to its neighbors. X 18, 800.

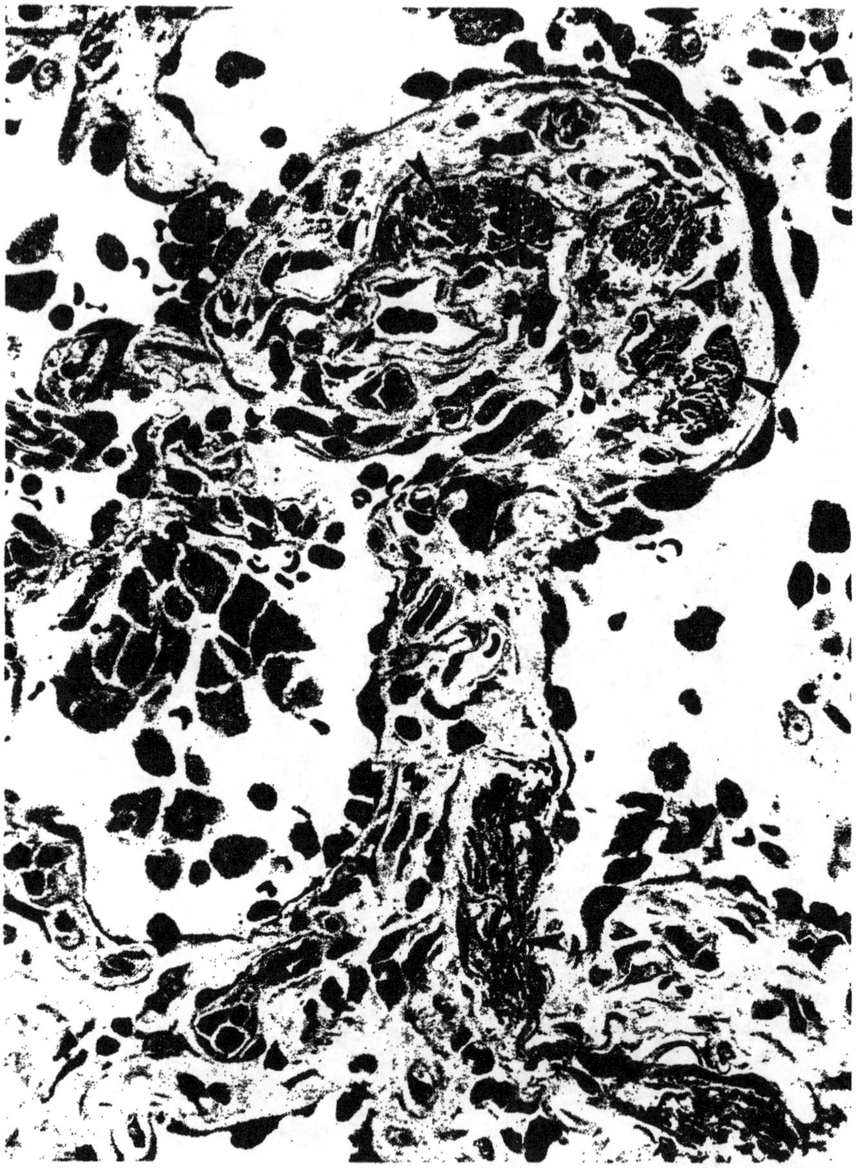

Fig. 9. Several clusters of smooth muscle cells (arrowheads) are present in widened, fibrotic pulmonary interstitium of patient with IPF. These smooth muscle cells are not related to blood vessels, from which they are clearly separated. The alveoli contain numerous macrophages and are lined by epithelial cells of various shapes. Half-micron-thick section of plastic-embedded tissue, alkaline toludine blue stain, X 1,000.

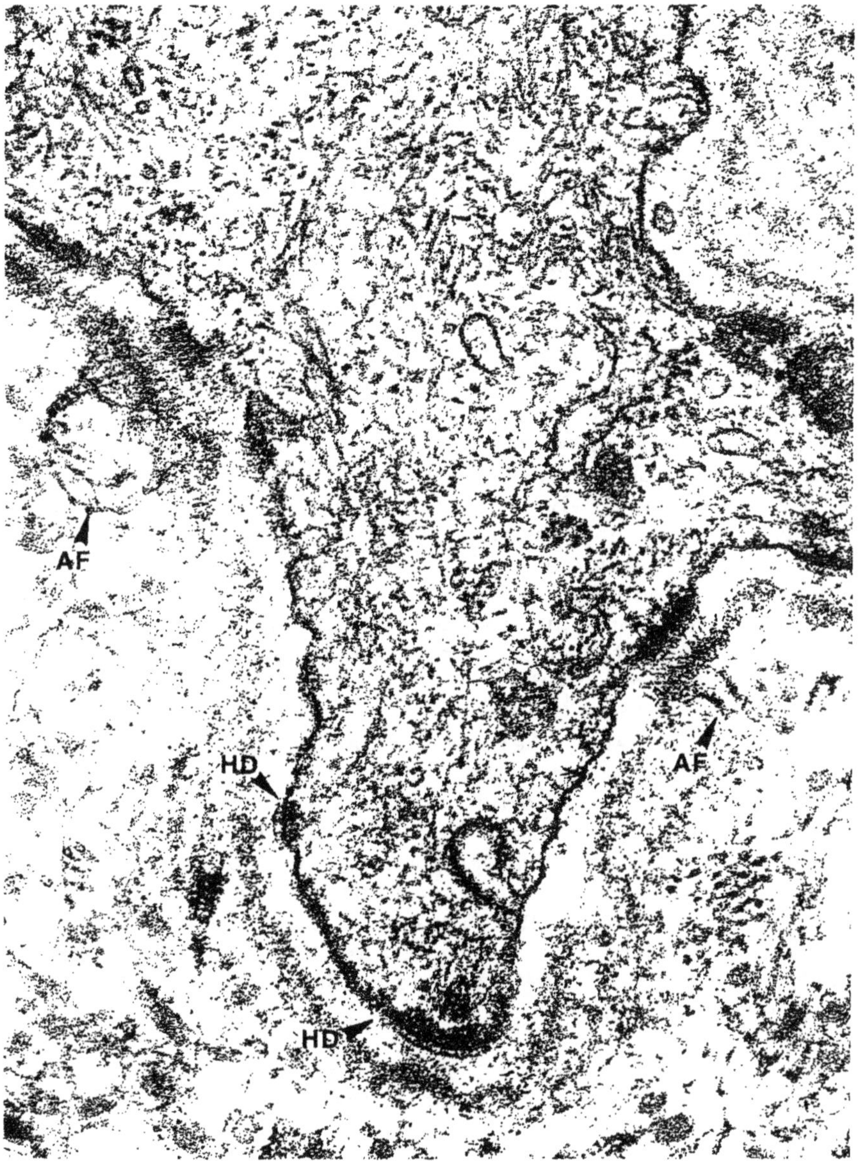

Fig. 10. Basal portion of cuboidal alveolar epithelial cell from patient with IPF shows abundant cytoplasmic filaments; several hemidesmosomes (HD) forming attachments between the plasma membrane and the basement membrane; anchoring fibrils (AF); and surrounding connective tissue containing collagen fibrils, connective tissue microfibrils and proteoglycan-like material. The anchoring fibrils [26] form arcs, the ends of which spread out fan-like and insert into the basement membrane; the banding pattern of anchoring fibrils differs from that of collagen fibrils. X 76,000.

alter collagen indirectly by affecting the parenchymal cells which normally synthesize and destroy collagen.

The effector cells that carry out these roles are present in the alveolar structures of the IPF lung in the following relative proportions: macrophages > lymphocytes and neutrophils > eosinophils and mast cells [4, 24, 34]. Although the relationship between these effector cells and the fibrosis of IPF has not been proven in all situations, convincing data have accumulated implicating certain dominant pathogenic processes. In many instances, the pathogenic process requires interdependence between different effector cells, but for convenience, we will discuss each cell separately.

Lymphocytes. The relative proportion of lymphocytes in the parenchyma of patients with IPF is normal, but since the number of inflammatory and immune effector cells is increased, the total number of lymphocytes (per alveolus) is also increased [4, 24, 34]. Although direct evaluation of the lymphocyte subpopulations in the IPF parenchyma has demonstrated that the proportions of T- and B-lymphocytes are normal, it is likely that at least certain lymphocyte subpopulations are different from those in normals. For example, there is some evidence that lymphocytes from patients with IPF recognize collagen as "non-self" and produce lymphokines such as macrophage migration inhibition factor (MIF) in response to it [29]. The mechanisms by which this occurs are not clear, but the T-lymphocyte is required in some fashion, since its removal completely obviates this phenomenon, at least in vitro.

Although completely untested, there are two additional roles that lymphocytes might play in relation to the fibrosis of IPF. First, there is evidence in guinea pigs that activated lymphocytes can "turn on" macrophages such that they secrete increased quantities of collagenase [37]. Second, evidence is accumulating that lymphocytes, in cooperation with monoclear phagocytic cells, produce factor(s) that suppress mesenchymal cell collagen synthesis by 30-40% [39]. Thus, it is theoretically possible that one fibrosis-related pathogenic mechanism in IPF is the loss of this suppressive effect and the resultant increased production of collagen by at least some mesenchymal cells.

Macrophages. As with lymphocytes, the relative proportion of macrophages in the IPF lung is not increased, but compared to normal lung, the total number of macrophages per alveolus is greatly elevated (Figs. 1-3, 9, 11) [4, 24, 34]. The reason why there are more macrophages present is not clear, but one possibility is that macrophages are induced to stay in affected alveoli by the influence of MIF produced by lymphocytes in the local area [29]. Since alveolar macrophages produce a collagenase capable of attacking types I and III collagen [20], one consequence of an increase in the numbers of macrophages per alveolus would be an imbalance in the maintenance of interstitial collagen toward collagen destruction. Further evidence that this might occur comes from the finding that 70% of patients with IPF have active collagenase in their lower respiratory tract while normals have none [28].

Recent evaluation of alveolar macrophages recovered from these patients suggests that the macrophage likely plays a critical role in the pathogenesis of IPF by recruiting neutrophils to the alveolar structures. This process is apparently mediated through the secretion by the macro-

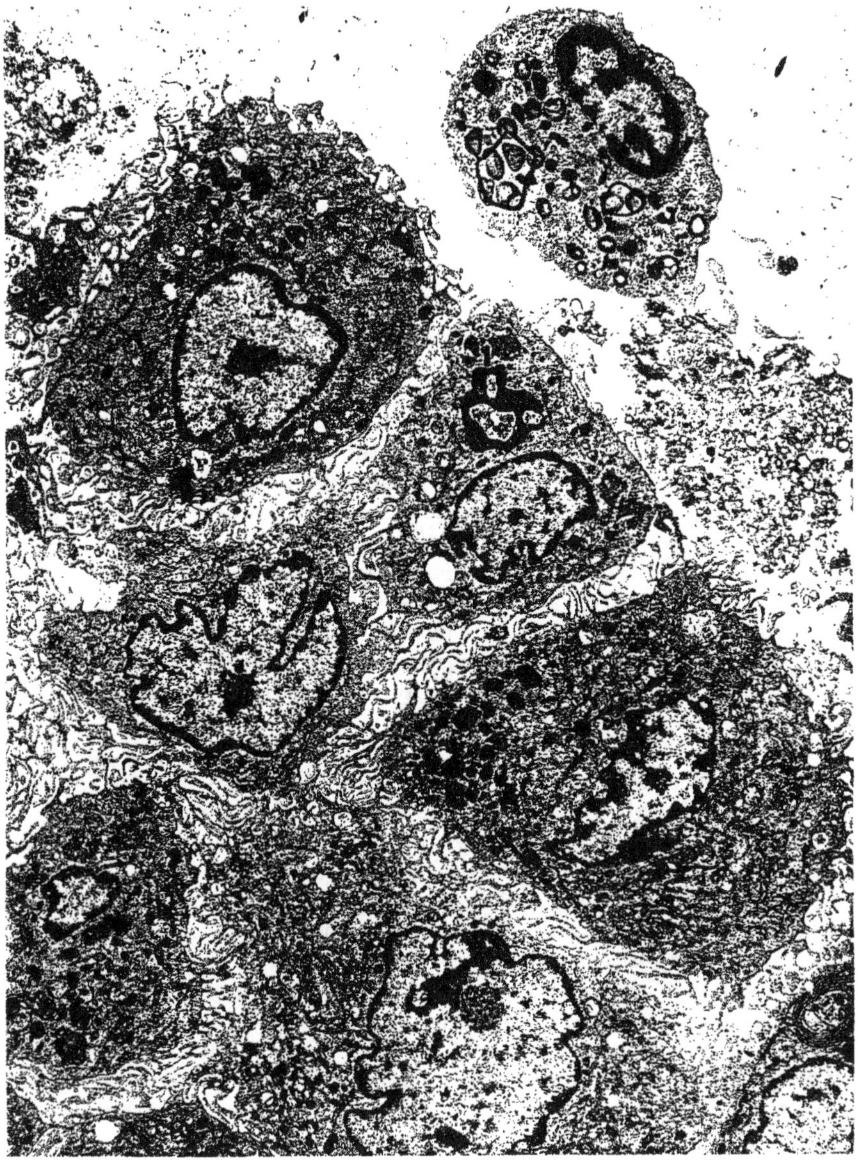

Fig. 11. View of cells in alveolar lumen in patient with IPF (compare with Figs. 1 and 2). The cell at upper right is an eosinophil leukocyte with typical cytoplasmic granules. The other cells are macrophages, characterized by marked irregularities of the contours of their plasma membranes (filopodia) and by their abundance of cytoplasmic dense bodies (lysosomes and residual bodies). X 5, 950.

phage of low-molecular-weight chemotactic factor which selectively attracts neutrophils [12, 23, 27]. Studies of IPF macrophages have shown that they are spontaneously secreting this neutrophil chemotactic factor, possibly mediated by the stimulation of immune complexes present in the lower respiratory tract of these patients [11]. As we will see, the recruitment of neutrophils to the alveoli is of particular importance, as the neutrophil is armed with a variety of proteases that can significantly influence the status of interstitial collagen.

Polymorphonuclear Leukocytes. Although eosinophils (Fig. 11) and mast cells are part of the chronic alveolitis of IPF, their role in the pathogenesis of the disease is unknown. In contrast, not only is there ample evidence that a significant number of neutrophils are present in the lung parenchyma of IPF patients (Fig. 12), but there is reason to believe the neutrophil may play an important role in the fibrosis of IPF.

There are two lines of evidence demonstrating a significant number of neutrophils in the lower respiratory tract of patients with IPF [24, 34]. First, analysis of cells recovered by bronchoalveolar lavage of these patients demonstrates that 10-20% of the cells recovered are neutrophils. Second, more definitive evidence comes from direct analysis of lung biopsies from these patients in which approximately 8% of the total inflammatory and immune effector cells recovered are neutrophils. Since these biopsies are sterile, and since they include rare airways relative to the number of alveoli, the neutrophils are undoubtedly part of the cells within the alveolar structures.

Unlike the macrophage, the neutrophil is a short-lived cell, suggesting neutrophil traffic in IPF from blood to alveoli must be large indeed. Since one consequence of neutrophil "death" is the release of proteolytic enzymes, it is likely that the presence of large numbers of neutrophils within the IPF parenchyma is associated with the release of relatively large quantities of collagenase, elastase and cathepsin-G, all of which are stored in neutrophil granules [25]. The consequences of having increased quantities of such enzymes within the interstitium are many, but two are particularly relevant to the disordered collagen that is part of the fibrosis of IPF. First, since neutrophil collagenase selectively attacks type I collagen over type III collagen [20], neutrophil collagenase may be responsible for some of the fraying of type I collagen seen on electron micrographs of the IPF interstitium. The finding that IPF patients have a collagenase in their lower respiratory tract active against type I collagen is consistent with this concept [28]. Second, there is recent evidence that fibronectin, a cell-surface macromolecule thought to be partially responsible for maintaining cell-cell and cell-connective tissue interactions, is particularly sensitive to destruction by neutrophil proteases such as elastase [33]. Thus, the presence of neutrophils in the IPF parenchyma may explain, in part, the mechanism by which parenchymal cells become topologically deranged in this disease, thus contributing to the disordering of collagen deposition that is so characteristic of the fibrosis of IPF.

The fact that IPF is a non-infectious disorder yet chronically associated with a significant number of neutrophils in the alveolar structures is so striking that IPF is now considered a chronic "neutrophil-accumulation" disorder of lung.

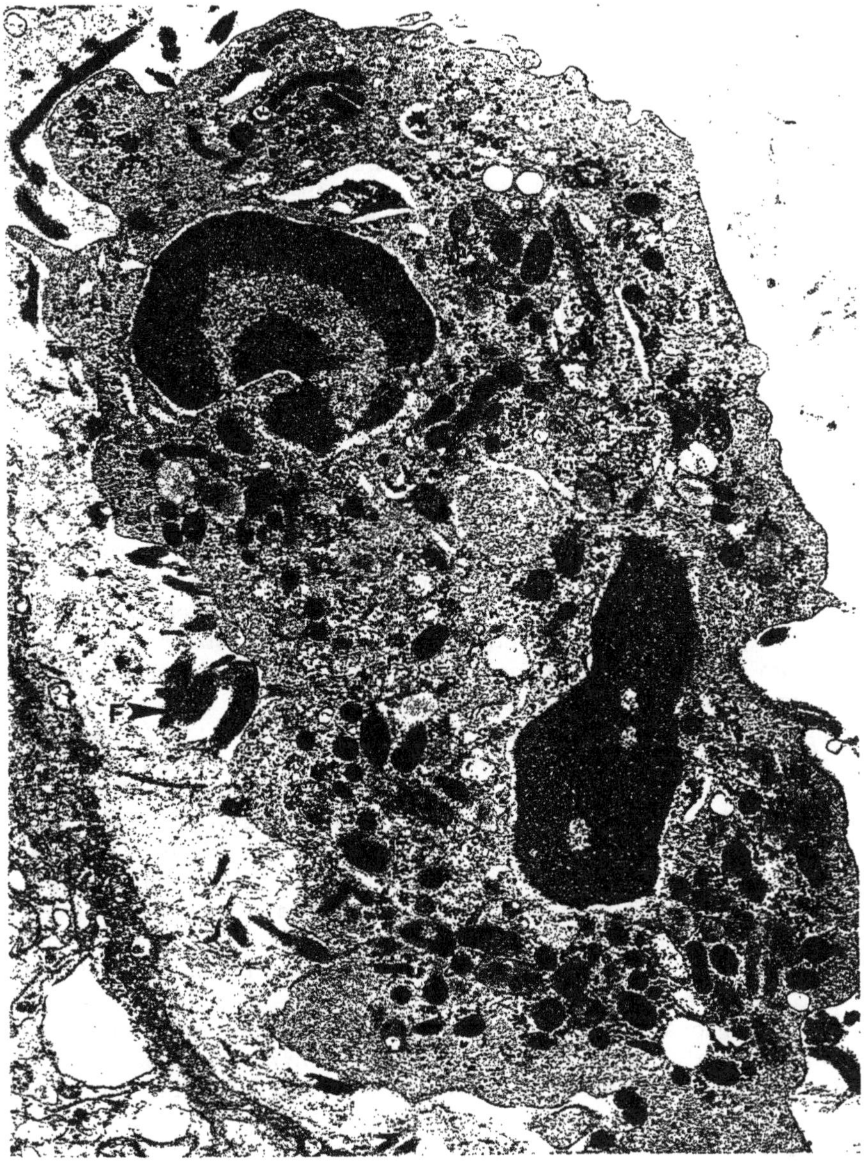

Fig. 12. Polymorphonuclear neutrophil leukocyte in fibrotic alveolar septum of patient with IPF is adjacent to collagen fibrils (upper right), strands of fibrin (F) and the basal portion of an alveolar epithelial cell (lower left). X 17, 600.

Clinical Considerations

It is clear from this discussion that, to stage and follow a patient with IPF, the clinician would like to have methods that independently and repeatedly assess the fibrosis, the alterations in parenchymal cells and the chronic alveolitis which are characteristic of this disease in mid-course. The open lung biopsy, of course, is one means of making these assessments, but biopsies are usually not performed sequentially, and it is difficult to quantitate the morphologic changes routinely. Although biopsy is currently the only method available to evaluate the alterations in parenchymal cells in IPF, recent methods have been developed to assess semiquantitatively the fibrosis and the alveolitis of this disease.

In a study of twenty-three patients with IPF in which the relative amount of fibrosis present in the biopsy was compared to a variety of physiologic monitors of the disease process, it became apparent that the results of traditional measurements such as volumes and diffusing capacity bore little relation to the degree of fibrosis [10]. In contrast, a number of parameters describing the deflation volume-pressure relationship of these patients (e.g., compliance at functional residual capacity, maximum transpulmonary pressure/total lung capacity), as well as parameters derived from steady-state exercise studies, did appear to correlate with the extent of fibrosis in each patient. Since exercise testing is the more routine of these two studies, it is probably the best available physiologic method to stage the fibrosis of IPF patients.

Two methods have been developed to stage and follow the degree of alveolitis of IPF, both of which are directly aimed at getting a semiquantitative measure of the number of neutrophils in the alveolar structures. The first is the analysis of the cells recovered by bronchoalveolar lavage [34]. As mentioned previously, the proportion of neutrophils found in lavage fluid closely parallels that found by direct analysis of open lung biopsies. The advantage of bronchoalveolar lavage is that it is easily performed, readily accepted by patients and carries little, if any, risk of morbidity if done carefully. Second, the relative number of neutrophils in the parenchyma of IPF patients can be assessed with gallium-67 rectilinear scans [31]. When conventional scanning methods are used, normal individuals do not accumulate gallium-67 in their lung parenchyma. In contrast, 70% of patients with IPF demonstrate significant quantities of this isotope within the parenchymal structures 48 h after administration. As with bronchoalveolar lavage, gallium-67 scanning is repeatable and carries little risk other than minor radiation exposure.

Therapy of IPF. The current concepts of the therapy of IPF involve attacking the disease in as early a stage as possible in the pathogenic process. Although it is theoretically attractive to think that at least some of the fibrosis of IPF could be prevented by agents that inhibit collagen synthesis, there is no agent available which will selectively provide this function in lung while sparing other organs [17]. Since collagen is the most abundant protein in the body, agents which inhibit collagen synthesis, secretion or maturation have significant "toxic" effects elsewhere, particularly in bone, where collagen is normally turning over at a rapid rate. Although some studies have suggested that such agents may be effective in experimental pulmonary fibrosis in animals [17], there is no evidence that these results can be directly transferred to the therapy of human disease.

More rational is the concept that IPF is vulnerable to attack by halting the chronic alveolits of the disorder. For several years, corticosteroids have been the mainstay of treatment of IPF [4, 6], and it is likely that their efficacy in slowing the progression of the disorder is through their anti-inflammatory properties. As evidence has accumulated that the alveolitis of IPF may also be mediated through immune mechanisms, clinicians have sought agents with broader anti-immune and anti-inflammatory actions than corticosteroids alone [6]. Although there are several anecdotal reports of the efficacy of immunosuppressive agents in IPF, there has only been one prospective double-blind study of corticosteroids alone vs. corticosteroids and azathioprine in the therapy of this disorder [9]. In the preliminary analysis of this data from twenty-seven patients followed over a one-year period, there was no additive effect of azathioprine in any of twenty-one parameters followed. This, together with the increased toxicity from an agent such as azathioprine, suggests that, at least for now, there is no proven role for immunosuppressive agents in the therapy of this disorder. In the Pulmonary Branch at the National Heart, Lung, and Blood Institute, we have several ongoing studies of other anti-inflammatory and anti-immune therapies in the treatment of these patients, but the results of these studies are not yet available.

References

1. Bradley, K., McConnell-Breul, S., Crystal, R. G.: Collagen in the human lung: Composition and quantitation of rates of synthesis. J. Clin. Invest. 55, 543-550 (1975)
2. Bradley, K. H., McConnell-Breul, S. D., Crystal, R. G.: Lung collagen composition and synthesis: Characterization and changes with age. J. Biol. Chem. 249, 2674-2683 (1974)
3. Bradley, K. H., McConnell-Breul, S. D., Crystal, R. G.: Lung collagen heterogeneity. Proc. Nat. Acad. Sci. 71, 2828-2832 (1974)
4. Crystal, R. G., Fulmer, J. D., Roberts, W. C., Moss, M. L., Line, B. R., Reynolds, H. Y.: Idiopathic pulmonary fibrosis: Clinical, histologic, radiographic, physiologic, scintigraphic, cytologic, and biochemical aspects. Ann. Int. Med. 85, 769-788 (1976)
5. Fulmer, J. D., Bienkowski, R. S., Cowan, M. J., Breul, S. D., Bradley, K. H., Ferrans, V. J., Roberts, W. C., Crystal, R. G.: Collagen concentration and rates of synthesis in idiopathic pulmonary fibrosis. (Unpublished ms.)
6. Fulmer, J. D., Crystal, R. G.: Interstitial Lung Disease. In: Current Pulmonology, vol. 1 (ed. D. H. Simmons), Pacific Palisades, California: Pinecliff Medical Publishing Company, 1978
7. Fulmer, J. D., Crystal, R. G.: The Biochemical Basis of Pulmonary Function. In: The Biochemical Basis of Pulmonary Function, pp. 419-466 (ed. R. G. Crystal). New York, Marcel Dekker, 1976
8. Fulmer, J., Elson, N., Bradley, K., Ferrans, V., Crystal, R. G.: Comparison of type-specific collagens synthesized by lung epithelial and mesenchymal cells. Clin. Res. 25, 416A (1977)

9. Fulmer, J., Elson, N., Von Gal, E., McLees, B., DeMets, D., Weinberger, S., Kelman, J., Crystal, R. G.: Treatment of idiopathic pulmonary fibrosis (IPF). Clin. Res. 26, 538A (1978)
10. Fulmer, J.D., Von Gal, E.R., Roberts, W.C., Crystal, R.G.: Morphologic-physiologic correlates of the severity of fibrosis in idiopathic pulmonary fibrosis. (Unpublished ms.)
11. Gadek, J., Hunninghake, G., Lawley, T., Kelman, J., Fulmer, J., Crystal, R. G.: Role of immune complexes in amplifying the alveolitis of idiopathic pulmonary fibrosis (IPF). Clin. Res. 26, 446A (1978)
12. Gadek, J., Hunninghake, G., Zimmerman, R., Crystal, R.: Mechanisms controlling release of neutrophil chemotactic factor by alveolar macrophages. Amer. Rev. Respir. Dis. 117 (Suppl.), 65 (1978)
13. Hamman, L., Rich, A. R.: Acute diffuse interstitial fibrosis of the lung. Bull. Johns Hopkins Hosp. 74, 177-212 (1944)
14. Hance, A. J., Bradley, K., Crystal, R. G.: Lung collagen heterogeneity. Synthesis of type I and type III collagen by rabbit and human lung cells in culture. J. Clin. Invest. 57, 102-111 (1976)
15. Hance, A. J., Crystal, R. G.: Collagen. In: The Biochemical Basis of Pulmonary Function, pp. 215-271 (ed. R. G. Crystal). New York, Marcel Dekker, 1976
16. Hance, A. J., Crystal, R. G.: Rigid control of the synthesis of collagen Types I and III by cells in culture. Nature 268, 152-154 (1977)
17. Hance, A. J., Crystal, R. G.: The connective tissue of lung. Amer. Rev. Respir. Dis. 112, 657-711 (1975)
18. Horwitz, A.L., Crystal, R. G.: Collagenase from rabbit pulmonary alveolar macrophages. Biochem. Biophys. Res. Commun. 69, 296-303 (1976)
19. Horwitz, A.L., Elson, N.A., Crystal, R.G.: Proteoglycans and Elastin. In: The Biochemical Basis of Pulmonary Function, pp. 273-311 (ed. R. G. Crystal). New York, Marcel Dekker, 1976
20. Horwitz, A.L., Hance, A.J., Crystal, R.G.: Granulocyte collagenase Selective digestion of type I over type III collagen. Proc. Nat. Acad. Sci., 1977, 74, 897-901 (1977)
21. Horwitz, A.L., Kelman, J.A., Crystal, R.G.: Activation of alveolar macrophage collagenase by a neutral protease secreted by the same cell. Nature 264, 772-774 (1976)
22. Howard, B.V., Macarak, E.J., Gunson, D., Kefalides, N.A.: Characterization of the collagen synthesized by endothelial cells in culture. Proc. Nat. Acad. Sci. 73, 2361-2364 (1976)
23. Hunninghake, G.W., Gallin, J.I., Fauci, A.S.: Immunologic reactivity of the lung. The in vivo and in vitro generation of a neutrophil chemotactic factor by alveolar macrophages. Amer. Rev. Respir. Dis. 117, 15-23 (1978)
24. Hunninghake, G.W., Kelman, J.A., Gadek, J.E., Elson, N.A., Fulmer, J.D., Crystal, R.G.: Comparison of inflammatory and immune effector cell populations in lavage fluid and lung biopsies of patients with pulmonary fibrosis. Amer. Rev. Respir. Dis. 117 (Suppl.), 68 (1978)

25. Janoff, A.: At least three human neutrophil lysosomal proteases are capable of degrading joint connective tissue. Ann. New York Acad. Sci. 256, 402-408 (1975)
26. Kawanami, O., Ferrans, V. J., Roberts, W. C, Crystal, R. G., Fulmer, J. D.: Anchoring fibrils: A new connective tissue structure in fibrotic lung disease. Amer. J. Pathol. 92, 127-148 (1978)
27. Kazmierowski, J. A., Gallin, J. I., Reynolds, H. Y.: Mechanism for the inflammatory response in primate lungs. Demonstration and partial characterization of an alveolar macrophage-derived chemotactic factor with preferential activity for polymorphonuclear leukocytes. J. Clin. Invest. 59, 273-281 (1977)
28. Kelman, J., Weinberger, S., Fulmer, J., Reynolds, H., Crystal, R. G.: Connective tissue specific enzymes of bronchoalveolar fluid in idiopathic pulmonary fibrosis (IPF). Clin. Res. 25, 503A (1977)
29. Kravis, T. C., Ahmed, A., Brown, T. E., Fulmer, J. D., Crystal, R. G.: Pathogenic mechanisms in pulmonary fibrosis: Collagen induced migration inhibition factor production and cytotoxicity mediated by lymphocytes. J. Clin. Invest. 58, 1223-1232 (1976)
30. Kuhn, C.: The cells of the lung and their organelles. In: The Biochemical Basis of Pulmonary Function, pp. 3-48 (ed. R. G. Crystal). New York, Marcel Dekker, 1976
31. Line, B. R., Fulmer, J. D., Reynolds, H. Y., Roberts, W. C., Jones, A. E., Harris, E. K., Crystal, R. G.: Gallium-67 citrate scanning in the staging of idiopathic pulmonary fibrosis: Correlation with physiology, morphology and bronchoalveolar lavage. Amer. Rev. Respir. Dis. 118, 355-365 (1978)
32. Mayne, R., Vail, M. S., Miller, E. J.: Characterization of the collagen chains synthesized by cultured smooth muscle cells derived from rhesus monkey thoracic aorta. Biochemistry 17, 446-452 (1978)
33. McDonald, J., Baum, B., Rosenberg, D., Kelman, J., Senior, R., Crystal, R. G.: Fibronectin, the major cell surface protein of cultured human lung fibroblasts: Destruction of structure and biological activity by human neutrophil proteinases. Amer. Rev. Respir. Dis. 117 (Suppl.), 170 (1978)
34. Reynolds, H. Y., Fulmer, J. D., Kazmierowski, J. A., Roberts, W. C., Frank, M. M., Crystal, R. G.: Analysis of broncho-alveolar lavage fluid from patients with idiopathic pulmonary fibrosis and chronic hypersensitivity pneumonitis. J. Clin. Invest. 59, 165-175 (1977)
35. Seyer, J. M., Hutcheson, E. T., Kang, A. H.: Collagen polymorphism in idiopathic chronic pulmonary fibrosis. J. Clin. Invest. 57, 1498-1507 (1976)
36. Spencer, H.: Chronic interstitial pneumonia. In: The Lung, pp. 134-150, (ed. A. A. Liebow and D. E. Smith). Baltimore: Williams and Wilkins, 1968
37. Wahl, L. M., Wahl, S. M., Mergenhagen, S. E., Martin, G. R.: Collagenase production by lymphokine-activated macrophages. Science 187, 261-263 (1975)

38. Weibel, E.R., Gehr, P., Haies, D., Gil, J., Bachofen, M.: The cell population of the normal lung. In: Lung Cells in Disease, pp 3-16 (ed. A. Bouhuys). New York: North-Holland, 1976
39. Weinberger, S., Fells, G., Bradley, K., Hunninghake, G., Gadek, J., Crystal, R.G.: Mononuclear cell-fibroblast interactions in the synthesis of lung collagen. Amer. Rev. Respir. Dis. 117 (Suppl.), 84 (1978)
40. Werb, Z., Reynolds, J.J.: Purification and properties of a specific collagenase from rabbit synovial fibroblasts. Biochem. J. 151, 645-653 (1975)

Accepted for publication:
28 April 1978

Ronald G. Crystal, M.D.
6D06, Building 10
National Institutes of Health
Bethesda, MD 20014, USA

Morphologic-Physiologic Correlates of the Severity of Fibrosis and Degree of Cellularity in Idiopathic Pulmonary Fibrosis

JACK D. FULMER, WILLIAM C. ROBERTS, EDWYNA R. VON GAL, and RONALD G. CRYSTAL, *Pulmonary Branch and Pathology Branch, National Heart, Lung, and Blood Institute, National Institutes of Health, Bethesda, Maryland 20014*

ABSTRACT Idiopathic pulmonary fibrosis (IPF) is a progressive disease of lung parenchyma characterized by a chronic inflammatory cellular infiltration and varying degrees of interstitial fibrosis. Current data indicate that the severity of fibrosis and the degree of cellularity determine, in part, the prognosis of IPF and the response to therapy. Whereas lung biopsy gives the best assessment of fibrosis and cellularity, physiologic studies are used to stage and monitor the disease process. To determine which physiologic studies correlate best with severity of fibrosis and degree of cellularity, these parameters were graded in lung biopsies of 23 patients with IPF and compared with a variety of physiologic studies.

Although vital capacity, total lung capacity, and diffusing capacity are commonly used as objective monitors of the disease process, none of these parameters correlated with either the severity of fibrosis or the degree of cellularity in biopsy specimens. In contrast, almost all parameters of lung distensibility correlated with the morphologic assessment of degree of fibrosis; compliance had the best correlation. Parameters of distensibility, however, correlated poorly with the degree of cellularity.

In comparison, gas exchange during exercise correlated with both morphologic parameters; the exercise-induced changes in arterial oxygen pressure per liter of oxygen consumed had a high correlation with the degree of fibrosis ($r = 0.89$; $P < 0.001$) and correlated to a lesser extent with the degree of cellularity ($r = 0.56$; $P = 0.009$). In contrast, neither the resting arterial oxygen tension nor the arterial oxygen tension at maximal exercise correlated with the morphologic assessment of degree of fibrosis or the degree of cellularity.

These morphologic-physiologic comparisons suggest that (*a*) lung volumes and diffusing capacity are poor monitors of both the degree of fibrosis and the degree of cellularity; (*b*) the fibrotic process contributes, at least in part, to parameters of lung distensibility, and both fibrosis and cellularity contribute to gas exchange alterations during exercise; and (*c*) parameters of lung distensibility and exercise-induced gas exchange alterations may be useful in staging the severity of disease in IPF.

Address reprint requests to Dr. Fulmer, Room 6D-06, Building 10, National Institutes of Health, Bethesda, Md. 20014.

Received for publication 25 November 1977 and in revised form 16 October 1978.

INTRODUCTION

Idiopathic pulmonary fibrosis (IPF)[1] is a progressive, generally fatal disease characterized by an interstitial and intra-alveolar inflammatory process, interstitial fibrosis, and revision of the distal lung architecture (1–12). Early in the disease, most patients with IPF present with exertional breathlessness, an alveolar filling pattern on chest roentgenogram, and reduced diffusing capacity. As the disease progresses, patients develop marked exertional dyspnea, a reticulonodular pattern on x-ray, and resting hypoxemia. Advanced IPF is characterized by breathlessness at rest and roentgenographically by a coarse reticular pattern with cystic lesions.

Current concepts of the pathogenesis of IPF are that

[1] *Abbreviations used in this paper*: A-aD_{O_2}, alveolar-arterial oxygen pressure gradient; CR, coefficient of retraction; DL_{CO}, diffusing capacity of the lungs; FRC, functional residual capacity; IPF, idiopathic pulmonary fibrosis; P_{50}, Pst at 50% of observed TLC; P_{70}, Pst at 70% of observed TLC; P_{max}, maximum transpulmonary pressure; Pst, static transpulmonary pressure during deflation; TLC, total lung capacity; VC, vital capacity.

the fibrosis is preceded by an inflammatory cellular infiltration. Early disease is characterized by minimal fibrosis and an active cellular response, whereas advanced disease is characterized by severe fibrosis and minimal cellularity (8, 11–13). Furthermore, correlative studies have shown that the prognosis and response to therapy in IPF is determined, in part, by the severity of fibrosis and the degree of cellularity (11, 13). Although the lung biopsy gives the best assessment of the severity of fibrosis and cellularity in IPF, it is generally performed only once in the course of the disease. It would, therefore, be useful to have monitors of the disease process that can be used repeatedly. In general, the currently accepted monitors of the overall severity of the disease in IPF are lung volumes, diffusing capacity, and arterial blood gases (14–17). There are, however, little data on the usefulness of physiologic tests in gauging either the severity of the fibrosis or the degree of cellularity.

To this end, the present study was designed to evaluate the usefulness of lung volumes, diffusing capacity, and arterial blood gases to guage the extent of fibrosis and cellularity in IPF, and to identify other physiologic studies that may be of use. To accomplish this, we have evaluated a group of patients with IPF by (*a*) grading the severity of fibrosis and cellularity in their lung biopsies; (*b*) characterizing the physiologic alterations in these patients by a number of tests, including lung volumes, diffusing capacity, tests of distensibility, and gas exchange at rest and exercise; and (*c*) comparing the results of the morphologic and physiologic data.

METHODS

Patient population

As part of a study of fibrotic lung disease, 250 patients were referred to the Pulmonary Branch of the National Heart, Lung, and Blood Institute, National Institutes of Health, Bethesda, Md. From this group, 75 were determined to have IPF by the following criteria (8–10).

Clinical. The 75 subjects revealed a history of progressive, exertional breathlessness; no history of exposure to inorganic, organic, gaseous, physical, or pharmacological agents known to cause pulmonary fibrosis; no history suggestive of hypersensitivity lung disease; no history of chronic bronchitis; no history of chronic pulmonary infection; and no history or clinical findings suggestive of left ventricular failure.

Roentgenographic. The presence of a diffuse interstitial pattern with no left ventricular enlargement.

Physiologic. There was presence of reduced lung volumes or diffusing capacity, exercise-induced hypoxemia, normal forced expiratory volume in 1 s/forced vital capacity, and normal airway resistance by body plethysmography.

Morphologic. A biopsy revealed varying degrees of interstitial fibrosis with interstitial and intra-alveolar cells consisting primarily of lymphocytes and macrophages, but including neutrophils and eosinophils; No vasculitis or granulomata was present, or significant inorganic material by polarized light microscopy, and negative cultures for bacteria, mycobacteria, and fungi.

Patients were included in this study if they met the diagnostic criteria for IPF, had a recent lung biopsy that was taken from a representative area as judged by the chest roentgenogram, and were able to participate in physiologic testing. If the lung biopsy demonstrated "end-stage lung" (see below), they were excluded.

From the initial 75 patients, 23 fit all of the above criteria. Patients who were excluded from the present study were done so because of failure to have a recent biopsy, failure to have a biopsy from an area on the film that was judged to be representative, or inability to participate in physiologic testing because of marked breathlessness or other medical problems. Of the 23 patients, 2 (M.C., V.J.) had rheumatoid arthritis, and 1 (O.N.) had an overlap connective tissue syndrome. These three patients all had lung biopsies that were indistinguishable from the other patients and had no evidence of lung or systemic vasculitis. 12 patients had open lung biopsy at our institution with physiologic testing performed 2–4 wk before biopsy; the other 11 patients had lung biopsies performed at an outside institution with physiologic testing performed at our institution an average of 4 mo after biopsy.

Morphologic grading of fibrosis and cellularity

All morphologic observations were made without knowledge of the results of physiologic testing. 22 of the biopsies were obtained by open thoracotomy; one was obtained by drill needle biopsy. For control tissue (no fibrosis), lung tissue was obtained at thoracotomy from patients with solitary nodules; in most cases, an entire lobe was removed. Parenchyma at least 1 cm in distance from the nodule was taken as representing normal lung. Before surgery, these patients underwent routine physiologic testing; only those with normal pulmonary function studies were accepted as controls.

All biopsy specimens were fixed in 10% neutral formalin, processed in alcohol and xylene, imbedded in paraffin, and serially sectioned at 6-μm intervals. Sections were stained with hematoxylin–eosin and Masson trichome. Grading of the degree of fibrosis in each biopsy was made with Masson trichome-stained sections and grading of the cellularity was made with hematoxylin–eosin stain. Grading of both the degree of fibrosis and degree of cellularity was made with an estimate of the increase in each compared with noninflated control lung. The grade of minimal (+1) was assigned when there was <10% increase; mild (+2) was assigned when there was a 10–25% increase; moderate (+3) was assigned when there was a 25–40% increase; and severe (+4) was assigned when there was >40% increase.

Each biopsy was graded an average of four times by three observers, and a mean grade of degree of fibrosis and degree of cellularity was determined. For each biopsy, an intra-observer and an inter-observer variability was computed.

Lung volumes, timed expiratory maneuvers, airway resistance and diffusing capacity

Lung volumes, standard-timed expiratory maneuvers, and single breath diffusing capacity for carbon monoxide were measured with a computerized modular lung analyzer (P-1200; Warren E. Collins, Inc., Braintree, Mass.) as previously described (10). Predicted values for vital capacity (VC), forced VC, and forced expiratory volume in 1 s were obtained from the predicted equations of Morris et al. (18); predicted residual volume and functional residual capacity (FRC) were taken from the data of Goldman and Becklacke (19).

Predicted total lung capacity (TLC) was obtained by adding predicted VC and predicted residual volume. The predicted values of diffusing capacity (DL_{CO}) of Gaensler and Wright (20) were used. Airway resistance was determined by the method of DuBois et al. (21) using a constant volume plethysmograph (Warren E. Collins, Inc.), as previously described (10). Normal airway resistance was considered to be 2.5 cm H_2O/liter per s (21).

Static volume-pressure relationship

Measurements of lung volume-pressure relationships were made as previously described (10). Balloon volume was corrected by the methods of Milic-Emili et al. (22) or Lemen et al. (23). A constant volume history was assured by having the patient hyperventilate and then inspire to TLC three times (24). Static transpulmonary pressure at the TLC (P_{max}) was recorded with glottis open while the subject maintained a maximum inspiration for 2–3 s (25–27). Static transpulmonary pressure during deflation (Pst) was measured as the pressure difference between mouth and esophageal balloon with glottis open and flow being interrupted by a solenoid-operated shutter. Static deflation volume-pressure curves were constructed using an average of 4 deflation maneuvers with 12–14 points per maneuver. Volume was corrected to body temperature, pressure saturated and required to be ±5% of VC as recorded by standard spirometry. From these data, the following parameters were quantitated.

Static deflation compliance (compliance). Compliance was measured as the change in volume per unit pressure change between FRC (liters) and FRC + 0.5 liter on the static deflation volume-pressure curve when volume was expressed as observed VC (liters) (Fig. 1A). Compliance was considered to be a monitor of lung distensibility in the tidal volume range. The normal range for compliance was considered to be 0.15–0.30 liters/cm H_2O (27).

Slope of the volume-pressure curve (comparative compliance). To compare compliance data between patients with a wide range of lung volumes, the volume-pressure data was plotted as a percent of predicted TLC vs. Pst (centimeters of H_2O) and the slope of the curve was measured between Pst at 50% observed TLC (P_{50}) and Pst at 70% observed TLC (P_{70}) using the formula: comparative compliance = (volume [as percent of predicted TLC] at P_{70} − volume [as percent of predicted TLC] at P_{50})/(P_{70}[centimeters of H_2O] − P_{50}[centimeters of H_2O]) (Fig. 1B, C). Comparative compliance was considered to be a measure of lung distensibility at mid-lung volumes that could be used to compare patient to patient; the units of comparative compliance are percentages of predicted TLC per centimeters of H_2O. Normal values are age related and range from 2.9 to 3.7%/cm H_2O (24).

Position of the volume-pressure curve (P_{70}). P_{70} was determined by recording the static transpulmonary pressure at 70% observed TLC (Fig. 1B). P_{70} provided an index as to whether the volume-pressure curve (when expressed as a percent of observed TLC) was normal or shifted to the right or left when compared with the normal data of Turner et al. (24). In addition, P_{70} was used as a measure of the pressure necessary to expand the lung at mid-range volume. Normal values are age related and range from 5.5 to 12.0 cm H_2O (24).

Maximum transpulmonary pressure (P_{max}). P_{max} was measured at TLC and expressed in centimeters of H_2O (Fig. 1A). P_{max} was used as an index of recoil pressure at maximum lung volume (TLC). Normal values are age dependent and range from 20 to 45 cm H_2O (24).

Coefficient of retraction (CR). Calculated by the formula of Schlueter et al. (26), CR = P_{max} (centimeters of H_2O)/ TLC (liters) (Fig. 1A). CR was used as an index of maximum recoil pressure when adjusted for the lung volume of the individual patient. Normal values range from 4.0 to 8.0 cm H_2O/liter (26, 28).

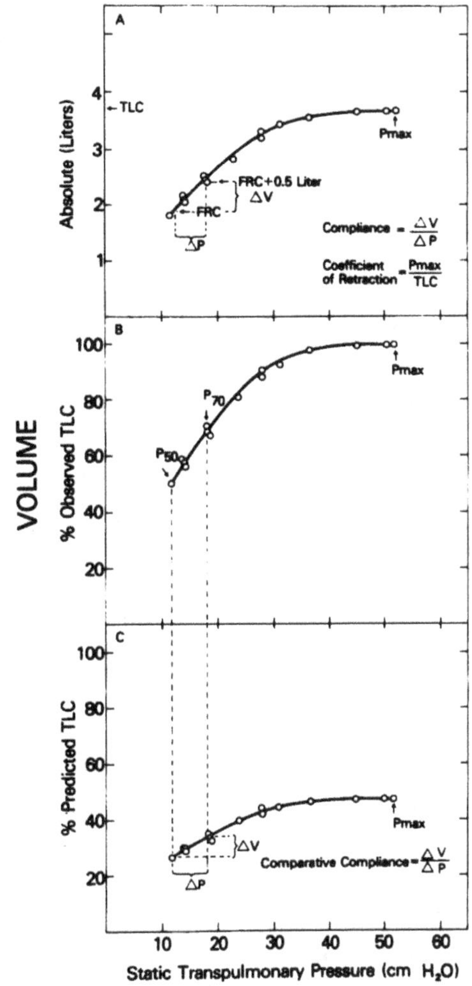

FIGURE 1 Analysis of the static deflation volume-pressure relationship. Illustration of the methods for (A) determining the measurement of compliance and CR, (B) determining the position of P_{70}, and (C) calculating comparative compliance. The data used for this example is from patient W.H.

Steady-state gas exchange and physiologic shunt

Steady-state gas exchange studies were performed at rest and, if possible, during graded exercise for a maximum of three levels of power output. Graded exercise was achieved using a motor-driven, variable speed and grade treadmill (model 18–94C, Quinton Instruments, Seattle, Wash.). A low-resistance, high-speed breathing valve (P-316, W. E. Collins) was used, and the gas collected in a 120-liter gasometer (P-1700, Warren E. Collins, Inc.). Breath-by-breath analysis of O_2, CO_2, and N_2 were monitored by a medical gas analyzer (model 1100; Perkin-Elmer, Pomona, Calif.) on line to an eight-channel universal recorder (Gould, Inc., Measurement Systems Div., Oxnard, Calif.). Expired gases in the gasometer were analyzed with the medical gas analyzer and checked against an infrared CO_2 analyzer (model LB-2, Beckman Instruments, Inc., Electronic Instruments Div., Schiller Park, Ill.) and paramagnetic O_2 analyzer (model OM-11, Beckman Instruments, Inc.). All gas analysis apparatus were calibrated before each study using room air and two gravimetrically determined gas mixtures (4% CO_2, 14% O_2, balance N_2; and 8% CO_2, balance O_2; Landsel Cryogenics, Hyattsville, Md.).

Arterial blood gas pressures were analyzed with a Radiometer blood micro-system (BMS 3-Mk2, The London Co., Cleveland, Ohio) and a direct reading acid base analyzer (PHM71-Mk, The London Co.). Calibration gases for the O_2 and CO_2 electrodes included four gases: 100% O_2, room air; 4% CO_2, balance N_2; and 8% CO_2, 21% O_2, balance N_2 (Liquid Carbonics, Baltimore, Md.). Gas mixtures were gravimetrically determined and checked by gas chromatography. The pH electrode was calibrated with certified Radiometer buffers (pH 6.841 and pH 7.383, The London Co.). The blood gas system was regularly checked against tonometered bloods (type 247; International Laboratories, Rockville, Md.).

After the patient was familiarized with the procedure and instructed in walking on the treadmill, a 20-gauge, thin-walled, Teflon catheter (Becton, Dickinson and Co., Rutherford, N. J.) was placed in the radial artery using local anesthesia. Cardiac monitoring was performed throughout the procedure.

All studies were done at steady state, defined as that point when end expiratory CO_2 and heart rate reached constant values (this usually took 3–6 min). The speed and incline of the treadmill were adjusted such that three levels of exercise could be attached based on the following target heart rates: stage 0, at rest in the sitting position; stage I, exercise with heart rate 110–120 beats/min; stage II, exercise with heart rate 130–140 beats/min; stage III; exercise with heart rate 140–160 beats/min. Patients rested between stages until their heart rates returned to stage 0 (resting level). Studies were terminated if any of the following occurred: (*a*) the electrocardiogram showed significant segment depression of >1 mV; (*b*) the electrocardiogram showed >10 premature ventricular contractions/min or >2 premature ventricular contractions in series; (*c*) the patient did not feel he could continue; or (*d*) if the arterial oxygen tension (P_{AO_2}) was <45 mm Hg in a patient >40 yr of age.

At each stage, once a steady state was achieved and expired gas had been used to flush the gasometer 3–5 times, expired gas was collected for 2 min. Midway during these 2 min, an arterial blood sample was taken. The collected expired gas was analyzed for the fraction of O_2, CO_2, and N_2; the arterial blood was analyzed for the partial pressure of O_2, and CO_2, and for pH. From these data, minute ventilation, alveolar ventilation, O_2 consumption ($\dot{V}O_2$), CO_2 production ($\dot{V}CO_2$), alveolar oxygen tension ($P_{A_{O_2}}$), and alveolar-arterial oxygen pressure gradient (A-aD_{O_2}), were calculated using standard equations (29). In addition, the following derived parameters were calculated.

Exercise parameter 1: the absolute change in Pa_{O_2} between rest and maximal exercise. Exercise parameter 1 = (Pa_{O_2} [maximal $\dot{V}O_2$ achieved] − Pa_{O_2} [stage 0]).

Exercise parameter 2: the absolute change in the A-aD_{O_2} between rest and exercise. Exercise parameter 2 = (A-aD_{O_2} [maximal $\dot{V}O_2$ achieved] − A-aD_{O_2} [stage 0]).

Exercise parameter 3: change in Pa_{O_2} per liter of oxygen consumed during exercise. Pa_{O_2} was plotted against $\dot{V}O_2$ for stages 0 through the maximal stage achieved; by the method of least squares, the slope ($\Delta Pa_{O_2}/\Delta\dot{V}O_2$) was computed (Fig. 2A). The normal range of $\Delta Pa_{O_2}/\Delta\dot{V}O_2$ in our laboratory is +5 to −3 mm Hg-min/liter which is in agreement with published data (30, 31).

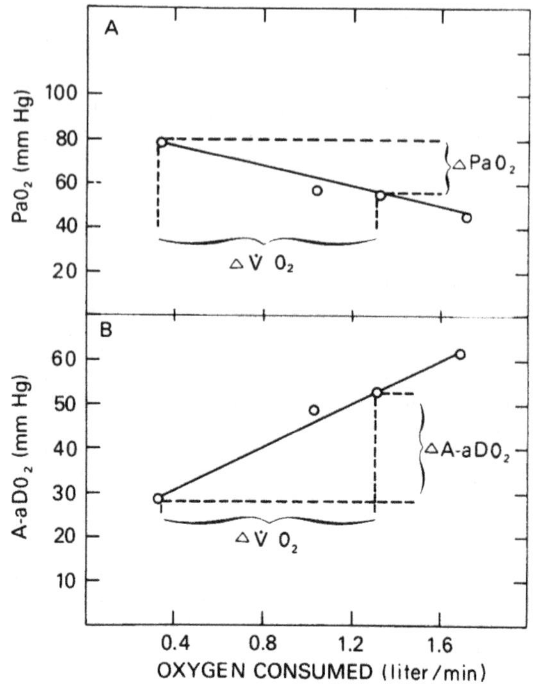

FIGURE 2 Method for calculation of (A) the change in Pa_{O_2} per liter oxygen consumed during exercise ($\Delta Pa_{O_2}/\Delta\dot{V}O_2$) and (B) the change in A-aD_{O_2} per liter oxygen consumed during exercise (ΔA-a$D_{O_2}/\Delta\dot{V}O_2$). The data used for this example is from patient W.H.

Exercise parameter 4: the change in A-aD_{O_2} per liter oxygen consumed during exercise. A-aD_{O_2} was plotted against $\dot{V}O_2$ for stage 0 through the maximal stage achieved; by the method of least squares, the slope (ΔA-a$D_{O_2}/\Delta\dot{V}O_2$) was computed (Fig. 2B). The normal range of ΔA-a$D_{O_2}/\Delta\dot{V}O_2$ in our laboratory is +4 to +8 mm Hg-min/liter which is in agreement with published data (30, 31).

Physiologic shunt was estimated using 100% O_2 after monitoring expired gases until no N_2 could be detected with a Valsava maneuver. Care was taken to periodically have the patient deep breathe to attempt to circumvent airway closure. The standard shunt equation was used with the arterial-venous oxygen content difference assumed to be 5 vol% (32).

Statistical analysis of data

Two-methods were used for data analysis: Spearman rank correlation and the two-tailed Student's *t* test. To facilitate discussion of the analysis, data were grouped as follows: (*a*) clinical data included age, sex, duration of symptoms, smoking history; (*b*) standard physiologic data included VC, TLC, FRC, and DL_{CO}; (*c*) distensibility data included compliance, comparative compliance, P_{70}, P_{max} and CR; (*d*) gas exchange data included resting and exercise Pa_{O_2}, resting and exercise A-aD_{O_2}, and exercise parameters 1–4 and physiologic shunt; and (*e*) morphologic data included the degree of fibrosis and the degree of cellularity assigned to each biopsy.

Spearman rank correlation was used to compare morphologic data to all other data because fibrosis and cellularity were ranked from minimal (+1) to severe (+4), and all other data were either continuous or ranked (33).

The two-tailed t test was used to compare mean values of gas exchange data between patients grouped by the extent of exercise achieved (stages I–III) (34). The Aspen correction was used for degrees of freedom when the variance of one mean value was >3 times the variance of the other mean value (35).

RESULTS

Clinical data

The study patients (16 male, 7 female) ranged in age from 27 to 67 yr (mean±SEM, 48.4±2.9 yr). Duration of symptoms ranged from 0.5 to 10 yr (mean±SEM, 2.0±0.5 yr) (Table I). Although some patients had a history of cough, none had clinical evidence of chronic bronchitis. Nine patients were taking prednisone at the time of evaluation and one patient was taking phenylbutazone (Table I).

Standard physiologic studies, timed spirometry, and airway resistance

Lung volumes were variable with mean values between 55 and 60% of predicted (Fig. 3). Total lung capacity ranged from normal (86% predicted) to severely reduced (33% predicted); DL_{CO} also ranged from normal (96% predicted) to severely reduced (15% predicted). With standard physiologic criteria based on percent predicted values of TLC (65–80% mild, 45–65% moderate, and <45% severe), 7 patients had mild restrictive disease, 12 had moderate disease, and 3 had severe disease. Applying the same criteria to the percent predicted values of DL_{CO}, 3 patients had a mild reduction, 12 had a moderate reduction, and 7 had a severe reduction in DL_{CO}.

Morphologic observations

The grading system used to estimate the degree of fibrosis, and the degree of cellularity in biopsy speci-

TABLE I

Clinical and Morphologic Data on 23 Patients with IPF

Clinical data							Morphologic data	
Patient	Symbol	Age	Sex	Duration of symptoms	Smoking history*	Drug history‡	Degree of fibrosis	Degree of cellularity
		yr		*yr*				
E.B.	○	48	M	1.5	Heavy	None	+1	+1
M.B.	●	60	F	2.0	Moderate	Prednisone	+3	+2
M.C.	◓	57	F	0.5	Nonsmoker	Phenylbutazone	+4	+3
R.C.	◒	66	M	0.5	Nonsmoker	Prednisone	+3	+3
R.I.C.	◐	32	M	0.5	Moderate	None	+2	+2
N.C.	◑	27	M	2.0	Light	Prednisone	+4	+2
A.D.	□	67	M	0.5	Moderate§	Prednisone	+4	+2
W.D.	■	43	M	0.5	Moderate§	None	+1	+1
G.F.	◧	51	M	2.0	Moderate§	Prednisone	+3	+2
A.H.	◨	27	F	2.0	Light§	None	+2	+2
W.H.	⬒	41	M	2.0	Light§	None	+3	+2
V.J.	⬓	27	F	0.5	Nonsmoker	None	+1	+1
W.L.	◪	67	M	10.0	Heavy§	None	+4	+2
O.N.	◩	27	F	1.5	Nonsmoker	Prednisone	+4	+2
P.R.	△	31	F	0.5	Moderate§	Prednisone	+2	+3
J.S.	▲	58	M	7.0	Moderate§	None	+4	+2
J.C.S.	◭	61	M	1.5	Heavy§	None	+4	+3
W.E.S.	◮	66	M	1.0	Cigars§	None	+4	+2
R.S.	⏶	52	M	2.0	Nonsmoker	Prednisone	+4	+2
J.K.S.	⏶	46	M	2.0	Moderate§	Prednisone	+4	+3
W.L.S.	▽	58	M	1.0	Moderate§	None	+2	+2
B.T.	▼	47	F	0.5	Nonsmoker	None	+4	+2
E.T.	⧨	55	M	5.0	Nonsmoker	None	+4	+2
Mean		48.4		2.0			+3.0	+2.0
±SEM		±2.9		±0.5			±0.2	±0.1

* Light <10 pack-yr; moderate = 10–25 pack-yr, heavy = >25 pack-yr.

‡ Only anti-inflammatory drugs are listed.

§ Stopped smoking >6 mo before study.

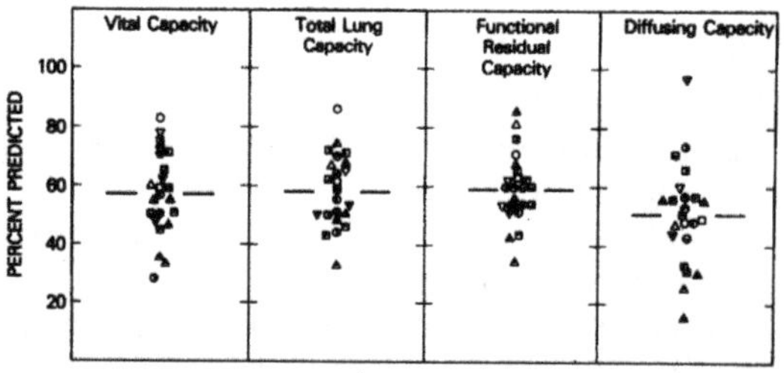

FIGURE 3 Distribution of lung volumes and diffusing capacity in 23 patients with IPF. Each symbol represents an individual patient; the key to the symbols is presented in Table I. Horizontal bars present the mean values.

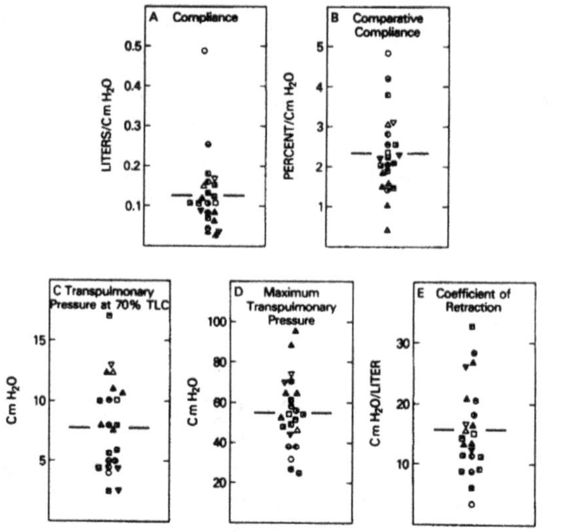

FIGURE 4 Distribution of (A) compliance, (B) comparative compliance, (C) P_{70}, (D) P_{max}, and (E) CR in 23 patients with IPF. Each symbol represents an individual patient; the key to the symbols is presented in Table I. Normal values are age dependent for compliance and comparative compliance and P_{70} (24, 27). The upper limits of normal for P_{max} and CR are 36 cm H_2O and 8 cm H_2O/liter, respectively (24, 26, 28).

mens was reproducible. Among three blinded observers, the average intra-observer coefficient of variation for grading of fibrosis was 6.2±1.2% and for the grading of cellularity was 8.0±1.5%. The mean inter-observer error was 8.0%.

3 biopsies (13%) demonstrated minimal fibrosis (+1); 4 biopsies had mild fibrosis (+2); 4 (17%) had moderate fibrosis (+3); and 12 had severe fibrosis (+4) (Table I). The average degree of fibrosis for all patients was moderate (+3). 3 (13%) biopsies had minimal cellularity (+1); 15 (65%) had mild cellularity (+2); 5 (22%) had moderate cellularity (+3); and none had severe cellularity (+4). The mean degree of cellularity was mild (+2).

Distensibility data

Compliance ranged from 0.03 to 0.49 liters/cm H_2O (mean 0.13±0.02 liters/cm H_2O). One patient (E.B.) had increased compliance, whereas 7 patients (R.C., R.I.C., W.D., G.F., A.H., P.R., W.L.S.) had normal or nearly normal compliance; the remaining 15 patients had reduced compliance (Fig. 4).

The volume-pressure curve, when expressed as a percent a predicted TLC, was shifted down and to the right in the majority of the patients (curves not shown). To quantitate the position of the curve when volume was expressed as a percent of observed TLC, P_{70} was computed (Fig. 1A). Whereas the average patient had a P_{70} of 7.6 cm H_2O (a value nearly normal for the mean age of these patients), seven patients (E.B., R.I.C., N.C., V.J., O.N., B.T., E.T.) had a reduced P_{70} (curves were shifted leftward). The remaining 10 patients had an increased P_{70}, indicating a rightward shift in their volume-pressure curves.

The comparative compliance of all patients ranged from 0.39 to 5.73% predicted TLC/cm H_2O. 74 percent (17 of 23) of the patients had values of comparative compliance that were reduced compared with those of age-matched controls; 4 patients (R.I.C., W.L.S., G.F., P.R.) had normal comparative compliance and 2 patients (E.B., R.C.) had increased comparative compliance (Fig. 4).

The maximum transpulmonary pressure at TLC (P_{max}) was increased in 78% of the patients (18 of 23) (Fig. 4); the average P_{max} of all patients was 54.4±3.8 cm H_2O. Of the 5 patients with normal P_{max}, 3 (V.J., R.C., P.R.) were between the ages of 25 and 35 yr.

CR was increased in 91% (21 of 23) patients; it was normal in 1 patient (W.D.) and was reduced in 1 patient (E.B.). In the entire group of patients, the average CR was 16.0±1.6 cm H_2O/liter compared with the normal range of 4.0–8.0 cm H_2O/liter.

Gas exchange data (Figs. 5 and 6)

Resting. In the entire group of 23 patients, the resting Pa_{O_2} ranged from 55.0 to 100.9 mm Hg (mean 73±3.0 mm Hg) and was normal (>80 mm Hg) in 8 patients (35%). The resting $A\text{-}aD_{O_2}$ ranged from 12 to 74 mm Hg (mean 38.8±3.7) but was normal (<15 mm Hg) in only 1 patient (M.C.) (4%). The average patient had mild alveolar hyperventilation (Pa_{CO_2}, 34.6±0.8 mm Hg) that was compensated to yield a normal pHa (7.42±0.09); no patient had CO_2 retention (data not shown). Assuming a normal arterial-venous oxygen content difference of 5 vol%, the average patient had a physiologic shunt of 10.9±1.4% (data not shown).

Exercise. Two patients were unable to exercise; M.B. had advanced osteoarthritis of the hips and W.L. required supplemental O_2 even with minimal exertion. Eight patients completed only stage I of the exercise protocol; four patients completed stages I and II: and nine patients completed all three stages. In general

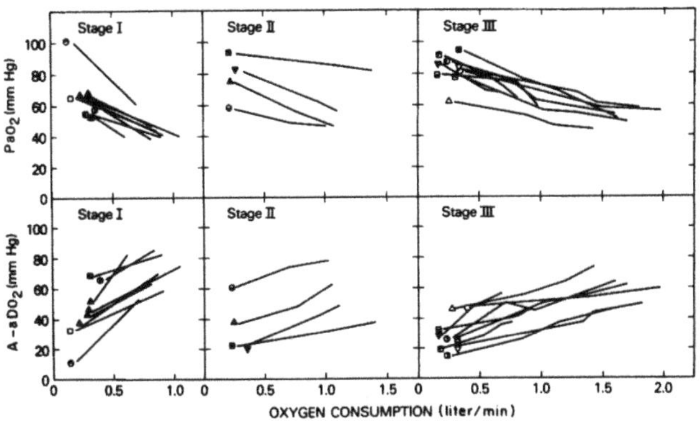

FIGURE 5 Resting and exercise gas exchange data in 23 patients with IPF. Each curve represents data from an individual patient; the key to the symbols presented to the left of each curve is shown in Table I. Values of Pa_{O_2} and $A\text{-}aD_{O_2}$ are plotted against power output ($\dot{V}_{O_2}$). Stage I presents all patients who could only exercise one stage, stage II presents all patients who exercise two stages, and stage III presents all patients who exercised all three stages.

the three stages of exercise reflected increasing $\dot{V}_{O_2}$. The average $\dot{V}_{O_2}$ at stage I for those who completed only stage I was 0.834±0.047 liters/min; this value did not differ significantly from the $\dot{V}_{O_2}$ at stage I (0.928 ±0.108 liters/min) for subjects who completed all three stages ($P > 0.1$). In addition, the average $\dot{V}_{O_2}$ at stage II for those who completed only stage II (1.140 liters/min) did not differ significantly from the average $\dot{V}_{O_2}$ at stage II for those who completed all three stages (1.104 liters/min, $P > 0.1$).

All 21 patients who completed stage I or greater demonstrated a fall in Pa_{O_2} and a rise in $A\text{-}aD_{O_2}$ with exercise. In general, exercise did not cause a significant alteration in Pa_{CO_2} or pHa except in the few patients who developed a mild metabolic acidosis at stage II or III.

For all patients, the Pa_{O_2} at the maximum stage of exercise achieved ranged from 38.3 to 81.8 mm Hg. The mean exercise Pa_{O_2} of patients who completed only stage I was 43.8±2.7 mm Hg, whereas the mean exercise Pa_{O_2} (at the highest $\dot{V}_{O_2}$) of patients who completed stage III was 59.0±3.0 mm Hg; these values were significantly different ($P = 0.002$). For all patients, the exercise $A\text{-}aD_{O_2}$ at the maximum stage of exercise ranged from 26.7 to 85.5 mm Hg. As a group, the maximum exercise $A\text{-}aD_{O_2}$ of those who completed only stage I (70.9±4.1 mm Hg) was significantly higher than the maximum exercise $A\text{-}aD_{O_2}$ of those who completed stage III (55.3±0.4 mm Hg) ($P = 0.016$).

For all patients, the absolute change in Pa_{O_2} between rest and exercise (exercise parameter 1) ranged from −9.6 to −39.9 mm Hg. Interestingly, even though the $\dot{V}_{O_2}$ of patients completing stage III (1.38±0.162 liters/min) was significantly greater than the $\dot{V}_{O_2}$ of patients completing only stage I of the exercise protocol (0.83 ±0.047 liters/min; $P = 0.004$), the mean values of exercise parameter 1 for groups I and III were not significantly different (stage I = −22.4 ±2.8 mm Hg; stage III = −20.8±2.3 mm Hg; $P = 0.64$). Similarly, for all patients, the absolute change in $A\text{-}aD_{O_2}$ between rest and exercise (exercise parameter 2) ranged from 13.0 to 48.2 mm Hg and there was no difference between the mean value of exercise parameter 2 for those completing only stage I compared with that of those completing stage III ($P = 0.39$).

In comparison to the absolute changes in Pa_{O_2} or $A\text{-}aD_{O_2}$ with exercise (exercise parameters 1 and 2), the change in Pa_{O_2} and $A\text{-}aD_{O_2}$ with increasing power output ($\dot{V}_{O_2}$) (exercise parameters 3 and 4) showed marked differences between the patients grouped according to the stage of exercise they were able to complete. Although $\Delta Pa_{O_2}/\Delta\dot{V}_{O_2}$ (exercise parameter 3) of the entire patient group varied from −9.2 to −78.1 mm Hg-min/liter, the mean value for those competing stage I (−43.8±6.1 mm Hg-min/liter) was significantly different from the mean value of those completing stage III (−21.5±3.3 mm Hg-min/liter, $P = 0.038$). In addition, although the $\Delta A\text{-}aD_{O_2}/\Delta\dot{V}_{O_2}$ (exercise parameter 4) of the entire patient group ranged from 8.0 to 106.6 mm Hg-min/liter), the mean value for patients completing stage I (53.6±10.6 mm Hg-min/liter) was

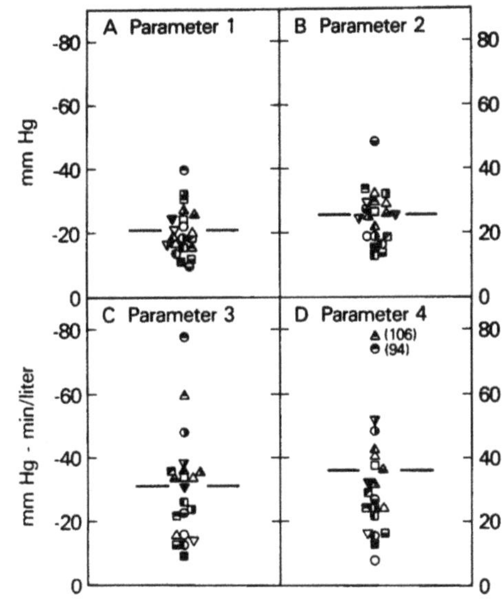

FIGURE 6 Derived exercise parameters in 23 patients with IPF. Each symbol represents an individual patient; the key is presented in Table I. All parameters are derived from the data presented in Fig. 4. A: exercise parameter 1 = Pa_{O_2} at maximal levels of exercise − resting Pa_{O_2}; B: exercise parameter 2 = $A\text{-}aD_{O_2}$ at maximal level of exercise − resting $A\text{-}aD_{O_2}$; C: exercise parameter 3 = change in Pa_{O_2} per liter oxygen consumed during exercise; D: exercise parameter 4 = change in $A\text{-}aD_{O_2}$ per liter oxygen consumed during exercise.

significantly different from the mean value of those completing stage II (24.4±4.5 mm Hg-min/liter, $P = 0.005$).

Comparison of morphologic data with clinical and standard physiologic data

The morphologic assessment of the degree of fibrosis and cellularity in lung biopsy specimens of the 23 patients did not correlate with age, sex, drug history, smoking history, or duration of symptoms (comparisons not shown). Of all clinical comparisons, only patient age had a trend toward correlation with the degree of fibrosis ($P = 0.054$); older patients tended to have more advanced fibrosis (+3 to +4).

Of the standard physiologic studies (V.C., T.L.C., F.R.C., and DL_{CO}), none correlated significantly with either the morphologic assessment of degree of fibrosis or degree of cellularity. Vital capacity did, however, show a trend toward correlation with the degree of fibrosis ($P = 0.05$), but could account for only ≅17% of the total variability ($r = 0.422$, $r^2 = 0.168$).

Similarly, when standard physiologic studies were ranked as mildly (+1), moderately (+2), or severely (+3) reduced compared with the predicted values (using Spearman rank correlation), there were no significant correlations with the morphologic data.

Comparison of the morphologic data with distensibility data (Table II)

Although almost all parameters derived from the static deflation volume-pressure curve correlated with the morphologic assessment of degree of fibrosis, compliance had the highest correlation coefficient ($r = 0.746$, $P = 0.001$). Comparative compliance, P_{max}, and CR also correlated significantly with the degree of fibrosis, but none could account for more than 42% of the observed variability (r^2 ranged from 0.31 to 0.42). In contrast, the morphologic assessment of degree of cellularity did not correlate with either compliance, comparative compliance, P_{max} or CR. There was a correlation between P_{70} and degree of cellularity ($r = 0.509$, $P = 0.013$); but this acounted for only 25% of the observed variability ($r^2 = 0.25$).

Comparison of morphologic data with gas exchange data (Table II)

There was no significant correlations between the morphologic assessment of either the degree of fibrosis or the degree of cellularity and either resting or exercise PaO_2 and $A\text{-}aDO_2$ or the absolute change in PaO_2 between rest and maximum exercise (exercise parameter 1). In contrast, there was a strong correlation between the morphologic assessment of degree of fibrosis with both the change in PaO_2 per liter oxygen consumed during exercise (exercise parameter 3, $r = 0.890$, $P < 0.001$) and the change in $A\text{-}aDO_2$ per liter oxygen consumed (exercise parameter 4, $r = 0.845$, $P < 0.001$). However, these latter two significant correlations were not selective for the degree of fibrosis; both exercise parameters 3 and 4 correlated with the degree of cellularity ($r = 0.556$ and $r = 0.449$; $P < 0.01$ for both). In addition, there was a significant negative correlation between $\dot{V}O_2$ at maximum exercise and the morphologic assessment of degree of fibrosis ($r = 0.692$; i.e., those patients with the most fibrosis were able to exercise the least). There was, however, no correlation between the degree of cellularity and $\dot{V}O_2$.

TABLE II
Comparisons of Morphologic Data with Distensibility and Gas Exchange Data in 23 Patients with IPF

Physiologic parameter	Morphologic comparisons*: Degree of fibrosis r	p	Degree of cellularity r	p
Distensibility data				
Compliance	−0.746	<0.001	−0.155	0.481
Comparative compliance	−0.583	0.004	−0.639	0.772
P_{70}	0.124	0.400	0.509	0.013
P_{max}	0.578	0.002	0.334	0.119
CR	0.655	<0.001	0.213	0.329
Gas exchange data				
Resting PaO_2	−0.231	0.288	−0.238	0.275
Resting $A\text{-}aDO_2$	0.377	0.735	0.095	0.667
Exercise PaO_2	−0.408	0.066	−0.362	0.107
Exercise $A\text{-}aDO_2$	0.208	0.367	0.383	0.087
$\dot{V}O_2$ (highest)	−0.692	<0.001	−0.200	0.385
Exercise parameter 1	0.356	0.113	−0.195	0.396
Exercise parameter 2	0.319	0.159	0.474	0.030
Exercise parameter 3	−0.890	<0.001	0.556	0.009
Exercise parameter 4	0.845	<0.001	0.449	0.041

* All comparisons were made with Spearman rank correlation.

Comparisons between the various physiologic studies

There was a significant correlation between compliance and the following: TLC ($r = 0.622$; $P = 0.002$), VC ($r = 0.582$; $P = 0.004$), P_{max} ($r = -0.538$; $P - 0.008$), and CR ($r = -0.661$; $P < 0.001$). In addition, compliance correlated with the change in PaO_2 per liter O_2 consumed during exercise (exercise parameter 3:

$r = -0.574$, $P = 0.007$) and the change in A-aDO_2 per liter O_2 consumed during exercise (exercise parameter 4: $r = -0.469$, $P = 0.032$). Similarly, there was a weak, but significant correlation between P_{max} and CR with exercise parameters 3 and 4 ($r < 0.4$; $P < 0.04$). There were no other remarkable correlations among the various physiologic studies.

DISCUSSION

To identify those physiologic studies that are most useful in staging and following the severity of the disease in IPF, we characterized the physiologic alterations in a relatively homogenous group of patients with this disease in mid-course and compared these data with the morphologic assessment of the degree of fibrosis and the degree of cellularity in their biopsies. These correlations demonstrate that (*a*) physiologic parameters assessing lung distensibility correlate very well with the morphologic assessment of the degree of fibrosis, but poorly with the degree of cellularity; (*b*) exercise-induced changes in gas exchange correlate with the degree of fibrosis and to a lesser extent with the degree of cellularity; and (*c*) lung volumes and diffusing capacity do not correlate with either morphologic parameter.

Physiologic alterations in IPF. The average patient in the current study had reduced lung volumes and diffusing capacity, reduced compliance, and hypoxemia that worsened with exercise. These physiologic alterations are classic for IPF and useful diagnostically (2, 4, 8–10).

All patients had either reduced lung volumes (V.C., T.L.C.) or reduced DL_{CO}, and the majority had a reduction in both. Lung compliance at FRC was, however, less sensitive to the presence of disease; only two-thirds of all patients had reduced compliance, whereas nearly one-third had normal or nearly normal compliance. Furthermore, the sensitivity of this measurement was only minimally improved by adjusting this value for the reduction in lung volume (comparative compliance).

P_{max} was increased in 80% of the study patients. Although the maximum value of P_{max} in the current study was higher than those previously recorded by Yernault et al. (28), the mean values were similar in both studies. It has been suggested that the discriminatory power of P_{max} in interstitial lung disease is greater when it is related to the measured lung volume as the CR (26). Our data support this; CR was increased in the majority of patients, being normal or reduced in only two patients (W.D., E.B.), both of whom had minimal fibrosis.

Although the average patient in the current study had mild resting hypoxemia, over one-third had normal values. In contrast only one patient (M.C.) had a normal A-aDO_2 at rest, suggesting that the A-aDO_2 is a sensitive test for the detection of interstitial lung disease.

Exercise gas exchange in IPF. Arterial hypoxemia that worsens during exercise is a well-documented and diagnostically useful feature of IPF (8, 38–40). Although the hypoxemia of IPF was initially thought to be the result of an oxygen diffusion defect, it has been shown that both resting and exercise-induced hypoxemia in this disease mainly results from ventilation-perfusion imbalance (36, 37). Uncommonly, patients with IPF exhibit an improvement in PaO_2 during exercise. This has been reported mainly in patients with co-existing obstructive lung disease (11). Other associated conditions that could result in improvement of PaO_2 during exercise include chronic bronchitis, and localized lower lobe on lobar diseae. All of these conditions would be expected to improve ventilation-perfusion imbalance during exercise by either mobilizing secretions or by improving ventilation to areas that are relatively hypoventilated at rest (40, 41). For this reason, to attempt to make the study population as homogeneous as possible, we only included IPF patients in the current study who had roentgenographic evidence of diffuse disease, no history of bronchitis, and a normal forced expiratory volume in 1 s/forced VC.

To help quantitate the changes in exercise-induced gas exchange alterations in IPF, four parameters were derived from the exercise data. Exercise parameters 1 and 2 quantitate the absolute changes in PaO_2 and A-aDO_2 from rest to maximum exercise. Although the study population varied in the clinical assessment of the severity of their disease and with the stage attained during exercise, there was no difference between the mean values of either exercise parameter 1 or exercise parameter 2 among those completing stage I compared with those completing stage III. It is evident, however, that exercise parameters 1 and 2 disregard the relative changes in power output ($\dot{V}O_2$) required to bring about these alterations. To circumvent this problem, we adjusted the absolute changes in PaO_2 and A-aDO_2 for the change in power output; exercise parameter 3 quantitates the change in PaO_2 during exercise per liter oxygen consumption, and exercise parameter 4 quantitates the change in A-aDO_2 during exercise per liter oxygen consumption. It is possible to do this because the changes in PaO_2 and A-aDO_2 during exercise in IPF are essentially linear (Fig. 2). In general, there was a good correlation between the value of exercise parameters 3 and 4 and the stage of exercise they were able to complete. Furthermore, those patients with clinically more severe disease and who completed only stage I, had a significantly higher value of exercise parameters 3 and 4 compared with those with less severe disease who completed all three stages of the exercise protocol.

Morphologic evaluation of IPF. Using current technology, the definitive assessment of fibrosis and cellularity in IPF must be based on morphologic standards. To use morphology to assess the usefulness of various physiologic parameters in IPF, we used specific morphologic criteria to semi-quantitate the degree of fibrosis and cellularity in biopsy specimens. With these criteria, the assessment of the degree of fibrosis and the degree of cellularity was reproducible with a small intra- and inter-observer variability.

Based on clinical presentation and duration of symptoms, the study population was judged to be mid-course in their disease (8–10, 42). This judgment was complemented by the morphology of the biopsy specimens. No patient had hyaline membranes (e.g., no early disease), none had honeycomb lung (13), and the average patient had moderate (+3) fibrosis and mild (+2) cellularity.

It could be argued that a lung biopsy is not representative of the overall morphologic alterations in IPF and that multiple samples from an inflated post-mortem lung are necessary to accurately assess the degree of fibrosis and cellularity. It is critical, however, that the evaluation of fibrosis and cellularity be done on biopsy specimens because (*a*) the assessment of fibrosis and cellularity in IPF is of most interest early and mid-course in the disease, at which time response to therapy is most likely to be best; (*b*) the most common cause of death in patients with IPF is overwhelming pulmonary infection (42). Such an insult is accompanied by large numbers of inflammatory cells that will alter the status of the overall cellularity grading, and inflammatory cells may release enzymes such as collagenase that may alter the status of interstitial fibrous tissue (43); and (*c*) for correlates to be made between morphologic and physiologic findings in IPF, the morphology must be obtained in proximity to the time of physiologic evaluation; this is impossible when relying on postmortem material.

Thus, to semi-quantitate the degree of fibrosis and cellularity in IPF in mid-course, it is mandatory that biopsy, and not autopsy material be used. To minimize error, the degree of fibrosis and the degree of cellularity were graded independently, using special stains for fibrous tissue (Masson) and hematoxylin–eosin for cells. In addition, only patients with diffuse disease were included in this study. Furthermore, to attempt to obtain tissue that is representative of the overall disease process, biopsies were performed in areas that appeared average on chest roentgenogram. This was complimented by direct vision at thoracotomy. Those biopsies from outside institutions were used in this study only when it was clear that they had been obtained from a representative area.

Morphologic-physiologic correlates in IPF. Although lung volumes and diffusing capacity are commonly used to stage and monitor patients with IPF, comparison of the morphologic data with VC, TLC, and DL_{CO} demonstrated no significant correlates. Whereas the comparison of VC and the morphologic grading of fibrosis approached significance, this correlation is at best a weak one. These findings are consistent with those of Gaensler et al. (44), who demonstrated a "fair correlation" between VC and the "overall severity of the anatomic lesion" among a group of patients with IPF, and no correlation with DL_{CO}. Thus VC, TLC, and DL_{CO} do not appear to be useful objective monitors of either the degree of fibrosis or the degree of cellularity in this disease. The reasons for the failure of these parameters to correlate with morphology are only speculative, but because TLC is largely determined by maximum inspiratory strength and by chest wall and lung recoil (45), it follows that fibrosis and(or) cellularity would contribute only to lung recoil and thus modulate only one of the factors that determines TLC. It also follows that the reduction in lung volumes allow for a greater mechanical advantage of inspiratory muscles such that the net inspiratory force can be increased beyond that normally attained, allowing for a greater distension of parenchyma at TLC (46). The fact that VC appeared to correlate more closely with the degree of fibrosis suggests that fibrosis contributes more toward determining residual volume than TLC. Possibly this is related to the increase in lung tissue volume and reduction in recoil pressure at functional residual capacity (46).

It is somewhat surprising that DL_{CO} fails to correlate with the morphologic assessment of either fibrosis or cellularity. This is possibly related to the number of factors that modulate the DL_{CO}, including ventilation-perfusion abnormalities, resistance to transport across the alveolar capillary bed, and capillary blood volume (47, 48).

Although standard physiologic studies did not correlate with the morphologic data, four of the five parameters used to assess lung distensibility correlated with the degree of fibrosis. Compliance was the best correlate, although comparative compliance, CR, and P_{max} also correlated with the degree of fibrosis. The fact that parameters of lung distensibility correlate with the degree of fibrosis is not surprising, because fibrous tissue is composed mainly of collagen, and collagen with its limited extensibility should affect lung distensibility (45). In contrast, the position of the volume pressure curve (P_{70}) did not correlate with the morphologic assessment of the degree of fibrosis, suggesting that many factors (e.g., cystic lung disease, lung tissue volume) also modulate the position of the volume pressure curve in this disease. In comparison to the significant correlates with the degree of fibrosis, only one parameter of lung distensibility (P_{70}) correlated with the morphologic assessment of degree of cellularity, and even this correlate was barely significant ($r^2 = 0.25$).

PaO_2 and $A\text{-}aDO_2$ at rest and at maximal levels of exercise are commonly used to evaluate patients with IPF. There were, however, no significant correlates between either the severity of fibrosis or degree of cellularity and these parameters. In contrast, Gaensler et al. (44), in a morphologic-physiologic correlative study of a variety of fibrotic lung diseases, found a significant correlation between $A\text{-}aDO_2$ at maximum exercise and an "overall histologic index." However, this latter study combined several different types of fibrotic lung disease with varying pathophysiology (4, 30, 49, 50) (IPF, asbestosis, silicosis, honeycomb lung) in the correlative morphologic-physiologic comparisons, whereas the current study used a homogeneous population of patients with IPF.

Whereas the PaO_2 and $A\text{-}aDO_2$ failed to correlate with morphologic data in our study patients, derived parameters from the exercise study did correlate with the morphologic data. Exercise parameters 3 and 4, which quantitate the changes in PaO_2 and $A\text{-}aDO_2$ in relation to power output, strongly correlated with the degree of fibrosis. These parameters were not, however, selective for fibrosis; both exercise parameters 3 and 4 also correlated to a lesser extent with the degree of cellularity. The failure of morphologic data to correlate with the resting and exercise PaO_2, $A\text{-}aDO_2$, and the absolute changes in PaO_2 and $A\text{-}aDO_2$ suggest that although fibrosis and cellularity may contribute to ventilation-perfusion imbalance, other factors apparently contribute more. This concept is supported by the recent studies in IPF demonstrating small airways disease, an alteration that may contribute to ventilation-perfusion imbalance (10). In addition, it has been suggested that pulmonary circulatory alterations can also contribute to ventilation-perfusion imbalance (51). Neither airways disease nor pulmonary vascular alterations appear to relate to the morphologic changes of fibrosis or cellularity (10, 52). However, when gas-exchange alterations are related to power output (exercise parameters 3 and 4), there are significant correlations with morphology, suggesting that both fibrosis and cellularity affect ventilation-perfusion imbalance and that the contribution of these morphologic features to gas exchange is constant during exercise.

Significance of anatomic-physiologic correlates in IPF. The demonstration of significant correlates between the morphologic grading of the degree of fibrosis and cellularity have important functional and clinical implications. First, these results suggest that the fibrotic process contributes, at least in part, to the physiologic alterations in IPF, especially those involving lung distensibility. Second, fibrosis and cellularity clearly contribute to gas exchange alterations during exercise in this disease. Third, because the prognosis and response to therapy is dependent upon the severity of fibrosis and degree of cellularity, these correlates may be useful in determining prognosis and response to chemotherapy. Preliminary data in our laboratory suggest that those parameters that correlate with fibrosis, particularly the parameters of distensibility, are good predictors of prognosis.

ACKNOWLEDGMENTS

The authors thank Doctors Byron McLees, Norton Elson, and John Bernardo for their helpful discussions; Dr. David Demets for statistical analysis of the data; Filippina Giacometti for her expert technical assistance; and Mrs. Exa Murray for her editorial assistance.

REFERENCES

1. Hamman, L., and A. R. Rich. 1944. Acute diffuse interstitial fibrosis of the lungs. *Bull. Johns Hopkins Hosp.* **74:** 177–212.
2. Austrian, R., J. H. McClement, A. D. Renzetti, Jr., K. W. Donald, R. L. Riley, and A. Cournand. 1951. Clinical and physiologic features of some types of pulmonary diseases with impairment of alveolar-capillary diffusion: the syndrome of "alveolar-capillary block." *Am. J. Med.* **11:** 667–685.
3. Rubin, E. H., and R. Lubliner. 1957. The Hamman-Rich syndrome: review of the literature and analysis of 15 cases. *Medicine (Baltimore).* **36:** 397–463.
4. Herbert, F. A., B. B. Nahmias, E. A. Gaensler, and H. E. MacMahon. 1962. Pathophysiology of interstitial pulmonary fibrosis: report of 19 cases and follow-up with corticosteroids. *Arch. Intern. Med.* **110:** 628–648.
5. Livingstone, J. L., J. G. Lewis, L. Reid, and K. E. Jefferson. 1964. Diffuse interstitial pulmonary fibrosis: clinical, radiological, and pathological study based on 45 patients. *Q. J. Med.* **33:** 71–103.
6. Liebow, A. A. 1968. New concepts and entities in pulmonary disease. *In* The Lung. A. A. Liebow and D. E. Smith, editors. The Williams & Wilkins Co., Baltimore. 332–365.
7. Scadding, J. G. 1974. Diffuse alveolar pulmonary fibrosis. *Thorax.* **29:** 217–281.
8. Crystal, R. G., J. D. Fulmer, W. C. Roberts, M. L. Moss, B. R. Line, and H. Y. Reynolds. 1976. Idiopathic Pulmonary Fibrosis: clinical, histologic, radiologic, physiologic, scintigraphic, cytological, and biochemical aspects. *Ann. Med. Intern.* **85:** 769–788.
9. Fulmer, J. D., and R. G. Crystal. 1976. The biochemical basis of pulmonary function, *In* The Biochemical Basis of Pulmonary Function. R. G. Crystal, editor. Marcel Dekker, New York. 419–466.
10. Fulmer, J. D., W. C. Roberts, E. R. von Gal, and R. G. Crystal. 1977. Small airways in idiopathic pulmonary fibrosis. Comparison of morphologic and physiologic observations. *J. Clin. Invest.* **60:** 595–610.
11. Carrington, C. B., E. A. Gaensler, R. E. Coutu, M. X. Fitzgerald, and R. G. Grupta. 1978. Natural history and treated course of usual and desquamative interstitial pneumonia. *N. Engl. J. Med.* **298:** 801–809.

12. Scadding, J. G., and K. F. W. Hinson, 1967. Diffuse fibrosing alveolitis (diffuse interstitial fibrosis of the lungs): correlation of histology at biopsy with prognosis. *Thorax.* **22:** 219–304.
13. Spencer, H. 1975. Pathogenesis of interstitial fibrosis of the lung. *Prog. Respir. Res.* **8:** 34–44.
14. Davies, D., J. S. Crowther, and A. MacFarlane. 1975. Idiopathic progressive pulmonary fibrosis. *Thorax.* **30:** 316–325.
15. Malmberg, R., E. Berglund, and L. Ader. 1965. Idiopathic interstitial fibrosis of the lungs: II reversibility of respiratory disturbances during steroid administration. *Acta. Med. Scand.* **178:** 59–66.
16. Brown, C. H., and M. Turner-Warwick. 1971. The treatment of cryptogenic fibrosing alveolitis with immunosuppressive drugs. *Q. J. Med.* **40:** 289–302.
17. Benson, M. K., and D. T. D. Hughes. 1972. Serial pulmonary function tests in fibrosing alveolitis. *Br. J. Dis. Chest.* **66:** 33–44.
18. Morris, J. F., A. Koski, and L. C. Johnson. 1971. Spirometric standards for healthy non-smoking adults. *Am. Rev. Respir. Dis.* **163:** 57–67.
19. Goldman, H. I., and M. R. Becklacke. 1959. Respiratory function tests: normal values at medium altitudes and the prediction of normal results. *Am. Rev. Tuberc. Pulm. Dis.* **79:** 457–467.
20. Gaensler, E. A., and G. W. Wright. 1966. Evaluation of respiratory impairment. *Arch. Environ. Health.* **12:** 146–189.
21. Dubois, A. B., S. Y. Botelho, and J. H. Comroe, Jr. 1956. A new method for measuring airway resistance in man using a body plethysmograph: values in normal subjects and in patients with respiratory disease. *J. Clin. Invest.* **35:** 327–335.
22. Milic-Emili, J., J. Mead, J. M. Turner, and E. M. Glauser. 1964. Improved technique for estimating pleural pressure from esophogeal balloons. *J. Appl. Physiol.* **19:** 207–211.
23. Lemen, R., M. Benson, and J. G. Jones. 1974. Absolute pressure measurements with hand-dipped and manufactured esophogeal balloons. *J. Appl. Physiol.* **37:** 600–603.
24. Turner, J. M., J. Mead, and M. E. Wohl. 1968. Elasticity of human lungs in relation to age. *J. Appl. Physiol.* **25:** 664–671.
25. Macklem, P. T., and M. R. Becklake. 1963. The relationship between mechanical and diffusing properties of lung in health and disease. *Am. Rev. Respir. Dis.* **87:** 47–56.
26. Schlueter, D. P., J. Immekus, and W. W. Stead. 1967. Relationship between maximal inspiratory pressure and total lung capacity (coefficient of retraction) in normal subjects and in patients with emphysema, asthma, and diffuse pulmonary infiltration. *Am. Rev. Respir. Dis.* **96:** 656–665.
27. Yernalt, J. C., and M. Englert. 1974. Static mechanical properties in young adults. *Bull. Eur. Physiopathol. Respir.* **10:** 435–450.
28. Yernalt, J. C., M. deJonghe, A. deCoster, and M. Englert. 1975. Pulmonary mechanics in diffuse fibrosing alveolitis. *Bull. Eur. Physiopathol. Respir.* **11:** 231–244.
29. Jones, N. L., E. J. M. Campbell, R. H. T. Edwards, and D. G. Robertson. 1975. Clinical Exercise Testing. W. B. Saunders Co., Philadelphia. 185–194.
30. Naimark, A., K. Wasserman, and M. D. McIlroy. 1964. Continuous measurement of ventrilatory exchange during exercise. *J. Appl. Physiol.* **19:** 644–652.
31. Whipp, B. J., and K. Wasserman. 1969. Alveolar-arterial gas tension differences during graded exercise. *J. Appl. Physiol.* **27:** 361–365.
32. Bendixen, H. H., L. D. Egbert, J. Hedley-Whyte, M. B. Laver, and H. Pontoppidan. 1965. Respiratory Care. The C. V. Mosby Co., St. Louis. 54.
33. Snedecor, C. W., and W. G. Cochran. 1967. Statistical Methods. Iowa State University Press, Ames, Iowa. 6th edition. 194–197.
34. Snedecor, G. W., and W. G. Cochran. 1967. Statistical Methods. Iowa State University Press, Ames, Iowa. 6th edition. 59–61.
35. Brownlee, K. A. 1960. Statistical Theory and Methodology in Science and Engineering. John Wiley and Sons, Inc., New York. 299–303.
36. Finley, T. N., E. W. Swenson, and J. H. Comroe, Jr. 1962. The cause of arterial hypoxemia at rest in patients with "alveolar-capillary block syndrome." *J. Clin. Invest.* **41:** 618–622.
37. Wagner, P. D., D. R. Dantzker, R. Dueck, J. L. DePolo, K. Wasserman, and J. B. West. 1976. Distribution of ventilation-perfusion ratios in patients with interstitial lung disease. *Chest.* **69**(Suppl): 256–257.
38. Stanek, V., J. Widimsky, J. Kasalicky, M. Nauratil, S. Daum, and L. Levinsky. 1967. The pulmonary gas exchange during exercise in patients with pulmonary fibrosis. *Scand. J. Respir. Dis.* **48:** 11–22.
39. Wasserman, K., and B. J. Whipp. 1975. Exercise physiology in health and disease. *Am. Rev. Respir. Dis.* **112:** 219–249.
40. Jones, N. L. 1977. The place of exercise testing in the investigation of patients with respiratory disorders. *Bull. Eur. Pathosiopath. Resp.* **13:** 425–439.
41. Jones, N. L. 1966. Pulmonary gas exchange during exercise in patients with chronic airway obstruction. *Clin. Sci. (Oxf.).* **31:** 39–50.
42. Stack, B. H. R., Y. F. J. Choo-Kang, and B. E. Heard. 1972. The prognosis of cryptogenic fibrosing alveolitis. *Thorax.* **27:** 535–542.
43. Horwitz, A. L., A. J. Hance, and R. G. Crystal. 1977. Granulocyte collagenase: selective digestion of Type I relative to Type III collagen. *Proc. Natl. Acad. Sci. U. S. A.* **74:** 897–901.
44. Gaensler, E. A., C. B. Carrington, R. E. Coutu, and M. X. Fitzgerald. 1975. Radiographic physiologic-pathologic correlations in interstitial pneumonias. *Prog. Respir. Res.* **8:** 223–241.
45. Mead, J. 1961. Mechanical properties of lungs. *Physiol. Rev.* **41:** 281–296.
46. Gibson, G. L., and N. B. Pride. 1977. Pulmonary mechanics in fibrosing alveolitis. *Am. Rev. Respir. Dis.* **116:** 637–647.
47. Hamer, J. 1964. Cause of low arterial oxygen saturation in pulmonary fibrosis. *Thorax.* **19:** 507–514.
48. Georges, R., G. Sauman, J. E. LaFosse, and J. Turiaf. 1975. Membrane-diffusing capacity and pulmonary capillary blood volume. *Prog. Respir. Res.* **8:** 198–212.
49. Seaton, A., N. L. Lapp, and W. K. C. Morgan. 1972. Lung mechanics and frequency dependence of compliance in coal miners. *J. Clin. Invest.* **51:** 1203–1211.
50. Lapp, N. L., A. Seaton, K. C. Kaplan, M. R. Hunsaken, and W. K. C. Mergm. 1941. Pulmonary hemodynamics in symptomatic coal miners. *Am. Rev. Respir. Dis.* **104:** 418–426.
51. McCarthy, D., and R. M. Cherniack. 1943. Regional ventilation-perfusion and hypoxia in cryptogenic fibrosing alveolitis. *Am. Rev. Respir. Dis.* **107:** 200–208.
52. McLees, B., J. Fulmer, N. Adair, W. Roberts, and R. Crystal. 1977. Correlative studies of pulmonary hypertension in idiopathic pulmonary fibrosis. *Am. Rev. Respir. Dis.* **115:** 354. (Abstr.)

Small Airways and Interstitial Pulmonary Disease

The concept of disease of the small airways was introduced in 1968 by Hogg and associates.[1] These workers defined the site and nature of obstruction of the airways in chronic obstructive pulmonary disease (COPD) at the small airways. Morphologically, small (less than 2 mm) airways were narrowed or obliterated by inflammation, mucus, or fibrosis. The concept of two components to disease of the small airways was introduced by them, *ie,* a reversible component due to acute inflammation or mucous plugging and an irreversible component due to fibrosis, distortion, and narrowing or obliteration of small airways. These findings suggested that disease of the small airways may be one of the earliest changes in COPD, and current data strongly support that suggestion.[2-4] The role of small airway disease in the eventual development of COPD, particularly emphysema, is unclear;[3,4] however, it is likely that small airway disease contributes to trapping of air and mechanical disruption of alveolar septae[4] and to the development of a distal chronic alveolitis. Once this last process has been initiated, the release of macrophagic or neutrophilic proteases may result in degradation of elastin and subsequent emphysema.[5]

In contrast to its occurrence in COPD, disease of the small airways was not considered to be a part of interstitial pulmonary disease until recently. Although grouped together because of common clinical, roentgenographic, physiologic, and morphologic features, interstitial pulmonary diseases are heterogeneous and have a variety of causes.[6] Just as COPD is characterized by an obstructive ventilatory defect with normal or increased pulmonary volumes, interstitial pulmonary disease has classically been characterized by a restrictive defect (reduced pulmonary volumes and compliance) without evidence of obstruction to airflow.[6] Because interstitial pulmonary disease is characterized morphologically by fibrosis of the supporting tissues of lung, primarily alveolar interstitium,[6] the concept of a restrictive ventilatory defect in this disorder is easy to accept. However, recent physiologic and morphologic observations indicate that disease of the small airways is not limited to COPD and that many of the morphologic and pathophysiologic features of COPD may be evident in interstitial pulmonary disease.

Although narrowing of small airways in acute idiopathic pulmonary fibrosis was mentioned by Hamman and Rich[7] in their original communication, only recently has emphasis been placed on small airways in interstitial pulmonary disease. Except for the "bronchiolitis obliterans interstitial pneumonia" described by Liebow and Carrington,[8] most reports have concentrated on alveolar pathologic abnormalities. The suggestion that functional alterations in interstitial pulmonary disease were consistent with small airway disease was made in 1973 by Ostrow and Cherniack[9] and subsequently by Yernalt et al.[10] Both groups found that some patients with interstitial pulmonary disease had evidence of increased resistance to airflow in small airways. In a study of 29 patients with idiopathic pulmonary fibrosis we[11] found small airways to be narrowed in 20 patients (70 percent). A detailed physiologic-morphologic correlative study of 18 of these 29 patients was made by obtaining pulmonary tissue and performing detailed testing of pulmonary function in the same patients.[12] Seventeen (94 percent) had peribronchiolar fibrosis or inflammation or bronchiolitis, and 12 (71 percent) of these 17 had narrowed small airways.[12] Furthermore, a good correlation was seen between the finding of narrowed small airways in the specimens from biopsy and two physiologic studies considered to be useful detectors of small-airway disease, *ie,* dynamic compliance and maximum expiratory flow-volume curves. Our study demonstrated that idiopathic pulmonary fibrosis is a disease that can involve small airways and that physiologic studies can define the function of small airways in this disease. Subsequent studies have shown that other diseases with pulmonary morphologic changes that can be indistinguishable from idiopathic pulmonary fibrosis (interstitial pulmonary disease associated with specific collagen vascular diseases and essential mixed cryoglobulinemia) may also have physiologic alterations consistent with disease of the small airways.[13-15]

Granulomatous interstitial pulmonary disease may also involve small airways. Young and associates[16] in 1967 demonstrated such an involvement by graulomata in patients with sarcoidosis. Although these workers noted no evidence of obstruction to airflow on simple spirometric testing, this publication preceded our current concepts of the relative insensitivity of this test to mild degrees of obstruction to airflow. Subsequent studies have shown that granulomata can involve small airways and that patients with sarcoidosis can have physiologic alterations consistent with disease of the small airways.[17-20]

At least three occupational or environmental interstitial diseases (hypersensitivity pneumonitis, asbestosis, and coal dust disease) have been shown to have physiologic alterations consistent with disease of the small airways.[21-23] A bronchiolo-alveolitis, the characteristic morphologic finding of hypersensitivity pneumonitis, is the morphologic equivalent of such functional abnormalities.[24] Similarly, the early morphologic change of coal dust disease is the coal macula which involves the small airways.[23]

Although many studies have now demonstrated its occurrence in interstitial pulmonary disease, small airway disease is not always present,[25-27] which suggests that several factors must determine its occurrence. These factors might include severity of the disease process, chronicity of the disease, susceptibility of the host, and certain environmental factors.[6,12,26,27] The functional significance of disease of the small airways is also variable. While it is likely that small airway disease is the earliest functional alteration in COPD, the significance of small airway disease in interstitial pulmonary disease is speculative. It is likely that disease of the small airways contributes to the ventilation-perfusion mismatching in interstitial pulmonary disease and hence to the hypoxemia of this disease.[6,12] In addition, small airway disease may be partly responsible for alterations in pulmonary recoil and pulmonary volumes[4] for example, trapping of air may mask the effects of alveolar fibrosis. Perhaps this is why pulmonary volumes correlate poorly or not at all with the severity of fibrosis in interstitial pulmonary fibrosis and in many of the inorganic dust diseases.[28,29] Disease of the small airways may also contribute to the development of chronic obstruction of airflow in interstitial pulmonary disease. Indeed, it is well documented but poorly recognized that some patients with interstitial pulmonary disease progress to show a pattern of chronic obstruction of airflow. The most notable example is chronic sarcoidosis, in which there may be functional evidence of chronic obstruction of airflow with an increased residual volume and normal or near normal total lung capacity.[30,31] Roentgenographically, there are dense areas of fibrosis with coexisting cystic lesions and hyperinflation.[31] Similarly, chronic obstruction of airflow may be present in patients with chronic hypersensitivity pneumonitis,[32] some of the inorganic dust diseases,[33] and chronic histiocytosis X of lung.[34] Although there are scant data on the mechanism of obstruction of airflow in these forms of interstitial pulmonary disease, both intrinsic narrowing of small airways and loss of elastic recoil probably contribute to the obstruction.[6,18]

In this issue (see page 473), McCarthy and associates describe two patients with idiopathic pulmonary fibrosis which rapidly progressed to COPD. Both patients initially had restrictive ventilatory defects (with normal timed spirometric data), but, in addition, both had evidence of increased resistance to airflow in small airways. Pulmonary biopsies in each showed an active alveolitis and either an obliterative bronchiolitis or endobronchiolar fibrosis. Both patients were treated with corticosteroids and improved initially. Six to 12 months later, both had physiologic, clinical, and radiographic findings typical of COPD. Pressure-flow studies indicated that a reduction in flow during maximum expiration was due mainly to reduced elastic recoil and increased dynamic compression. These data would be consistent with emphysema.[35] The report of McCarthy et al and the data cited in this editorial strongly support the concept that there are distinctive similarities between the interstitial and obstructive pulmonary diseases. The report by McCarthy et al also raises questions on the possibility of acute interstitial injury as a cause for COPD. It is well documented that acute bronchiolar injury can lead to COPD, for example, that resulting from acute inhalation of smoke.[36] Could an acute viral alveolitis and bronchiolitis or subclinical idiopathic pulmonary fibrosis do the same? Current data suggest that lobar emphysema is associated with acute viral pneumonias.[37] Certainly, influenza can be associated with physiologic alterations consistent with disease of the small airways.[38] This type of injury in the susceptible person may lead to classic COPD or to chronic obstructive disease of the small airways, as described by Macklem and colleagues.[39] Recently, Miller et al[40] suggested that sarcoidosis may cause diffuse bullous emphysema.

The report by McCarthy and associates also raises important therapeutic questions. Whereas Ostrow and Cherniack[9] and we[12] observed improvement in the physiologic abnormalities of small airways on treatment with corticosteroids, the two patients of McCarthy et al developed obstructive pulmonary disease despite corticosteroid treatment. This suggests that most small airways were irreversibly damaged, perhaps with fibrosis. Could agents that interfere with collagen synthesis, secretion, or cross-linking have altered the disease process? Of even greater importance is the question of the overall significance of small airway disease in interstitial pulmonary disease. Clearly, we should be actively investigating mechanisms of alveolar and bronchiolar injury and repair in both the "interstitial" and "obstructive" pulmonary diseases. The functional distinction between these two classes of diseases becomes less distinct as our knowledge of them increases.

*Jack D. Fulmer, M.D., F.C.C.P.**
Birmingham, Ala
*and William C. Roberts, M.D., F.C.C.P.***
Bethesda, Md

*Veterans Administration Medical Center and Department of Medicine, University of Alabama.
**Pathology Branch, National Heart, Lung, and Blood Institute.
Reprint requests: Dr. Fulmer, Department of Medicine (Pulmonary), University of Alabama Medical Center, Birmingham 35294

References

1 Hogg JC, Macklem PT, Thurlbeck WM. Site and nature of airway obstruction in chronic obstructive lung disease. N Engl J Med 1968; 278:1355-60.
2 Cosio M, Ghezzo H, Hogg JC, et al. The relations between structural changes in small airways and pulmonary function tests. N Engl J Med 1977; 298:1277-81.
3 Thurlbeck WM. Changes in lung structure. In: Macklem PT, Permutt S, eds. The lung in the transition between health and disease. New York: Marcel Dekker, Inc, 1979:17-41.
4 Macklem PT. Changes in lung mechanics: pressure-volume and pressure-flow relations. In: Macklem PT, Permutt S, eds. The lung in the transition between health and disease. New York: Marcel Dekker, Inc, 1979:53-71.
5 Kuhn C, Senior RM. The role of elastases in the development of emphysema. Lung 1978; 155:185-97.
6 Fulmer JD, Crystal RG. Interstitial lung diseases. In Simmons DE, ed. Current pulmonology. Boston: Houghton Mifflin Professional Publishers, 1979; 1:1-65.
7 Hamman L, Rich AR. Acute diffuse interstitial fibrosis of the lungs. Bull Johns Hopkins Hosp 1944; 74:177-212.
8 Liebow AA, Carrington CB. Alveolar diseases: the interstitial pneumonias. In: Simon M, Potchen EJ, LeMay M, eds. Frontiers of Pulmonary Radiology. New York: Grune and Stratton, Inc, 1967: 102-41.
9 Ostrow D, Cherniack RM. Resistance to airflow in patients with diffuse interstitial lung disease. Am Rev Respir Dis 1973; 108:205-10.
10 Yernalt JC, Dejoinghe M, DeCoster A, et al. Pulmonary mechanics in diffuse fibrosing alveolitis. Bull Physiopathol Respir 1975; 11:231-44.
11 Roberts WC. Histologic observations in idiopathic pulmonary fibrosis. (pp 773-776). In: Crystal RG (moderator). Idiopathic pulmonary fibrosis: clinical, histologic, radiographic, physiologic, scintigraphic, cytologic, and biochemical aspects. Ann Intern Med 1976; 85:769-88.
12 Fulmer JD, Roberts WC, Von gal ER, et al. Small airways in idiopathic pulmonary fibrosis: comparison of morphologic and physiologic observations. J Clin Invest 1977; 60:595-610.
13 Guttadauria M, Ellman H, Emmanuel G, et al. Pulmonary function in scleroderma. Arthritis Rheumatism 1977; 20:1071-9.
14 Wohlgelernter D, Loke J, Matthay RA, et al. Systemic and discoid lupus erythematosis: analysis of pulmonary function. Yale J Biol Med 1978; 51:157-64.
15 Bombardieri S, Paoletti P, Ferri C, et al. Lung involvement in essential mixed cryoglobulinemia. Am J Med 1979; 66:748-55.
16 Young RC Jr, Carr C, Shelton TG, et al. Sarcoidosis: relationship between changes in lung structure and function. Am Rev Respir Dis 1967; 95:224-38.
17 Young RC Jr, Headings VE, Bose S, et al. Alpha-1 antitrypsin levels in sarcoidosis: relationship to disease activity. Chest 1973; 64:39-45.
18 Kaneko K, Sharma OP. Airway obstruction in pulmonary sarcoidosis. Bull Eur Physiopathol Respir 1977; 13:231-40.
19 Levinson RS, Metzger LF, Stanley NN, et al. Airway function in sarcoidosis. Am J Med 1977; 62:51-9.
20 Carrington CB, Gaensler EA, Mikus JP, et al. Structure and function in sarcoidosis. NY Acad Sci 1976; 278: 265-83.
21 Allen DH, Williams GV, Woolcock AJ. Bird breeders' hypersensitivity pneumonitis: progress studies of lung function after cessation of exposure to the provoking antigen. Am Rev Respir Dis 1976; 114:555-66.
22 Jodoin G, Gibbs GW, Macklem PT, et al. Early effects of asbestos exposure on lung function. Am Rev Respir Dis 1971; 104:525-35.
23 Seaton A, Lapp NL, Morgan WKC. Lung mechanics and frequency dependence of compliance in coal miners. J Clin Invest 1972; 51:1203-11.
24 Seal RME, Hapke EJ, Thomas GO, et al. The pathology of the acute and chronic stages of farmers lung. Thorax 1968; 23:469-89.
25 Schofield NM, Davies RJ, Cameron IR, et al. Small airways in fibrosing alveolitis. Am Rev Respir Dis 1976; 113:729-35.
26 DeTroyer A, Yernalt JC, Dierekx P, et al. Lung and airways mechanics in early pulmonary sarcoidosis. Bull Eur Physiopathol Respir 1978; 14:299-310.
27 Bjerke RD, Tashkin DP, Clements DJ, et al. Small airways in progressive systemic sclerosis. Am J Med 1979; 66:201-9.
28 Fulmer JD, Roberts WC, Von Gal ER, et al. Morphologic-physiologic correlates of the severity of fibrosis and degree of cellularity in idiopathic pulmonary fibrosis. J Clin Invest 1979; 63:665-76.
29 Gaensler EA, Carrington CB, Coutu RE, et al. Radiographic physiologic-pathologic correlates in interstitial pneumonias. Prog Respir Res 1975; 8:223-41.
30 Miller A, Teirstein AS, Jackler I, et al. Airway function in chronic pulmonary sarcoidosis with fibrosis. Am Rev Respir Dis 1974; 109:179-89.
31 DeRemee RA, Andersen HA. Sarcoidosis: a correlation of dyspnea with radiographic stage and pulmonary function changes. Mayo Clin Proc 1974; 49:742-5.
32 Braun SR, doPico GA, Tsiatis A, et al. Farmer's lung

disease: long-term clinical and physiologic outcome. Am Rev Respir Dis 1979; 119:185-91.

33 Morgan WKC, Seaton A. Occupational lung diseases. Philadelphia: WB Saunders Co, 1975: 132-4, 174-92.

34 Basset F, Corrin B, Spence H, et al. Pulmonary histiocytosis X. Am Rev Respir Dis 1978; 118:811-20.

35 Leaver DG, Tattersfield AE, Pride NB. Contributions of loss of lung recoil and of enhanced airways collapsibility to the airflow obstruction of chronic bronchitis and emphysema. J Clin Invest 1973; 52:2117-34.

36 Kirkpatrick MB, Bass JB. Severe obstructive lung disease after smoke inhalation. Chest 1979; 76:108-10.

37 Fraser RG, Paré JAP. Diagnosis of diseases of the chest. Philadelphia: WB Saunders Co, 1979; 3:1431.

38 Little JW, Hall WJ, Douglas RG, et al. Amantadine effect on peripheral airways abnormalities in influenza. Ann Intern Med 1976; 85:177-82.

39 Macklem PT, Thurlbeck WM, Fraser RG. Chronic obstructive disease of small airways. Ann Intern Med 1971; 74:167-77.

40 Miller A, Teirstein AS, Chuang MT. The sequence of physiologic changes in pulmonary sarcoidosis: correlation with radiographic stages and response to therapy. Mt Sinai J Med 1977; 44:852-65.

Self-Induced Pulmonary Granulomatosis*

A Consequence of Intravenous Injection of Drugs Intended for Oral Use

Bruce F. Waller, M.D.; William J. Brownlee, M.D.; and William C. Roberts, M.D., F.C.C.P.

Dr. William C. Roberts: Herein we will discuss pulmonary and cardiac findings in a girl who injected into her systemic veins dissolved drugs originally intended for oral use. Dr. Brownlee will describe the patient.

*From the Pathology Branch, National Heart, Lung, and Blood Institute, National Institutes of Health, Bethesda, Md, and the District of Columbia Medical Examiner's Office, Washington, DC.
Reprint requests: Dr. Roberts, National Institutes of Health, Bldg 10A, Room 3E30, Bethesda 20205

Dr. William J. Brownlee: An 18-year-old white woman began injecting heroin intravenously at the age of 15 years, about 30 months before her death.

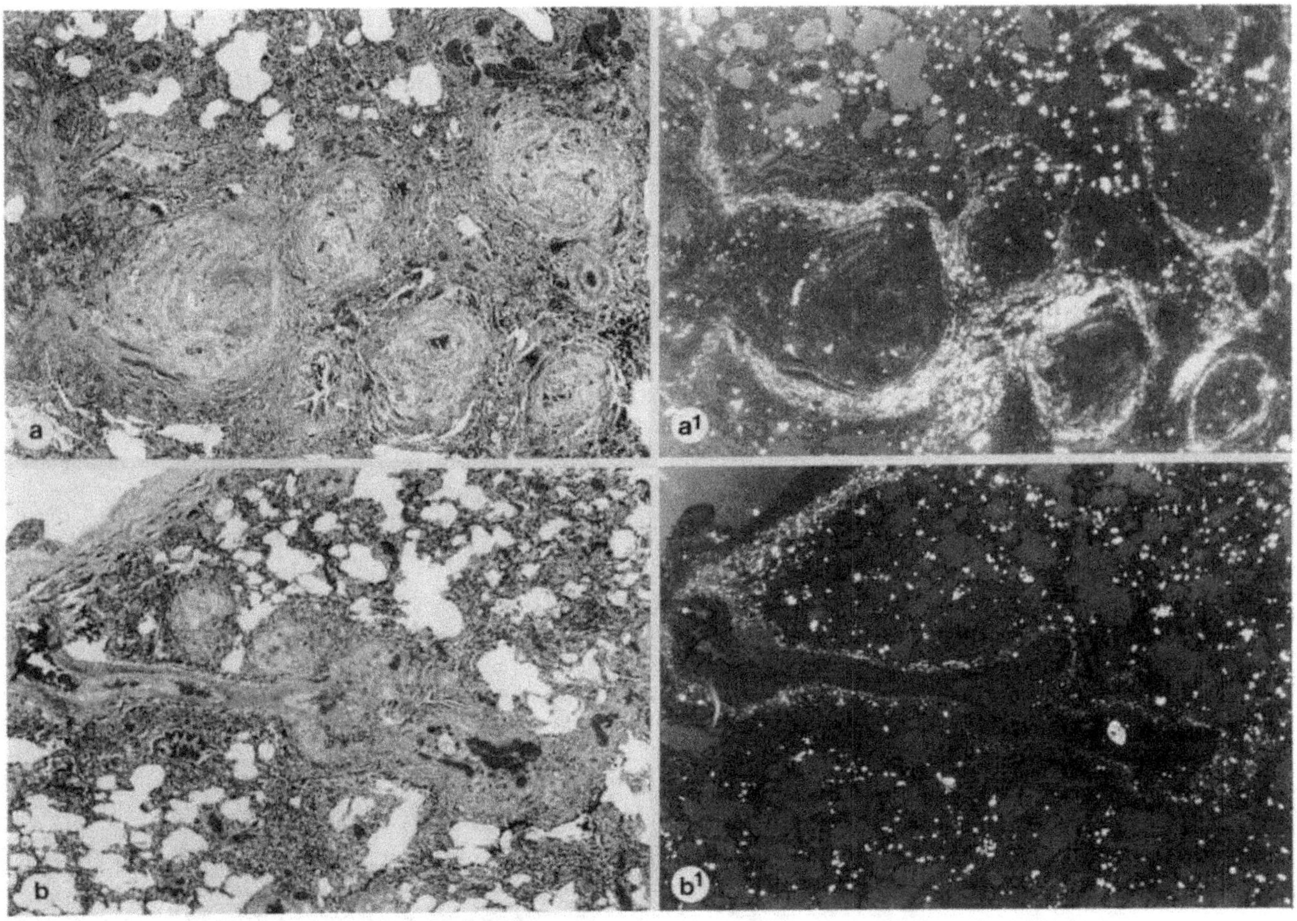

FIGURE 1. Multiple talc granulomas in pulmonary interstitium (*a* and *a*¹) and within lumen of pulmonary artery (*b* and *b*¹). Polarized sections (*a*¹ and *b*¹) are from the same areas shown in *a* and *b*, respectively. Refractile material, for most part, represents talc (hematoxylin-eosin, original magnifications × 60 [*a* and *a*¹] and × 22 [*b* and *b*¹]).

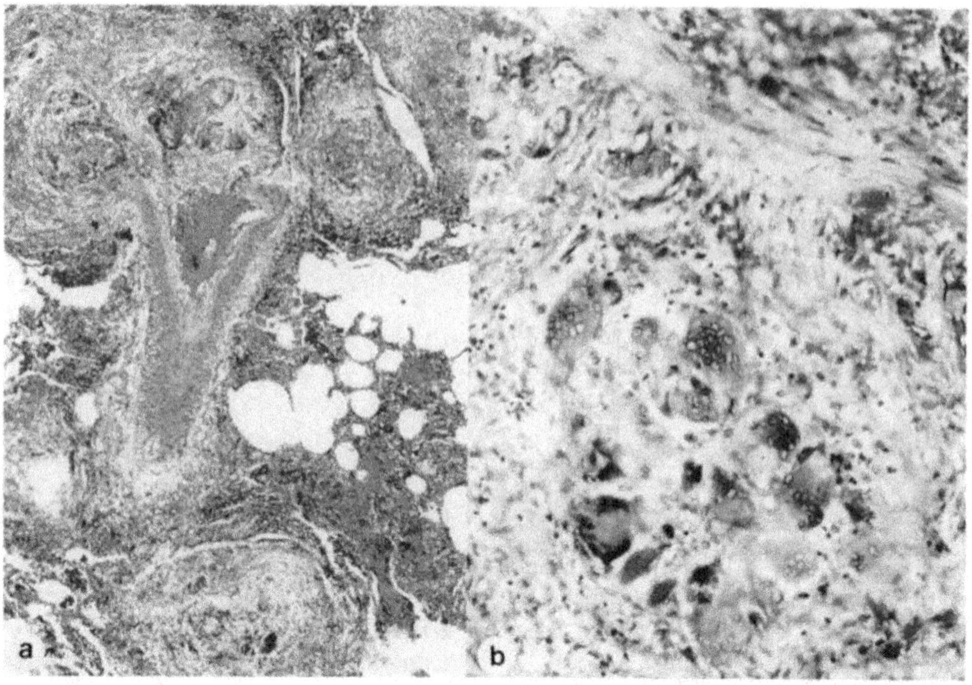

FIGURE 2. Talc granulomas located within pulmonary artery (*a*) and close-up of large granuloma adjacent to pulmonary artery (*b*) (hematoxylin-eosin, original magnifications × 100 [*a*] and × 220 [*b*]).

About six months later, she began injecting regularly into her systemic veins various other drugs, including methylphenidate (Ritalin), after dissolving them in liquids. She noted periodic wheezing and exertional dyspnea about 12 months before death, and these symptoms gradually progressed thereafter. The patient died suddenly at home after an episode of severe dyspnea. She had never sought medical care.

At necropsy, the surfaces of both lungs appeared normal; but on sectioning, multiple small (about 1 to 2 mm) relatively firm lesions were present throughout all lobes. Histologically, these little nodules were granulomas containing refractile material typical of talc (Fig 1 and 2). The alveolar septa contained similar refractile material and also numerous inflammatory cells (Fig 3). In addition, the media and intima of many pulmonary arteries

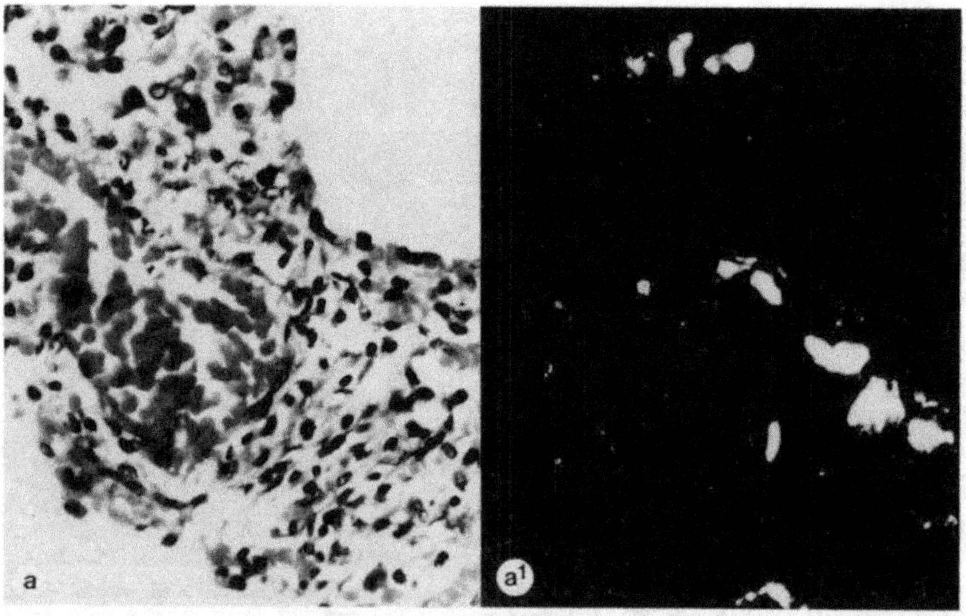

FIGURE 3. Alveolar septum containing many mononuclear inflammatory cells producing "active-appearing" alveolitis (*a*). Same section polarized is shown (*b*). Lumina of septal capillaries contain birefringent particles typical of talc (*b*) (hematoxylin-eosin, original magnification × 500).

were thickened, and many small pulmonary arteries were totally obstructed by talc-containing granulomas (Fig 2). The heart, which weighed 440 gm, was typical of that observed in cor pulmonale; both the right atrial and right ventricular cavities were dilated, and their walls were quite thickened; the tricuspid valvular anulus was dilated.

Dr. Roberts: This girl obviously died from self-induced pulmonary granulomatosis, causing morphologic evidence of severe pulmonary hypertension. Because it holds the components of the pill together, talc is present in virtually all tablets; and, consequently, if tablets of nearly any variety are dissolved in a fluid and injected into systemic veins, rather than swallowed, pulmonary talc granulomas are the expected consequence. If few talc granulomas form, no functional consequence ensues. If numerous talc granulomas develop, the consequence is either obstruction of the lumina of many pulmonary arteries, producing pulmonary hypertension and cor pulmonale or interstitial pulmonary fibrosis or both. Although nearly all contain talc, the tablets most commonly used for intravenous injection after crushing and dissolving are methylphenidate (Ritalin) (as in our patient), methadone, tripalennamine (Pyribenzamine), propoxyphene hydrochloride (Darvon), phenmetrazine (Preludin), and amphetamines.

Dr. Waller, would you summarize the findings in previously reported necropsies of patients with pulmonary talc granulomatosis?

Dr. Bruce F. Waller: From 1950 to June 1979, at least 16 necropsies of patients with pulmonary talc granulomas from intravenous injection of dissolved tablets were reported (Table 1).[1-12] All patients were known to have repeatedly injected intravenously drugs intended for oral use for periods ranging from 2 to 20 years (average, ten years). In each patient, foreign material consistent with talc was present in the pulmonary granulomas. The 16 patients ranged in age from 22 to 52 years (average, 31 years); 13 were men, and three were women. In all 16 patients the granulomas were present in both pulmonary interstitium and in the lumina of the

Table 1—*Data from 16 Necropsies of Patients with Pulmonary Talc Granulomas from Intravenous Injection of Dissolved Tablets*

		Duration of Addiction, yr*			Pulmonary Granuloma**		Alveolitis†				Pulmonary Arteries‡			Weight of Heart,	RV Wall
Reference	Patient's Sex and Age (yr)	IV	Oral	Total	PA	I	Leu	PC	Lym	AH	MT	IT	PL	gm	>5 mm§
Spain[1]	M, ...	...	...	...	+	++	−	−	−	−	0	0	0	...	+
Wendt et al[2]	F, 32	← 2→		2	++	+	+	−	+	+	+	+	+	720	+
Burton et al[3]	M, 25	...	...	...	+	++	−	−	−	+	0	0	0	400	+
Butz[4]	M, 29	...	...	...	++	+	+	−	+	+	+	+	+	375	+
Hahn et al[5]	M, 30	...	...	...	+	++	−	−	−	−	0	0	0	...	−
Hahn et al[5]	F, 28	...	...	...	+	++	−	−	−	−	0	0	+	...	−
Bainborough and Jerico[6]	M, 35	...	...	...	+	++	−	−	−	−	0	0	0	...	+
Douglas et al[7]	M, 52	←30→		30	+	++	−	−	−	−	0	0	0	...	+
	F, 28	←10→		10	+	++	−	−	−	−	0	0	0	...	−
	M, 42	← 5→		5	+	+	−	−	−	−	+	+	+	...	−
Lewman[8]	M, 30	← 7→		7	++	+	−	−	−	−	+	+	+	400	+
Groth et al[9]	M, 40	5	?	5	+	++	−	−	+	−	−	−	−	...	+
Genereux and Emson[10]	M, 52	←25→		25	+	++	−	−	−	−	0	0	0	...	+
	M, 32	←"Many"→		...	+	++	−	−	+	−	0	0	0	...	0
Arnett et al[11]	M, 22	← 7→		7	++	+	−	−	−	−	+	+	+	550	+
Paré et al[12]	M, 25	5	1.5	6.5	+	++	−	−	−	−	−	−	−	...	−

*IV, intravenous.
**PA, pulmonary arteries; and I, interstitium.
†Leu, leukocytes; PC, plasma cells; Lym, lymphocytes; and AH, alveolar hemorrhage.
‡MT, medial thickening; IT, intimal thickening; and PL, plexiform lesion.
§RV, right ventricular.

pulmonary arteries. In 11 patients the interstitium appeared to be the predominant location; in four, the pulmonary arteries were the predominant location; and in one patient, it was not mentioned. The interstitial location led to pulmonary interstitial fibrosis, and the arterial location led to pulmonary arterial narrowing with changes consistent with pulmonary hypertension. The patients who had been taking dissolved tablets intravenously the longest tended to have the talc granulomas located primarily in the pulmonary interstitium, and those with the shortest duration of addiction tended to have the granulomas predominantly in the lumina of the pulmonary arteries. Morphologic evidence (right ventricular hypertrophy or pulmonary arterial changes or both) of pulmonary arterial hypertension was present in 13 of the 16 patients. In addition to the 16 necropsies, at least 13 living patients[1,5,11,13,14] have been reported to have talc granulomas in pulmonary biopsies. Of them, seven had pulmonary arterial changes indicative of pulmonary hypertension. Thus, of 29 previous reports of cases of pulmonary talc granulomas, 20 had morphologic evidence of pulmonary hypertension, and six had plexiform lesions indicating that the pulmonary hypertension was severe.[15]

Dr. Roberts: Dr. Waller, what does the roentgenogram of the chest disclose in patients with pulmonary talc granulomatosis?

Dr. Waller: The roentgenographic changes appear, to some extent at least to be dependent on the stage of the process at which the patient is examined. When the pulmonary granulomas are few in number, the pulmonary parenchyma is normal by radiographic examination. When the pulmonary granulomas are widespread and fatal, the pulmonary parenchyma by roentgenographic examination may still be normal.[4,12,16] Thus, a normal roentgenogram of the chest does not rule out the presence of extensive pulmonary talc granulomatosis. In a study of 17 living patients who administered intravenously at least 2,500 to 50,000 dissolved tablets of methadone during periods ranging from one to nine years, ten patients had normal and seven had abnormal chest roentgenograms.[12] The abnormalities consisted of widespread nodules measuring 1 mm or less in diameter (seven patients) and diminished pulmonary volumes (two patients). Surprisingly, pulmonary infarcts appear to be infrequent, despite the frequent total obliteration of the lumina of many pulmonary arteries. Of course, the patients with pulmonary hypertension may have dilated pulmonary trunks and right ventricular and right atrial cavities. The electrocardiogram in the latter patients also may provide evidence of right ventricular hypertrophy and right atrial abnormality.

Dr. Roberts: Dr. Waller, what alterations in pulmonary function occur in patients with pulmonary talc granulomatosis?

Dr. Waller: Relatively few reported necropsies of cases of fatal pulmonary granulomatosis were from patients who had pulmonary function tests during life, and most patients with pulmonary function tests have not had the pulmonary granulomatosis confirmed anatomically (biopsy or necropsy). Nevertheless, several patients who took dissolved tablets intravenously for long periods have undergone tests of pulmonary function.[12,14] The major functional abnormality is a slowed diffusion of air from the alveolar spaces to the alveolar capillaries (decreased diffusing capacity). A second abnormality described is an increased period of time to expel a certain amount of pulmonary air (diminished forced expiratory volume in one second and diminished midexpiratory flow rate). These latter disturbances may result in an increased pulmonary volume (*ie*, hyperinflation). Whether or not this diminished expiratory flow rate and increased residual pulmonary volume are the result of the pulmonary granulomatosis or whether they are the result of associated cigarette smoking, which is extremely common in the drug addicts, is unclear. Surprisingly, despite the extensive distribution of the pulmonary talc granulomas, systemic arterial hypoxia is usually absent; or at least, cyanosis, except terminally, is uncommon. *Dyspnea* is the usual symptom resulting from the pulmonary talc granulomatosis. Again, clinical evidences of pulmonary infarcts are not reported.

Dr. Roberts: I have a few comments regarding pulmonary morphologic findings in patients with talc granulomatosis. As shown in Figure 1, numerous birefringent particles may be present throughout the pulmonary parenchyma. These birefringent particles are more numerous in alveolar septa not containing granulomas than in the granulomas *per se*. The alveolar septa usually contain many mononuclear inflammatory cells, producing a very "active"-appearing diffuse *alveolitis* as a consequence of the talc granulomatosis (Fig 3). The inflammatory cells generally consist of lymphocytes, plasma cells, and eosinophils; or at least, this was the finding in our patient. In our patient, large numbers of plasma cells and eosinophils were present in many alveolar septa. The alveolitis is consistent with the pulmonary functional abnormality of slowed perfusion of air from alveolar space to alveolar capillary. There has been

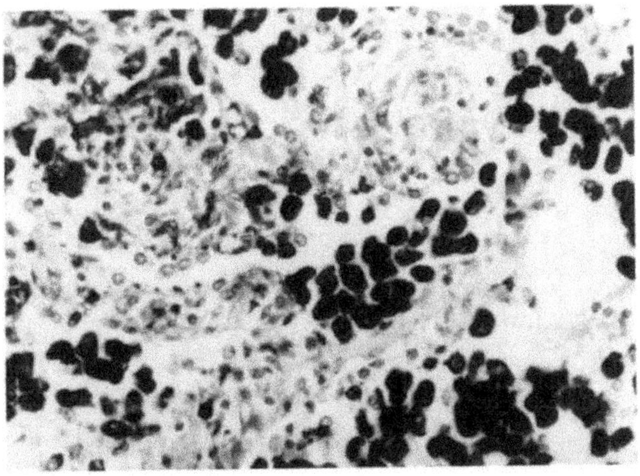

FIGURE 4. Hemosiderin-laden macrophages located within alveolar spaces (Mallory's stain for iron, original magnification × 400).

very little comment regarding alveolitis in previous reports on pulmonary talc granulomatosis. Another infrequently mentioned abnormality in the lungs of these patients is the presence of hemosiderin-laden macrophages within the alveolar spaces. We interpret this abnormality, which was quite extensive in our patient, as resulting from a rupture of the membranes of alveolar capillaries, allowing extravasation of erythrocytes and other blood products into the alveolar spaces (Fig 4). Thus, it might be possible to find hemosiderin or iron deposits in the pulmonary expectorates; however, talc spicules or granulomas are infrequent in the alveolar spaces.

I have one final comment regarding diagnosis. Some patients with pulmonary talc granulomatosis initially have evidence of severe pulmonary hypertension. A male patient with pulmonary talcosis, who was previously studied by us,[11] was initially diagnosed as having primary or idiopathic pulmonary hypertension. The finding of evidence of severe pulmonary hypertension in a man should arouse suspicion of the possibility of pulmonary talc granulomatosis as the cause of the pulmonary hypertension, because most patients with primary pulmonary hypertension are women, and most patients with pulmonary talc granulomatosis are men.

REFERENCES

1 Spain DM: Patterns of pulmonary fibrosis as related to pulmonary function. Ann Intern Med 33:1150-1163, 1950

2 Wendt VE, Puro HE, Shapiro J, et al: Angiothrombotic pulmonary hypertension in addicts: "Blue velvet" addiction. JAMA 188:755-757, 1964

3 Burton JF, Zawadzki ES, Wetherell HR, et al: Mainliners and blue velvet. J Forensic Sci 10:466-472, 1965

4 Butz WC: Pulmonary arteriole foreign body granulomata associated with angiomatoids resulting from the intravenous injection of oral medications, e.g., propxyphene hydrochloride (Davron®). J Forensic Sci 14:317-325, 1969

5 Hahn HH, Schweid AL, Beaty HN: Complications of injecting dissolved methylphenidate tablets. Arch Intern Med 123:656-659, 1969

6 Bainborough AR, Jerico KWF: Cor pulmonale secondary to talc granulomata in the lungs of a drug addict. Can Med Assoc J 103:1297-1298, 1970

7 Douglas FG, Kafilmont KJ, Patt NL: Foreign particle embolism in drug addicts. Ann Intern Med 75:865-872, 1971

8 Lewman LV: Fatal pulmonary hypertension from intravenous injection of methylphenidate (Ritalin) tablets. Hum Pathol 3:67-70, 1972

9 Groth DH, Mackay GR, Crable JV, et al: Intravenous injection of talc in a narcotics addict. Arch Pathol 94:171-178, 1972

10 Genereux GP, Emson HE: Talc granulomatosis and angiothrombotic pulmonary hypertension in drug addicts. J Can Assoc Radiol 25:87-93, 1974

11 Arnett EN, Battle WE, Russe JV, et al: Intravenous infection of talc-containing drugs intended for oral use: A cause of pulmonary granulomatosis and pulmonary hypertension. Am J Med 60:711-717, 1976

12 Paré JAP, Fraser RG, Hogg JC, et al: Pulmonary "mainline" granulomatosis; Talcosis of intravenous methadone abuse. Medicine 58:229-239, 1979

13 Szwed JJ: Pulmonary angiothrombosis caused by "blue velvet" addiction. Ann Intern Med 73:771-774, 1970

14 Robertson CH, Reynolds J, Wilson JE III: Pulmonary hypertension and foreign body granulomatosis, in intravenous drug abusers: Documentation by cardiac catheterization and lung biopsy. Ann J Med 61:657-663, 1976

15 Virmani R, Roberts WC: Pulmonary arteries in congenital heart disease: A structure-function analysis. Cardiovasc Clin 10:455-499, 1979

16 Hopkins GB, Taylor DG: Pulmonary talc granulomatosis. Ann Rev Respir Dis 101:101-108, 1970

Collagen Concentration and Rates of Synthesis in Idiopathic Pulmonary Fibrosis[1-2]

JACK D. FULMER,[3] ROBERT S. BIENKOWSKI,[4] MORTON J. COWAN,[5] SALLY D. BREUL, KATHRYN M. BRADLEY, VICTOR J. FERRANS, WILLIAM C. ROBERTS, and RONALD G. CRYSTAL

SUMMARY

To define the biochemical correlates of the apparent morphologic increase in lung interstitial collagen in idiopathic pulmonary fibrosis (IPF), collagen content was quantitated, and the morphologic degree of fibrosis was assessed in 9 patients with IPF and 6 control subjects. There were no significant differences in the collagen content among patients with IPF compared with that of control subjects. In addition, there was no correlation between collagen content and the morphologic assessment of the degree of fibrosis. Analysis of the collagen content from multiple sites made from base to apex of postmortem material from 3 patients with IPF and 2 control subjects demonstrated a wide, but similar, variation in collagen content in both groups; no definite pattern of anatomic distribution was found in either the patients with IPF or the control subjects. Furthermore, the rates of collagen and noncollagen protein synthesis in explants of lung of patients with IPF demonstrated no significant differences compared with those of the control subjects. The results of this study are consistent with the concept that IPF is a disease of an alteration in quality, form, and location of collagen rather than simply a disease of increased interstitial collagen.

Introduction

Idiopathic pulmonary fibrosis (IPF) is a fatal disorder of the lung associated with a progressive loss of lung volume and functioning alveolar-capillary units (1-11). It is grouped with the fibrotic lung disorders because patients with IPF have characteristic restrictive physiologic and morphologic findings of apparent increased fibrous tissue within the alveolar interstitium (5, 9, 10-12). The deposition of fibrous tissue is generally assumed to be an active process resulting from an increased synthesis of connective tissue components in response to injury (13).

"Fibrous tissue" is composed mostly of collagen, a group of heterogeneous but well defined macromolecules, characterized biochemically by distinct amino acid composition and relative resistance to proteolysis, and mechanically by limited distensibility (14, 15). Because patients with IPF have reduced lung compliance and apparent increased amounts of interstitial fibrous tissue, it would be expected that quantitation of collagen per unit amount of parenchymal tissue would reveal increases compared with that found in normal persons.

(Received in original form February 7, 1980 and in revised form April 16, 1980)

[1] From the Pulmonary Branch and Pathology Branch, National Heart, Lung and Blood Institute, National Institutes of Health, Bethesda, Maryland 20205.

[2] Requests for reprints should be addressed to Ronald G. Crystal, M.D., Building 10, Room 6DO6, National Institutes of Health, Bethesda, MD 20205.

[3] Present address: Department of Medicine, Veterans Administration Hospital, University of Alabama, Birmingham, Alabama.

[4] Present address: Pulmonary Division, Department of Pediatrics, Albert Einstein College of Medicine, Bronx, New York.

[5] Present address: Department of Pediatrics, University of California, San Francisco, California.

To evaluate the biochemical correlates of the implied morphologic and physiologic increases of interstitial collagen in this disease, we have compared collagen concentration in lung biopsy and autopsy specimens of patients with IPF and control subjects. To assess one aspect of the processes that regulate collagen deposition in the lungs of these patients, we have also quantitated the rates of synthesis of collagen in short-term explants of pulmonary parenchyma obtained at open lung biopsy.

Methods

Study population. The 11 patients (6 men and 5 women) included in this study met all of the criteria for IPF (5, 6, 8–11) (table 1). Their ages ranged from 27 to 66 yr with an average of 55 ± 5 SEM. The average duration of exertional breathlessness at the time of physiologic testing and open lung biopsy was 1.4 ± 0.2 yr. None of the patients had been on chemotherapy prior to, or at the time of, lung biopsy. Patients were judged to be mid-course in their disease; none had "end-stage lung" at the time of biopsy. All but one patient had reduced total lung capacity (mean, 54.2 ± 4.7% of predicted); all had reduced diffusing capacity (mean, 53.2 ± 3.9% of predicted); and all had a normal FEV_1% (mean, 109.2 ± 3.0% of predicted). Eight patients had resting hypoxemia, and all demonstrated a fall in arterial oxygen tension during exercise.

Biochemical studies were performed on open lung biopsies in 9 of the 11 patients, and on autopsy specimens in 3 who died as a result of their disease. One patient (WES) had a biopsy of all 3 lobes of the right lung; biochemical studies were performed on these specimens and also on autopsy specimens available 7 months later.

Patients used as controls were selected using the following criteria: (*1*) Patients having lobectomy or wedge resection for removal of a primary lung tumor or metastases of a distant tumor, but without clinical or radiographic evidence of diffuse lung disease, and no morphologic evidence of disease in the tissue sample used for biochemical analysis. (*2*) Patients who died of causes unrelated to lung disease in whom there was no prior history of lung disease.

There were a total of 8 patients (6 men and 2 women) in the control group (table 2). Their ages ranged from 15 to 70 yr (mean, 33.5 ± 6.4 yr). Histologic evaluation of all tissue from these control subjects showed normal lung.

Initial handling of tissue specimens. Lung samples obtained at open biopsy weighed 3 to 5 g (wet). Immediately after resection, the tissue was placed in sterile phosphate buffered saline (PBS; pH, 7.4, NIH Media Unit) at 4° C. Portions were taken for light and electron microscopy, as well as for bacterial, mycobacterial, and fungal culture. The remaining material was used for quantitation of collagen concentration (collagen/dry wt), DNA concentration (DNA/dry wt), and rates of collagen and noncollagen protein synthesis (see below).

TABLE 1

CLINICAL, PHYSIOLOGIC AND MORPHOLOGIC DATA OF PATIENTS WITH IDIOPATHIC PULMONARY FIBROSIS

Patient	Age (Yr)	Sex	Duration of Symptoms (Yr)	Vital Capacity* (% Pred.)	Total Lung Capacity* (% Pred.)	Diffusing Capacity* (% Pred.)	FEV_1% (% Pred.)	PaO_2* (mmHg)	PaO_2† (mmHg)	Biopsy Site	Degree of Fibrosis	Symbol
MB	60	F	2.0	50	51	57	124	71.8	55.8	LLL	+3	○
EB	48	M	1.5	83	86	48	96	80.5	56.8	LUL	+1	●
AH	27	F	2.0	75	71	66	98	93.3	54.0	LUL	+2	◐
WH	41	M	2.0	50	46	52	112	79.2	49.0	LUL	+3	◒
VJ	27	F	0.5	50	50	71	114	79.0	67.3	RLL	+1	◐
CM	27	F	1.0	45	60	54	96	—	—	RML	+2	◑
ON	27	F	1.5	42	43	57	104	89.5	71.0	LUL	+4	◔
WLS	58	M	1.0	78	68	60	114	80.2	59.0	RLL	+2	◔
WES	66	M	1.0	35	49	58	104	74.2	46.0	RUL, RML, RLL‡	+2, +4§	◔
BS	53	M	0.5	32	38	37	119	67.5	—	‖	+4	◕
RS	52	M	2.0	33	34	25	120	55.5	39.0	‖	+4	◕
Mean	44.2		1.4	52.1	54.2	53.2	109.2	77.1	55.3			
SEM	± 4.5		± 0.2	± 5.5	± 4.7	± 3.9	± 3.0	± 3.4	± 3.3			

Definition of abbreviations: LLL = left lower lobe; LUL = left upper lobe; RLL = right lower lobe; RML = right middle lobe; RUL = right upper lobe. See figures 1-5 for definition of symbols used.

* Methods used are described in reference (6).

† Arterial oxygen tension at maximal degree of exercise.

‡ Multiple samples from right lung obtained at autopsy were also analyzed.

§ The degree of fibrosis varied from lobe to lobe: RUL +4, RML +2, RLL +4.

‖ Open lung biopsy performed, but biochemical data available only from multiple samples of right lung obtained at autopsy.

In some cases, not all analyses could be performed because of the limited amount of tissue.

Quantitation of collagen and DNA concentration in tissue samples. Samples of lung tissue (biopsy or autopsy) were homogenized (30 s at 10,000 rpm) in 0.5 M of acetic acid using a Polytron (Brinkmann Instruments, Westbury, N.Y.) equipped with a microtip. To reduce foam, a drop of octanoic acid was added to each sam-

TABLE 2

CLINICAL AND MORPHOLOGIC DATA OF CONTROLS

Patient	Age (Yr)	Sex	Major Clinical Diagnosis	Biopsy Site*	Degree of Fibrosis*	Symbol
GC	27	F	Cervical carcinoma	RML	0	□
RE	70	F	Adenocarcinoma	RML	0	■
JF	30	M	Ewing's sarcoma	LLL	0	■
DH	15	M	Osteogenic sarcoma	RLL	0	■
NL	35	M	Osteogenic sarcoma	RLL	0	■
RL	16	M	Osteogenic sarcoma	RML	0	■
NO	45	M	Head trauma	Left†	0	■
NT	46	M	Myocardial infarction	Right†	0	■
Mean ± SEM	35.5 ± 6.4					

Definition of abbreviations: RML = right middle lobe; RLL = right lower lobe; LLL = left lower lobe. See figures 1, 3, 4, and 5 for definition of symbols used.

* Portion of lung used for these studies had normal morphologic findings.

† Multiple samples of lung obtained at autopsy were used for biochemical studies.

ple. After homogenization, aliquots of known volume were taken and lyophilized for measurement of dry weight, hydroxyproline, and DNA (16, 17). Dry weight was measured directly on an analytical balance, and hydroxyproline was quantitated by a modification of the method of Juva and Prockop (18), and DNA was quantitated by a modification of the method of Burton (19). The quantity of collagen in each aliquot was determined using the formula: collagen (μg) = [7.5] × [hydroxyproline (μg)] (17). From these measurements, the following were calculated: collagen/dry wt, DNA/dry wt, and collagen/DNA.

Histologic evaluation of degree of fibrosis in lung tissue. Tissue specimens were fixed in 10% buffered formalin, processed in alcohols and xylene, embedded in paraffin, serially sectioned at a thickeness of 6 microns, and stained with hematoxylin/eosin and Masson trichrome. Grading of the degree of fibrosis in each biopsy was made using sections stained with Masson trichrome, as follows:

No fibrosis (0). Normal lung.

Minimal fibrosis (+1). Areas of normal and nearly normal alveolar septums, but with areas showing interstitial fibrosis; no loss of alveoli or revision of parenchymal architecture; less than 10% increase in total collagen fibers compared with that of normal lung.

Mild fibrosis (+2). Mildly thickened alveolar septums; some areas of nearly normal alveoli; no loss of alveoli or revision of parenchymal architecture; 10 to 25% increase in collagen fibers compared with that of normal lung.

Moderate fibrosis (+3). Moderately thickened alveolar septums; rare areas of normal alveoli; scattered areas of disrupted parenchymal architecture; 25 to 40% increase in collagen fibers compared with that of normal lung.

Severe fibrosis (+4). All alveolar septums thickened to varying degrees, but recognizable alveoli still present; many areas of revised architecture with loss of normal parenchymal structure; greater than 40% increase in collagen fibers compared with that of normal lung.

Each biopsy sample was graded an average of 4 times, and the closest mean grade assigned.

Evaluation of biochemical methods used to quantitate collagen concentration. Two approaches were used to evaluate the reproducibility of the methods used to quantitate collagen/dry wt in lung samples: (*1*) To evaluate the precision of the entire assay, a large portion of lung was homogenized, multiple aliquots were taken from the homogenate, and collagen/dry wt was determined in each aliquot; and (*2*) to evalulate the accuracy of the assay for collagen, multiple aliquots were taken from a standard solution of hydroxyproline, and the content of hydroxyproline was determined in each aliquot.

Quantitation of the rates of collagen and noncollagen protein synthesis. Open lung biopsy specimens were minced in PBS (4° C) to pieces ≤ 1 mm, rinsed with PBS, and divided into portions weighing approximately 200 to 300 mg (wet). These aliquots of minced lung were then incubated in 2 ml of culture medium (equal parts of Dulbecco's modified Eagle's medium and PBS, supplemented with 0.5 mM ascorbic acid and 0.6 mM β-aminopropionitrile) (16, 17). All incubations were carried out in a Dubnoff metabolic shaker (Fisher Scientific, Pittsburgh, Pa.) at 40 cycles/min at 37° C, in an atmosphere of 95% O_2-5% CO_2. After a period of 45 min, the culture medium was replaced with fresh medium containing 5 μCi/ml of [^{14}C]proline (260 mCi/mmole, Schwarz-Mann, Orangeburg, N.Y.). Incubations were done in duplicate for 1, 2, 3, and 4 h. When the amount of tissue available was limited, the incubations were done in duplicate for 1 h and for 4 h.

After incubation, the tissue sample was rinsed 3 times with 10 ml of PBS (4° C) and homogenized in 5 ml of 0.5 M of acetic acid, as described above. Aliquots of the

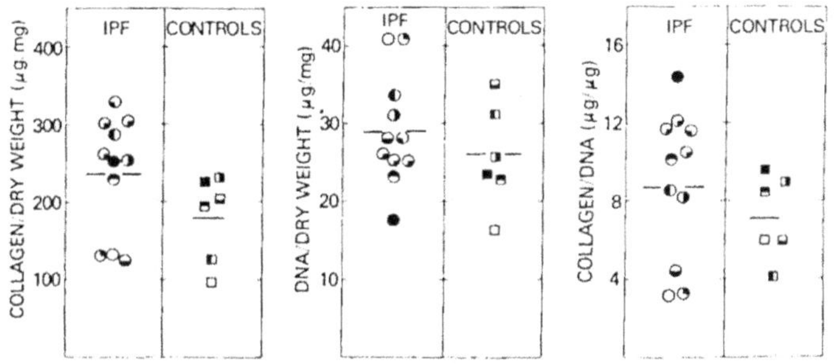

Fig. 1. Quantitation of collagen and DNA in lung parenchyma of patients with idiopathic pulmonary fibrosis (IPF) compared with control subjects. The mean value for all patients in each group is indicated by the horizontal bars. Each patient is identified by a symbol (to identify patient, see tables 1 and 2). Each symbol shown on the graph represents the mean value for all analyses on a single biopsy specimen; on the average, there were 7 analyses performed on each. Patient WES (◒) had biopsies of the right upper, middle, and lower lobes. Comparisons of the IPF and control groups demonstrated no significant differences in any category: collagen/dry wt (μg/mg): IPF, 237 ± 22; control, 180 ± 22, p = 0.16. DNA/dry wt (μg/mg): IPF, 29.0 ± 2.3; control, 25.8 ± 2.9, p = 0.38. Collagen/DNA (μg/μg): IPF, 8.9 ± 1.1; control, 7.2 ± 0.9, p = 0.42.

homogenate were taken for determination of DNA, [^{14}C]hydroxyproline, and [^{14}C]proline labeled noncollagen protein (16, 17). Because the rate of protein synthesis is dependent on the pool size of the isotope, the specific activity of free [^{14}C]proline in the lung explants was determined as previously described (16, 17). From these data, the following were quantitated: the rate of collagen synthesis (nmole of hydroxyproline synthesized/mg DNA-hour), the rate of noncollagen protein synthesis (nmol of protein incorporated into noncollagen protein/mg DNA-hour), and the percentage of collagen synthesis (the relative amount of protein synthesis by the explant that was devoted to collagen synthesis) (17).

Statistical methods. Two statistical tests were used, the two-tailed *t* test and Spearman's correlation. The former was used to compare mean values of biochemical data between and within patients with IPF and control subjects. The Spearman's correlation procedure was used to compare the morphologic ranking of severity of fibrosis with the concentration of collagen in lung biopsy specimens.

Results

Collagen and DNA in biopsy samples. The collagen concentration in open biopsy samples of lung parenchyma was quantitated in 11 biopsy specimens from 9 patients with IPF. Collagen/dry wt (μg/mg) varied from 120 to 330 μg/mg (mean, 237 ± 22 μg/mg) (figure 1). In comparison, the collagen concentration of 6 biopsy specimens from 6 control subjects did not vary as widely (90 to 245 μg/mg), but the mean value of 180 ± 22 μg/mg was not significantly different from that in the IPF group (p = 0.10).

The relative number of cells per unit of tissue (DNA/dry wt) from the patients with IPF varied over a twofold range (22 to 42 μg/mg), with an average of 29.0 ± 2.3 μg/mg. The number of cells per unit of tissue from the control subjects also varied over a twofold range (18 to 36 μg/mg). As with the values for collagen/dry wt, the mean control values for DNA/dry wt (25.8 ± 2.0 μg/mg) were not significantly different from those in the IPF group (p = 0.38).

Similarly, when the amount of collagen in a biopsy specimen was compared with the amount

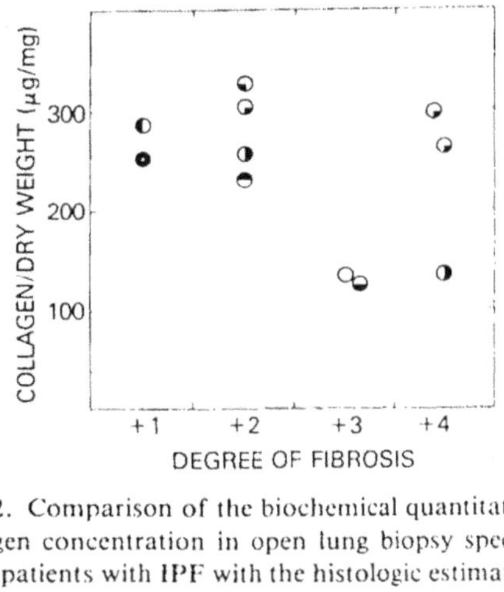

Fig. 2. Comparison of the biochemical quantitation of collagen concentration in open lung biopsy specimens from patients with IPF with the histologic estimation of "degree of fibrosis" on the same biopsy specimens. Each patient is identified by symbols defined in table 1; Patient WES (◒) had biopsies of the right, upper, and middle and lower lobes. The histologic estimate of "degree of fibrosis" was made using Masson trichrome stain. There was no significant correlation between the biochemical and histologic data (Spearman's correlation r = 0.52, p = 0.10).

TABLE 3

EVALUATION OF THE ASSAY USED TO QUANTITATE COLLAGEN PER DRY WEIGHT IN HUMAN LUNG SAMPLES*

Patient	Diagnosis	Source of Lung	Number of Aliquots of Homogenate	Collagen/Dry Wt in Each Aliquot (μg/mg)
WES	IPF	RML†	15	143 ± 7‡
NO	Control	RML	16	141 ± 21
NT	Control	RML	17	135 ± 15

* Lung tissue obtained at autopsy was homogenized and aliquoted; collagen/dry wt was then quantitated in each aliquot. The coefficient of variation of these assays ranged from 5 to 15% (mean, 12.8%).
† RML = right middle lobe.
‡ Mean ± SEM.

of DNA in the same sample (collagen/DNA), there were no differences between the patients with IPF (8.9 ± 1.1 μg/μg) and the control subjects (7.2 ± 0.9 μg/μg) (p = 0.42).

Comparison of biochemical and morphologic estimates of collagen concentration. The morphologic estimate of collagen concentration ("degree of fibrosis") in the open lung biopsies from patients with IPF demonstrated a broad range from minimal (+1) to severe (+4). One patient (WES) underwent multiple biopsies because the presentation of the disease was atypical, with the chest roentgenogram showing dense interstitial infiltrates in the right upper and lower lobes, but only sparse infiltration in the right middle lobe. Morphologic evaluation of the biopsies showed severe fibrosis in the upper and lower lobes and mild fibrosis in the middle lobe (table 1). Although the quantitative biochemical measurement of collagen concentration of the biopsies from these 9 patients also demonstrated a broad range of values (figure 1), there was no significant correlation between the morphologic and biochemical estimates of collagen concentration (r = 0.52, p = 0.10) (figure 2).

Evaluation of the assay used to quantitate collagen concentration. Quantitation of collagen/dry wt in a sample of lung tissue was accomplished by homogenizing the tissue in 0.5 M of acetic acid, and taking aliquots for measurement of hydroxyproline and dry wt. There are 3 potential sources of error in this assay: (*1*) the chemical assay for hydroxyproline; (*2*) measurement of dry wt; (*3*) the reproducibility of sampling a homogenate of tissue, a portion of which exists in an insoluble form. However, evaluation of the assay demonstrated little variability in the assay itself.

The coefficient of variation was 5.9% for the chemical assay of hydroxyproline, 1.9% for the measurement of dry wt, and 12.8% for the precision of sampling of the homogenate (table 3).

Variation of collagen concentration in autopsy

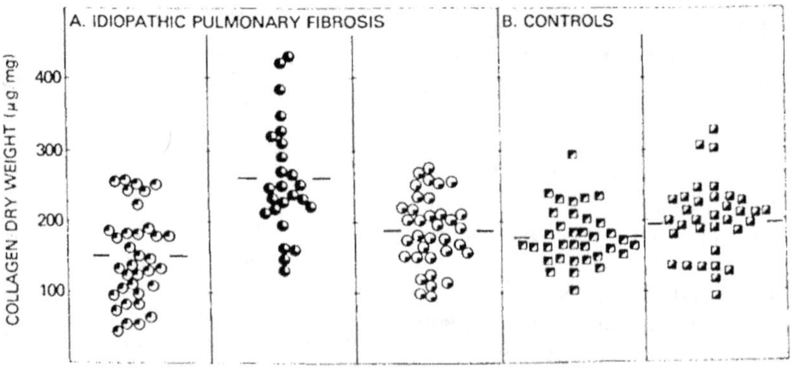

Fig. 3. Collagen concentration in multiple tissue samples taken from fibrotic and control lungs at autopsy. A. Patients with IPF (BS ◐, RS ◐, WES ◑); B. Control subjects (NO ◩; NT ◪). All data are expressed as collagen/dry wt (μg/mg). Mean values are shown by the bars. Comparison of the data demonstrated significant differences at p < 0.01 for the following: Patient RS compared with each of the 4 other patients, and Patient BS compared with Patients WES and NT. All other comparisons were not significant at 95 %.

TABLE 4

ANATOMIC DISTRIBUTION OF COLLAGEN IN LUNGS OF PATIENTS WITH IDIOPATHIC PULMONARY FIBROSIS COMPARED WITH CONTROL SUBJECTS*

		Collagen/Dry Wt† ($\mu g/mg$)		
Patient	Diagnosis	Upper Zone	Middle Zone	Lower Zone
BS	IPF	155 ± 41‡ (n = 4)	161 ± 31 (n = 6)	133 ± 21 (n = 11)
RS	IPF	301 ± 24 (n = 12)	274 ± 24 (n = 12)	231 ± 24 (n = 12)
NO	Control	177 ± 17 (n = 10)	64 ± 10 (n = 13)	179 ± 14 (n = 15)
NT	Control	266 ± 14 (n = 12)	191 ± 15 (n = 12)	160 ± 15 (n = 12)

* Multiple samples were taken from each lung with a number-8 cork borer. A portion was used for histologic evaluation, and the remainder for biochemical analysis. All samples from patients with IPF demonstrated +4 fibrosis; all samples from control subjects demonstrated normal lung.

† Comparisons between zones within the same patients demonstrated significant differences at $p < 0.05$ for the following: Patient RS, upper versus lower; Patient NO, upper versus middle; Patient NT, upper versus lower. Comparisons of the same zones between patients demonstrated some significant differences, but these were randomly distributed between the patients with IPF and the control subjects.

‡ Mean ± SEM.

specimens. There was a wide variation in the collagen concentration in multiple lung samples from patients with IPF and from control subjects (figure 3). The collagen concentration in patients with IPF varied over a threefold range in 2 patients and over a sevenfold range in a third. In comparison, collagen concentration varied over approximately a threefold range in both control subjects. These variations were vastly greater than the variations induced by the assay itself. Although there were some significant differences in the distribution of these values, the differences were random and were independent of whether or not the patients had IPF.

Anatomic distribution of collagen concentration in autopsy specimens. There was a broad range in the values of collagen concentration in the upper, middle, and lower zones of the lungs of both fibrotic patients and control subjects (table 4). For 1 patient with IPF (RS) and 1 control subject (NT), there were significant differences between the collagen concentrations in upper and lower zones. There were no other significant differences between zones among either patients with IPF or control subjects. Comparisons of the same zones in different patients demonstrated some significant differences, but these were randomly distributed between patients with IPF and control subjects.

Comparison of collagen concentration in biopsy and autopsy specimens. In 1 patient with IPF (WES), collagen concentration was determined in the right middle and right upper lobes, both at open lung biopsy and at autopsy 7 months later (table 4). For both lobes, the collagen concentration was significantly higher at the time of biopsy than at autopsy ($p < 0.001$). In addition, the average collagen concentration in the biopsy sample from the right middle lobe was significantly higher than that in the biopsy sample from the right upper lobe; at biopsy, the deviations between lobes were also significantly different, but at that time, the right upper lobe had a higher concentration of collagen than the right middle lobe.

Protein synthesis in biopsy specimens. Biopsy samples from patients with IPF and control subjects actively incorporated [^{14}C]proline into collagen (represented by [^{14}C]hydroxyproline) over at least 4 h (figure 4). The rates of collagen synthesis (averaged over the number of cells in the sample) varied more than sixfold in the patients with IPF and twofold to threefold in the control subjects; there were, however, no significant differences between these 2 groups (figure 5A). The rate of noncollagen protein synthesis also showed a wide variation in both patients with IPF and control subjects (figure 5B). As with the rate of collagen synthesis, the differences were not significant. Collagen represented 1.3 to 3.4% of all proteins synthesized by the biopsy samples of patients with IPF (figure 5C). In comparison, collagen represented from 1.2 to 5.4% of all proteins synthesized by biopsy samples from the control subjects; there was no difference between the 2 groups.

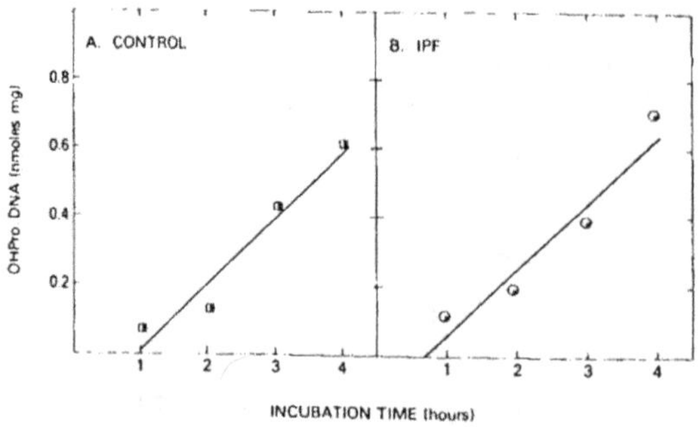

Fig. 4. Quantitation of the rate of collagen synthesis per cell in biopsy specimens from control and fibrotic lungs. Collagen synthesis is represented by the incorporation of [^{14}C]proline into collagen as [^{14}C]hydroxyproline; the number of cells in the sample is represented by DNA. The rate of collagen synthesis was calculated by fitting the best straight line to the data determined at 1 to 4 h of incubation. A. Example of a control patient (NL ◨); the rate of collagen synthesis was 0.18 nmol hydroxyproline (OHPro)/mg DNA-hour (least squares fit, r = 0.97). B. Example of a patient with IPF (WES ◒); the rate of collagen synthesis was 0.19 nmol hydroxyproline/mg DNA-hour (r = 0.96).

Discussion

Quantitation of the concentration of collagen in lung parenchyma of patients with IPF has demonstrated that: (*1*) collagen/dry wt in the IPF lung is the same as in the normal lung; (*2*) collagen/dry wt in multiple sites within the lung of a patient with IPF varies over a several-fold range, similar to the variation found in normal persons; (*3*) collagen/dry wt in IPF biopsy specimens does not correlate with the light microscopic evaluation of the degree of fibrosis in the same sample. Detailed evaluation of the methods used to quantitate collagen concentration showed that the assays used in these studies are a valid representation of the collagen concentration in lung and not an artifact of the chemical assay, the measurement of dry wt, or of the method used to homogenize and aliquot the tissue samples. In addition, evaluation of the relative activity of cells of lung parenchyma from patients with IPF indicates that under the conditions used in these experiments, on the average, these cells are synthesizing collagen at a normal rate.

The classic concept of IPF is that the parenchyma of the patients is stiff and noncompliant, at least in part due to the accumulation of interstitial collagen (1–11, 20). In a recent correlative study of the morphologic and physiologic characteristics of IPF, this concept was validated by demonstrating that the reduced compliance, elevated elastic recoil, and exercise-induced fall in Pa_{O_2} noted in IPF all correlate with the degree of interstitial fibrosis found on biopsy (11). Hence, the physiologic assessment of parenchymal collagen in IPF agrees with the light microscopic assessment of parenchymal collagen in this disease.

In this context, the finding that parenchymal collagen concentration in IPF is the same as that in normal persons is unexpected. However, assessment of the current morphologic concepts of inter-

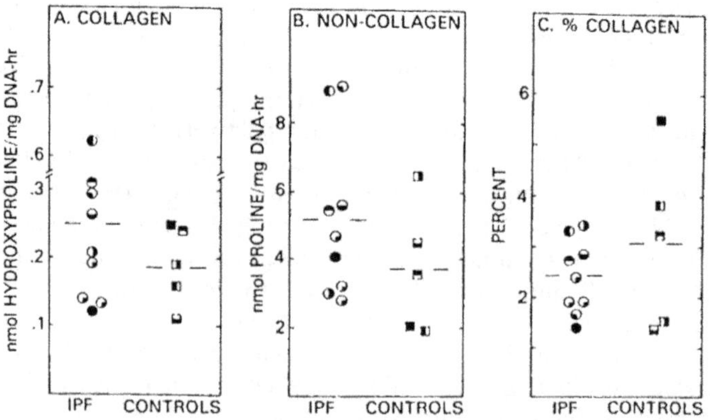

Fig. 5. Comparison of rates of collagen synthesis, rates of noncollagen protein synthesis and the percentage of collagen synthesis in open lung biopsy specimens of patients with IPF and control subjects. Each symbol represents a patient (to identify patient, see tables 1 and 2). Patient WES had biopsies of all 3 lobes of the right lung; these data are given separately. Mean values are shown as horizontal bars. There were no significant differences between the patients with IPF and the control subjects for any of these parameters. A. Rate of collagen synthesis (nmol hydroxyproline/mg DNA-hour): IPF, 0.25 ± 0.02; control, 0.19 ± 0.02; p = 0.16. B. Rate of noncollagen protein synthesis (nmole proline/mg DNA-hour): IPF, 5.2 ± 0.8; control, 3.7 ± 0.8; p = 0.26. C. Percentage of collagen synthesis (the relative amount of protein synthesis devoted to collagen): IPF, 2.4 ± 0.2 %; control, 3.1 ± 0.8 %; p = 0.31.

stitial collagen in normal lung and in IPF suggests that the biochemical, physiologic, and morphologic concepts of this disease can be reconciled.

Current morphologic concepts of interstitial collagen in normal subjects and in patients with IPF. To the histologist working with light microscopy, the term "collagen fibers" suggests parallel arrays of extracellular fibers staining pink with a hematoxylin and eosin stain and blue with a Masson trichrome stain. The term "reticulin" refers to the randomly arrayed extracellular fibers that are seen with silver stains (15).

By electron microscopy, there are at least 3 morphologic forms of collagen found in the normal alveolar interstitium (15): (*1*) most prominent are the parallel arrays of 500 to 1,000 å-thick, crossbanded fibers; (*2*) the randomly arrayed 160 to 350 å-thick fibrils, which differ from the 100 to 150 å-thick microfibrillar component of elastic fibers (the former are larger, randomly arrayed, and show crossbanding, whereas the latter are smaller, usually found on the periphery of amorphous elastin, and are not crossbanded); (*3*) basement membrane collagen, which usually appears amorphous or very finely filamentous.

The biochemical correlates of these morphologic structures are just beginning to be understood. There are at least 4 distinct types of collagens in the alveolar interstitium: Type I, Type III, Type IV, and Type V (15, 21–25). The composition of Type IV collagen (epithelial and endothelial basement membrane collagen) is still controversial; it may consist of at least 2 separate collagen types (24). Likewise, the composition of Type V collagen (smooth muscle and, possibly, other basement membrane collagen) is still under active investigation (24). It also may be comprised of 2 distinct collagen types.

It is likely that in the normal adult lung, more than 90% of the collagen is of Types I and III, but this has not been definitely proved (15). Types I and III are normally found in a ratio of approximately 1.5 to 2.5 to 1 (22). By analogy to other tissues, it is now believed that most of the parallel arrays of fibers seen by light microscopy and the crossbanded fibers seen by electron microscopy are Type I collagen (26). Reticulin may be, in part, Type III collagen; in other tissues, reticulin appears to correspond to the randomly arrayed 150 to 350 å-thick fibrils seen by electron microscopy (26). It is currently believed, but not definitely proved, that Types III, IV, and V collagens within the lung parenchyma are not detected by stains such as Masson trichrome.

Morphologic evaluation of the connective tissue in IPF has demonstrated thickening of alveolar interstitium with fibrous tissue, and basement membrane disruption and thickening (5, 9, 10, 27–30). In addition (figures 6 and 7), the interstitium of the lung in IPF shows: (*1*) some areas with accumulations of thick, crossbanded collagen fibers; (*2*) rearrangement of interstitial collagen with focal accumulation in some areas, loss of interstitial structure in others, as well as alterations in fiber form and orientation; (*3*) over-all, more collagen, but there also appears to be more other noncellular as well as cellular parenchymal constituents present.

Reconciliation of physiologic, morphologic, and biochemical data in IPF. The morphologic, physiologic, and biochemical findings in IPF can be reconciled by considering 3 concepts: (*1*) IPF is a disease associated with changes in collagen types. Seyer and associates (22) have demonstrated that IPF is a disease in which there is a shift in ratio of interstitial collagens toward more Type I collagen; in IPF, Type I collagen represents approximately 80% of the lung collagen. Such a shift would be characterized by an increase in the thick, crossbanded fibers on light and electron microscopy. Because Type I collagen fibers are less compliant than the fibers of other collagen types, the parenchyma would be less compliant compared with that of normal lung. Thus, a shift in collagen types without a change in total collagen/dry wt would be consistent with the morphologic and physiologic alterations found in IPF. (*2*) IPF is associated with a derangement of the form of interstitial collagen and rearrangement of its location (figures 6 and 7). The processes that are responsible for these changes are not known, but they may be associated with the presence of collagen-specific proteolytic enzymes in the IPF lung (31). In addition, alterations in the number, types, and location of collagen synthesizing cells, as seen in IPF, may significantly influence the location of collagen fibers within the interstitium. Independent of their cause, such changes in collagen form and location likely have a profound influence on lung mechanical properties. However, changes in form and location are not detected by a biochemical measurement of collagen content of a biopsy sample. In this context, the finding that collagen/dry wt in the IPF lung is similar to normal lung is consistent with the morphologic and physiologic findings. (*3*) The biochemical quantitation of collagen is based on the amount of collagen in a biopsy relative to the amount of other parenchymal constituents; if the latter are altered, changes in collagen

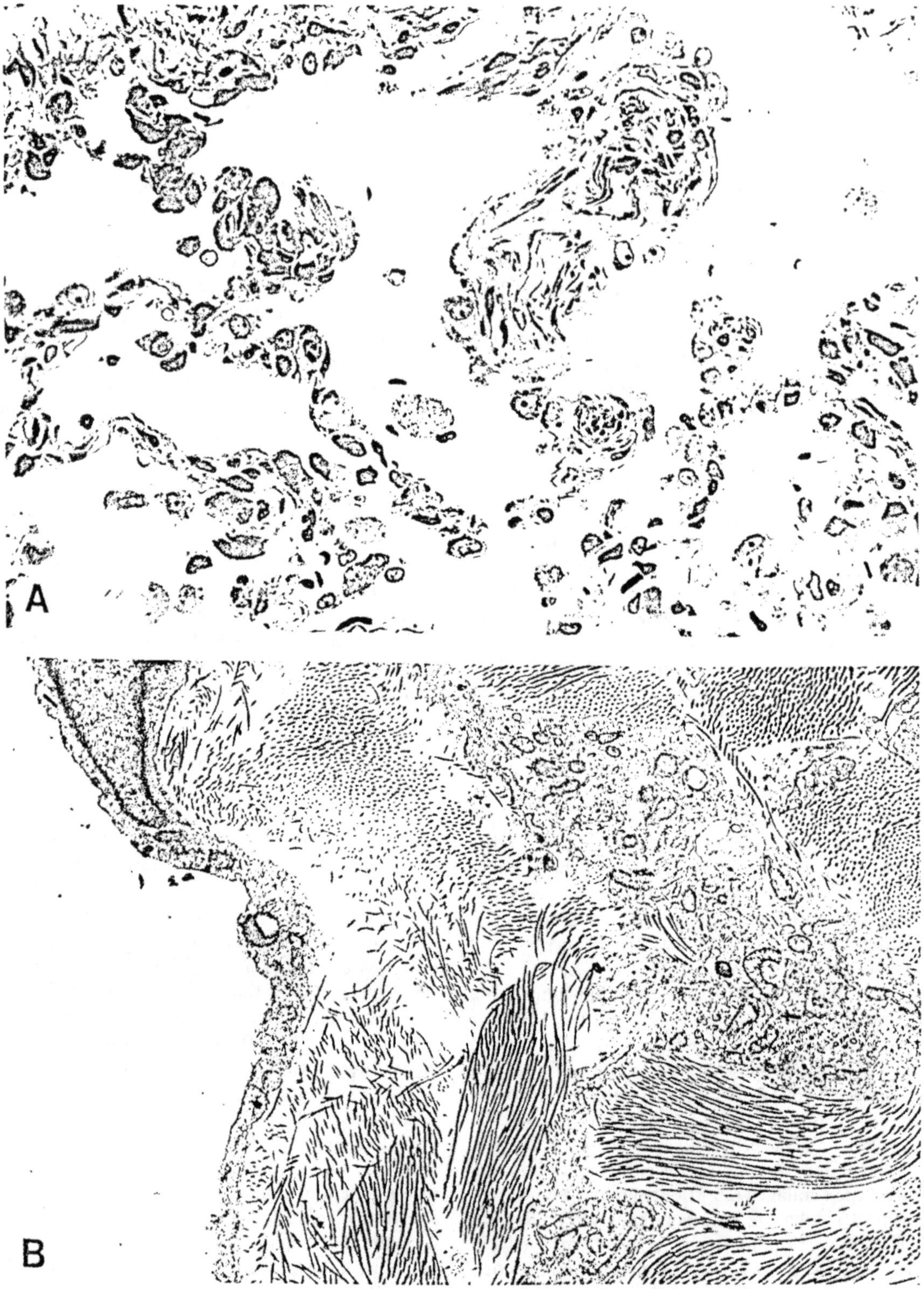

Fig. 6. Open lung biopsies of patients with IPF demonstrating focal accumulation of collagen. A. Medium power light photomicrograph of parenchyma in Patient WH; some interstitial areas are normal, whereas others are markedly thickened with collagen fibers and other constituents (1-μ section, toluidine blue stain; original magnification: ×375). B. Transmission electron micrograph of the same patient demonstrating accumulation of thick, cross-banded collagen fibers (probably Type I collagen) and rearrangement of interstitial collagen. Some fibers have a twisted, tortuous appearance. A Type I epithelial cell is on the left and an interstitial mesenchymal cell is in the middle (uranyl acetate stain; original magnification: ×8,500).

may not be detectable. There is evidence that the percentage of lung occupied by tissue (cells and interstitium) is increased in IPF, whereas the percentage of lung occupied by air is decreased (32). Thus, although interstitial collagen fibers may be increased in number in this decrease, other extracellular and cellular constituents may be increased as well. These constituents probably include serum proteins, other as yet unidentified macromolecules, and cells (including the abundant inflammatory cells that are characteristic of the histology of IPF). Evidence for this is provided by a comparison of the biochemical data from open lung biopsy and autopsy of the same patient (table 5). In both lobes, the collagen/dry wt in both biopsy material samples was higher than that in autopsy samples 7 months later. Although it is possible that parenchymal collagen was destroyed in the interval, a more likely explanation is that cellular components (particularly inflammatory cells) and serum proteins contributed to the increased dry weight of the autopsy samples, thereby lowering collagen/dry wt. In this context, it is not difficult to conceptualize how IPF might be a disease in which not only interstitial collagen is increased, but other parenchymal components are increased as well, so that in the mid-course of the disease, collagen/dry wt is normal, but at death, collagen/dry wt could even be decreased. As with rearrangement of collagen fibers, a proportional increase in collagen as well as other constituents might cause significant

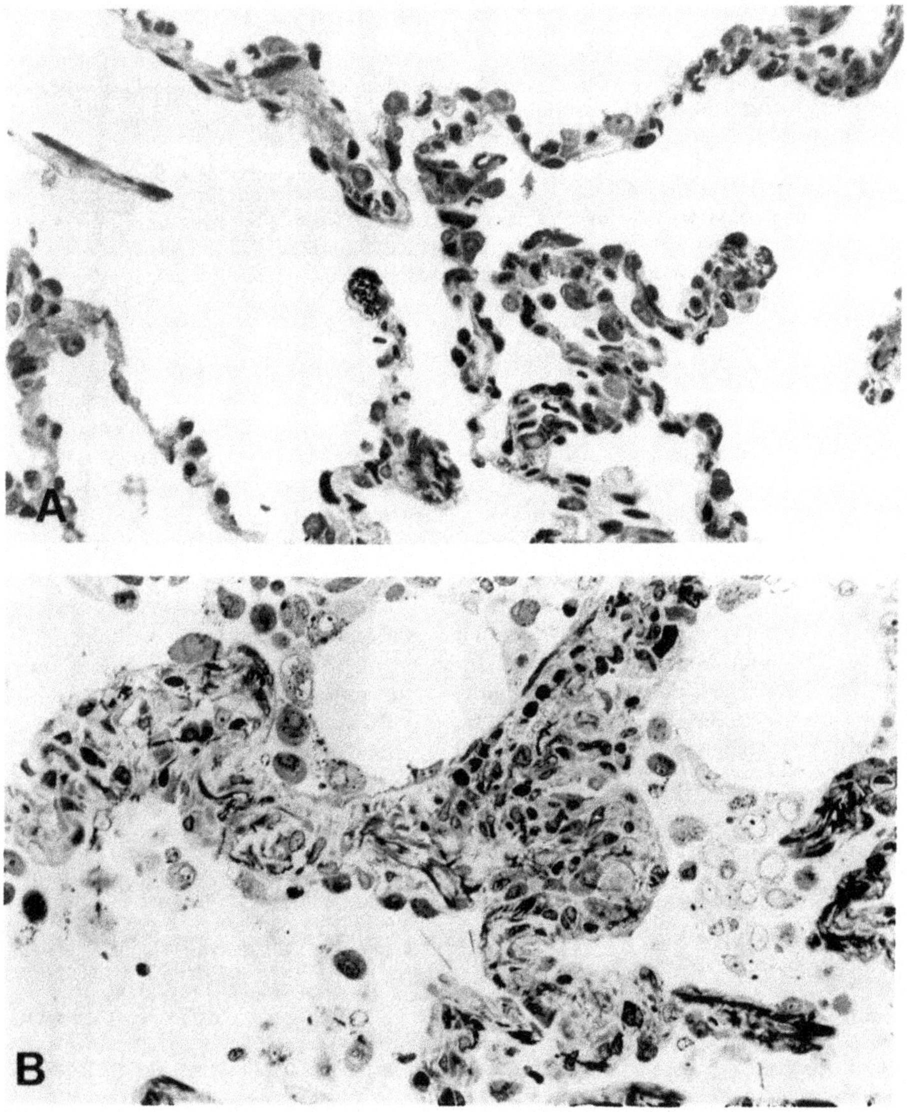

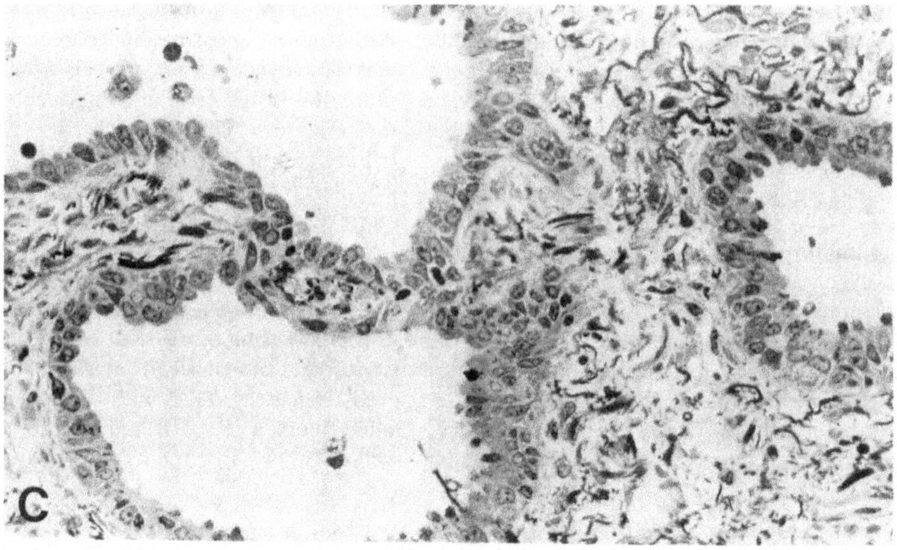

Fig. 7. Comparison of cellular and connective tissue components in the normal alveolar interstitium with those of 2 patients with IPF. All sections are 1 μ thick. A. Normal lung (toluidine blue stain; original magnification: ×320). B. Medium power view of the alveolar interstitium in Patient MB demonstrating a rearrangement of interstitial collagen with a thickened interstitium. The intra-alveolar spaces are filled with cells, and the interstitial spaces have an abnormal accumulation of cells. Because cells contribute to dry wt, collagen/dry wt of this region may be normal, even though there is an increased amount of interstitial collagen (toluidine blue stain; original magnification: ×300). C. Medium power view of the alveolar septums from the biopsy of the right upper lobe in Patient WES revealing thickened interstitium with increased interstitial collagen and cells, and hyperplasia of the alveolar lining cells. As in B, the cells contribute to dry wt, thus reducing the determination of collagen/dry wt for this region (toluidine blue stain; original magnification: ×300).

alterations of parenchymal volume-pressure relationships.

Implications for the pathogenesis of IPF. These physiologic-morphologic-biochemical correlates suggest that rather than resulting from a generalized accumulation of interstitial collagen fibers, IPF is more likely a complex disease in which parenchymal cells are altered and in which inflammatory cells play an important role.

Changes in collagen types require active cellular processes of production and/or degradation. Although normal lung interstitial fibroblasts rigidly control the types of collagen they produce (33, 34), there could be changes in their differentiated state so that each cell might shift the types of collagen that it synthesizes. For example, it has been shown that under certain conditions, chondrocytes can shift from production of Type II collagen to the production of Type I collagen (35, 36). Alternatively, since the ratio of collagen types produced by each cell appears to be cell-specific (34, 35–37), alteration of the types of collagen in the interstitium might result from alterations in the cellular populations of the parenchyma. Consistent with this concept is the recent observation that in the IPF lung, macrophages direct neutrophils to injure interstitial fibroblasts (38).

Rearrangement of interstitial collagen implies

TABLE 5

COMPARISON OF COLLAGEN PER DRY WEIGHT IN BIOPSY AND AUTOPSY SPECIMENS FROM PATIENT WES

Site	Source	Number of Samples Analyzed	Collagen/Dry Wt (μg/mg)	p Value
Right middle lobe	Biopsy	8	300 ± 14	< 0.001
	Autopsy	15	143 ± 2	
Right upper lobe	Biopsy	8	261 ± 13	< 0.001
	Autopsy	14	167 ± 2	

initial destruction of collagen in its normal anatomic location. Collagen is an unusual macromolecule in that it is resistant to attack by most proteolytic enzymes; under the physiologic conditions of the extracellular space, only collagenase can destroy it. Thus, to rearrange collagen, it is first necessary to have a specific enzyme present that will destroy it. Recent studies (31) suggest that patients with IPF do have active collagenase in their lower respiratory tract, thus giving a mechanism by which the initial disordering of interstitial collagen might occur.

Rearrangement of interstitial collagen also implies that collagen is laid down in abnormal locations. The most likely mechanism for this is that the cells that produce collagen are in abnormal locations. There is increasing evidence that the normal topologic arrangement of tissue is dependent on cell-cell and cell-matrix interactions. These processes involve large macromolecules that cause cells to adhere to each other and to their extracellular matrix. Studies by McDonald and co-workers (39) suggest that proteases released by inflammatory cells may specifically destroy these macromolecules, such that cellular order is disrupted. Thus, even though the rate of collagen production by lung cells may be normal in IPF, if cellular order is disrupted, there would be deposition of collagen in abnormal areas. This could result in the morphologic finding of focal accumulations of collagen seen in IPF.

Unification of the concepts derived from physiologic, morphologic, and biochemical methods suggest that IPF is a disease in which interstitial collagen is changed, disordered, and rearranged; and in which the cells of the lower respiratory tract are changed in numbers, type, function, or location.

Acknowledgment

The writers thank Drs. Byron McLees and Steve Weinberger for their helpful criticisms; Filippina Giacometti for her expert technical assistance; and Ellen Wright for her editorial assistance.

References

1. Hamman L, Rich AR. Acute diffuse interstitial fibrosis of the lungs. Bull Johns Hopkins Hosp 1944; 74:177-212.
2. Ruben EH, Lubliner R. The Hamman-Rich syndrome: review of the literature and analysis of 15 cases. Medicine (Baltimore) 1957; 36:397-463.
3. Herbert FA, Nahmias BB, Gaensler EA, MacMahen HE. Pathophysiology of interstitial pulmonary fibrosis: report of 19 cases and follow-up with corticosteroids. Arch Intern Med 1962; 110:628-48.
4. Livingstone JL, Lewis JG, Reid L, Jefferson KE. Diffuse interstitial pulmonary fibrosis: clinical, radiologic and pathologic study based on 45 patients. Q J Med 1964; 33:71-104.
5. Crystal RG, Fulmer JD, Roberts WC, Moss ML, Line BR, Reynolds HY. Idiopathic pulmonary fibrosis: clinical, histologic, radiologic, physiologic, scintigraphic, cytologic and biochemical aspects. Ann Intern Med 1976; 85:769-88.
6. Fulmer JD, Roberts WC, von Gal ER, Crystal RG. Small airways in idiopathic pulmonary fibrosis: comparisons of morphologic and physiologic observations. J Clin Invest 1977; 60:595-610.
7. Crystal RG, Gadek JE, Hunninghake GW, Fulmer JD, Line BR, Ferrans VJ. Interstitial lung disease: current concepts of pathogenesis, staging, and therapy Am J Med (in press).
8. Reynolds HY, Fulmer JD, Kazmierowski JA, Roberts WC, Frank MM, Crystal RG. Analysis of bronchoalveolar lavage fluid from patients with idiopathic pulmonary fibrosis and chronic hypersensitivity pneumonitis. Am Rev Respir Dis 1977; 59:165-75.
9. Fulmer JD, Crystal RG. Interstitial lung disease. In: Simmons DH, ed, Current pulmonology. Vol. 1. Boston: Houghton Mifflin, 1979:1-65.
10. Crystal RG, Fulmer JD, Baum BJ, *et al*, Cells, collagen and idiopathic pulmonary fibrosis. Lung 1978; 155:199-224.
11. Fulmer JD, von Gal ER, Roberts WC, Crystal RG. Morphologic-physiologic correlates of the severity of fibrosis in idiopathic pulmonary fibrosis. J Clin Invest 1979: 63:665-76.
12. Fulmer JD, Crystal RG. The biochemical basis of pulmonary function. In: Crystal RG, ed, Biochemical basis of pulmonary function. New York: Marcel Dekker, 1976:419-66.
13. Bachofen M, Weibel ER. Basic pattern of tissue repair in human lungs following unspecific injury. Chest 1974; Suppl 65:185-7.
14. Crystal RG. Lung collagen: definition, diversity and development. Fed Proc 1974; 33:2248-55.
15. Hance AJ, Crystal RG. The connective tissue of lung. Am Rev Respir Dis 1975; 112:657-711.
16. Bradley KH, McConnell SP, Crystal RG. Lung collagen composition and synthesis: characterization and changes with age. J Biol Chem 1974; 249:2674-83.
17. Bradley K, McConnell-Breul S, Crystal RG. Collagen in the human lung, quantitation of rates of synthesis and partial characterization of composition. J Clin Invest 1975; 55:543-50.
18. Juva K, Prockop DJ. Modified procedure for the assay of ^{3}H or ^{14}C-labeled hydroxyproline. Annal Biochem 1966; 15:77-83.
19. Burton K. A study of the conditions and mechanisms of the diphenylamine reaction for the colorimetric estimation of deoxyribonucleic acid. Biochem J 1956; 62:315-23.
20. Austrian R, McClement JH, Renzetti AD Jr, Donald KW, Riley RL, Cournand A. Clinical and physiologic features of some types of pulmonary diseases

with impairment of alveolar-capillary diffusion: the syndrome of "alveolar-capillary block." Am J Med 1951; 11:667-85.

21. McLees BD, Schleiter G, Pinnell SR. Isolation of Type III collagen from human adult parenchymal lung tissue. Biochemistry 1977; 16:185-90.
22. Seyer JM, Hutcheson ET, Kang AH. Collagen polymorphism in idiopathic pulmonary fibrosis. J Clin Invest 1976; 57:1498-1507.
23. Madri HA, Furthmayr H. Isolation and tissue localization of Type AB₂ collagen from normal lung parenchyma. Am J Pathol 1979; 94:323-32.
24. Bornstein P, Traub W. In: Neurath H, Hill RL, eds, The proteins. 3rd ed, vol IV. New York: Academic Press, 1979:411-632.
25. Madri JA, Furthmayr H. Collagen polymorphism in the lung. Immunochemical study of pulmonary fibrosis. Hum Pathol 1980 (in press).
26. Gay S, Müller PK, Meigel WN, Kuhn K. Polymorphie des Kollagens. Neue Aspekte für Strukter und Funktion des Bindegewebes. Der Hautarzt 1976; 27:196-205.
27. Brody AR, Craighead JE. Interstitial associations of cells lining air spaces in human pulmonary fibrosis. Virchows Arch [Pathol Anat] 1976; 372:39-49.
28. Cassan SM, Divertie MD, Brown AL. Fine structural morphometry on biopsy specimens of human lung, 2, diffuse idiopathic pulmonary fibrosis. Chest 1974; 65:275-8.
29. Kawanami O, Ferrans VJ, Roberts WC, Crystal RG, Fulmer JD. Anchoring fibrils: a new connective tissue structure in fibrotic lung disease. Am J Pathol 1978; 92:127-48.
30. Kawanami O, Ferrans VJ, Fulmer JD, Crystal RG. Nuclear inclusions in alveolar epithelium of patients with fibrotic lung disorders. Am J Pathol 1979; 94:301-22.
31. Gadek JE, Kelman JA, Fells GA, *et al.* Collagenase in the lower respiratory tract of patients with idiopathic pulmonary fibrosis. N Engl J Med 1979; 301:737-42.
32. Bignon J, Hem B, Molinier B. Morphometric and angiographic studies in diffuse interstitial pulmonary fibrosis. Prog Respir Res 1975; 8:141-160.
33. Hance AJ, Crystal RG. Rigid control of synthesis of collagen Types I and III by cells in culture. Nature 1977; 268:152-4.
34. Breul SD, Bradley KH, Hance AJ, Schafer MP, Berg RA, Crystal RG. Control of collagen production by human diploid lung fibroblasts. J Biol Chem 1980; 255:5250-60.
35. Gay S, Müller PK, Lemmen C, Remberger K, Matzen K, Kühn K. Immunohistological study on collagen in cartilage-bone metamorphosis and degenerative osteoarthritis. Klin Wochenschr 1976; 54:969-76.
36. Mayne R, Vail MS, Mayne PM, Miller EJ. Changes in types of collagen synthesis as clones of chick chondrocytes grow and eventually lose division capacity. Proc Natl Acad Sci USA 1976; 73:1674-8.
37. Crystal RG, Bradley K, McConnell-Breul S, Collins J, Hance A, Cowan M. Collagen in the lung: development of a technology applicable to human lung disease. Chest 1975; 67(Suppl:30-1).
38. Hunninghake G, Szapiel S, Fulmer J, Keogh B, Crystal RG. Neutrophil-mediated fibroblast destruction in idiopathic pulmonary fibrosis (IPF). Am Rev Respir Dis 1979; 119:72.
39. McDonald JA, Baum BJ, Rosenberg DM, Kelman JA, Brin SC, Crystal RG. Destruction of a major extracellular adhesive glycoprotein (fibronectin) of human fibroblasts by neutral proteases from polymorphonuclear leukocyte granules. Lab Invest 1979; 40:350-7.

Pulmonary Sarcoidosis: A Disease Characterized and Perpetuated by Activated Lung T-Lymphocytes

Moderator: RONALD G. CRYSTAL, M.D. *Discussants:* WILLIAM C. ROBERTS, M.D.; GARY W. HUNNINGHAKE, M.D.; JAMES E. GADEK, M.D.; JACK D. FULMER, M.D.; and BRUCE R. LINE, M.D.; Bethesda, Maryland

The alveolitis of pulmonary sarcoidosis is characterized by an intense, mononuclear cell infiltrate that probably precedes granuloma formation. Pathogenic mechanisms underlying pulmonary sarcoidosis can be shown by study of the mononuclear cells composing the alveolitis. Bronchoalveolar lavage has shown that the sarcoid lung is characterized by increased numbers of "activated" T-lymphocytes within the alveolar structures. In contrast to normal control cells, the lung T-lymphocytes of patients with sarcoid release the mediator, monocyte chemotactic factor, that probably contributes to the pathogenesis of sarcoidosis by recruiting blood monocytes to the lung, thus providing cellular building blocks for granuloma formation. Conventional monitors of the activity of pulmonary sarcoidosis, such as blood studies, pulmonary function testing, and chest roentgenograms, show little relation to the intensity of the T-lymphocyte alveolitis as assessed by bronchoalveolar lavage or by histopathologic studies. In contrast, quantification of lavage T-lymphocyte populations and ^{67}Ga scintigraphy of the chest provide a sensitive and specific means of assessing the activity of the alveolitis in pulmonary sarcoidosis and may provide a rational basis for therapy.

DR. RONALD G. CRYSTAL (Chief, Pulmonary Branch, National Heart, Lung, and Blood Institute): Sarcoidosis is a multisystem disease of undetermined cause characterized by the presence of noncaseating granulomas in many organs (1-6). Although the cause is unknown and the morphologic findings nonspecific, the combination of clinical, roentgenographic, histologic, and physiologic findings are so characteristic that in modern clinical practice the diagnosis of sarcoidosis is usually unambiguous (6-11). Sarcoidosis has been described in most tissues of the body, but for most patients lung involvement has the most serious consequences. At least 90% of all patients have pulmonary manifestations (1, 3-6, 12-14). Of these, 20% to 25% will have permanent loss of lung function, and 5% to 10% will die from the disease (1, 3, 4, 14-18).

The presence of granulomas in the alveolar structures in pulmonary sarcoidosis has long been considered histologic evidence that there are heightened cellular immune processes. However, many studies have documented a nonspecific depression of cellular immunity in this disorder. For example, most patients with active sarcoidosis have anergy to skin tests (12, 19, 20), impairment of the in-vitro proliferative response of blood mononuclear cells to antigens and mitogens (21-23), and a peripheral blood T-lymphocytopenia (24-28).

One explanation for this apparent paradox is that studies of uninvolved tissues such as skin and blood do not reflect the ongoing immune processes at the site of granuloma formation. The development of methods to directly evaluate the inflammatory and immune effector systems within the human lung has led to remarkable insights into the pathogenesis of this disease. Specifically, by 1978 it had become obvious that pulmonary sarcoidosis is characterized and perpetuated by increased numbers of activated T-lymphocytes within the alveolar structures (28-34).

To show the importance and ramifications of lung T-lymphocytes in this disease, we have used a study population of 45 persons with biopsy proven pulmonary sarcoidosis. Included were 20 males and 25 females, with an average age of 37 ± 5 years (all data are presented as the mean ± SE). By conventional clinical criteria, 19 were classified as having "active" disease.

First, we will define the disease morphologically, stressing the temporal sequence of the histologic findings. Second, we will detail the types, numbers, and function of lung inflammatory and immune effector cells, emphasizing the critical role of lung T-lymphocytes. Third, we will evaluate the tests available for staging sarcoidosis in terms of the sensitivity and specificity of these methods in staging the activity of the disease within the alveolar structures. Finally, we will review the therapy of pulmonary sarcoidosis, emphasizing the importance of using measures of inflammatory and immune activity within the lung as criteria for making decisions.

Morphologic Aspects

Dr. William C. Roberts (Chief, Pathology Branch, National Heart, Lung, and Blood Institute): The characteristic morphologic feature of pulmonary sarcoidosis is the presence of multiple noncaseating granulomas in the lung (Figure 1, *upper left*). The granulomas are always present in the alveolar septa (Figure 1, *upper right*) and usually in the walls of bronchi, pulmonary arteries, and veins (Figure 1, *lower left* and *right*) (1-3, 7, 35, 36).

COMPOSITION OF THE SARCOID GRANULOMA

The sarcoid granuloma is usually sharply circumscribed. Its central follicle consists of tightly packed cells,

▶ An edited transcription of a Combined Clinical Staff Conference at the Clinical Center, Bethesda, Maryland, 29 June 1978, by the National Institutes of Health, U.S. Department of Health, Education, and Welfare.

▶ Authors who wish to cite a section of the conference and specifically indicate its author can use this example for the form of reference:
ROBERTS WC. Morphologic aspects of pulmonary sarcoidosis, pp. 73-6. In: CRYSTAL RG, moderator. Pulmonary sarcoidosis: a disease characterized and perpetuated by activated lung T-lymphocytes. *Ann Intern Med.* 1981;**94**:73-94.

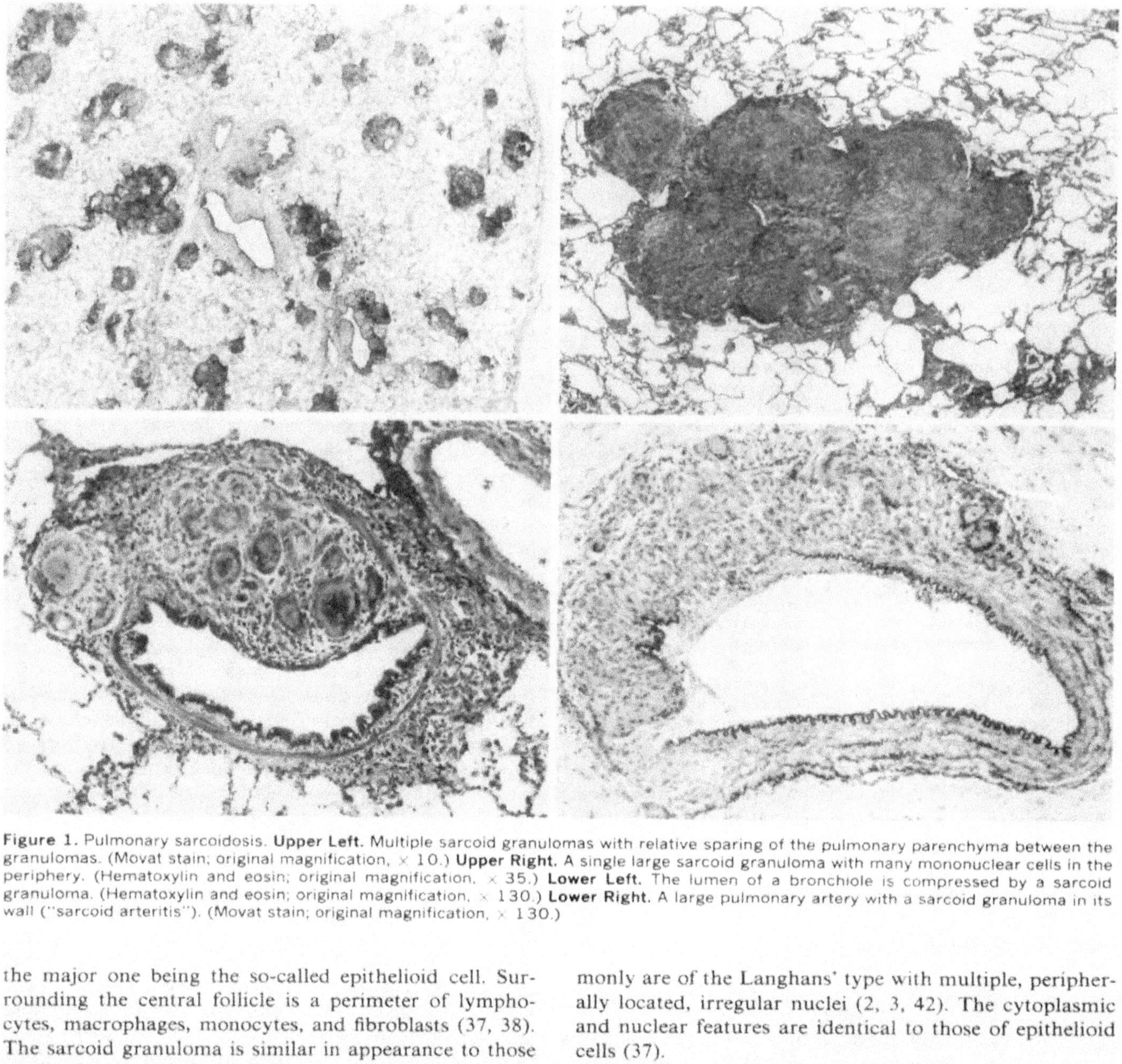

Figure 1. Pulmonary sarcoidosis. **Upper Left.** Multiple sarcoid granulomas with relative sparing of the pulmonary parenchyma between the granulomas. (Movat stain; original magnification, × 10.) **Upper Right.** A single large sarcoid granuloma with many mononuclear cells in the periphery. (Hematoxylin and eosin; original magnification, × 35.) **Lower Left.** The lumen of a bronchiole is compressed by a sarcoid granuloma. (Hematoxylin and eosin; original magnification, × 130.) **Lower Right.** A large pulmonary artery with a sarcoid granuloma in its wall ("sarcoid arteritis"). (Movat stain; original magnification, × 130.)

the major one being the so-called epithelioid cell. Surrounding the central follicle is a perimeter of lymphocytes, macrophages, monocytes, and fibroblasts (37, 38). The sarcoid granuloma is similar in appearance to those in all other types of granulomatous disease with the exception of tuberculosis (1-6).

Epithelioid cells occupy the body of the follicle as nodular collections of tightly packed cells. The term *epithelioid* was originally used because the size and arrangement of the cells were similar to the cells of epithelium; the epithelioid cell is now known, however, to be derived from the mononuclear-phagocyte system (39). Because epithelioid cells do have abundant cytoplasmic organelles, it has been suggested that they have secretory capabilities (40-42). Several populations of epithelioid cells have been described, but these "subclasses" are now believed to represent stages in the development of one cell type (6, 42-44).

Multinucleated giant cells, often up to 150 μm in diameter, are frequently found among the epithelioid cells within the granuloma follicle. The giant cells most commonly are of the Langhans' type with multiple, peripherally located, irregular nuclei (2, 3, 42). The cytoplasmic and nuclear features are identical to those of epithelioid cells (37).

The macrophages within the follicle are 10 to 25 μm in diameter and have numerous cytoplasmic processes that interdigitate with those of adjacent cells. The nuclei are indented and contain finely dispersed chromatin. The macrophages are rich in cytoplasmic organelles; but like epithelioid cells, the macrophages have a paucity of phagosomes or phagolysosomes, suggesting that they are not actively involved in phagocytosis (37). However, the macrophages within the granulomas do have numerous electron-dense lysosomes, suggesting that they are secretory cells (45).

The monocytes of the sarcoid follicle have a smoother surface then the macrophages (37). The nuclei are dark, and the cytoplasm has fewer organelles then the macrophage or epithelioid cell. Many of the lymphocytes of the follicle have the morphologic features of *activated* lymphocytes (37, 42, 43, 46). They are larger than the usual

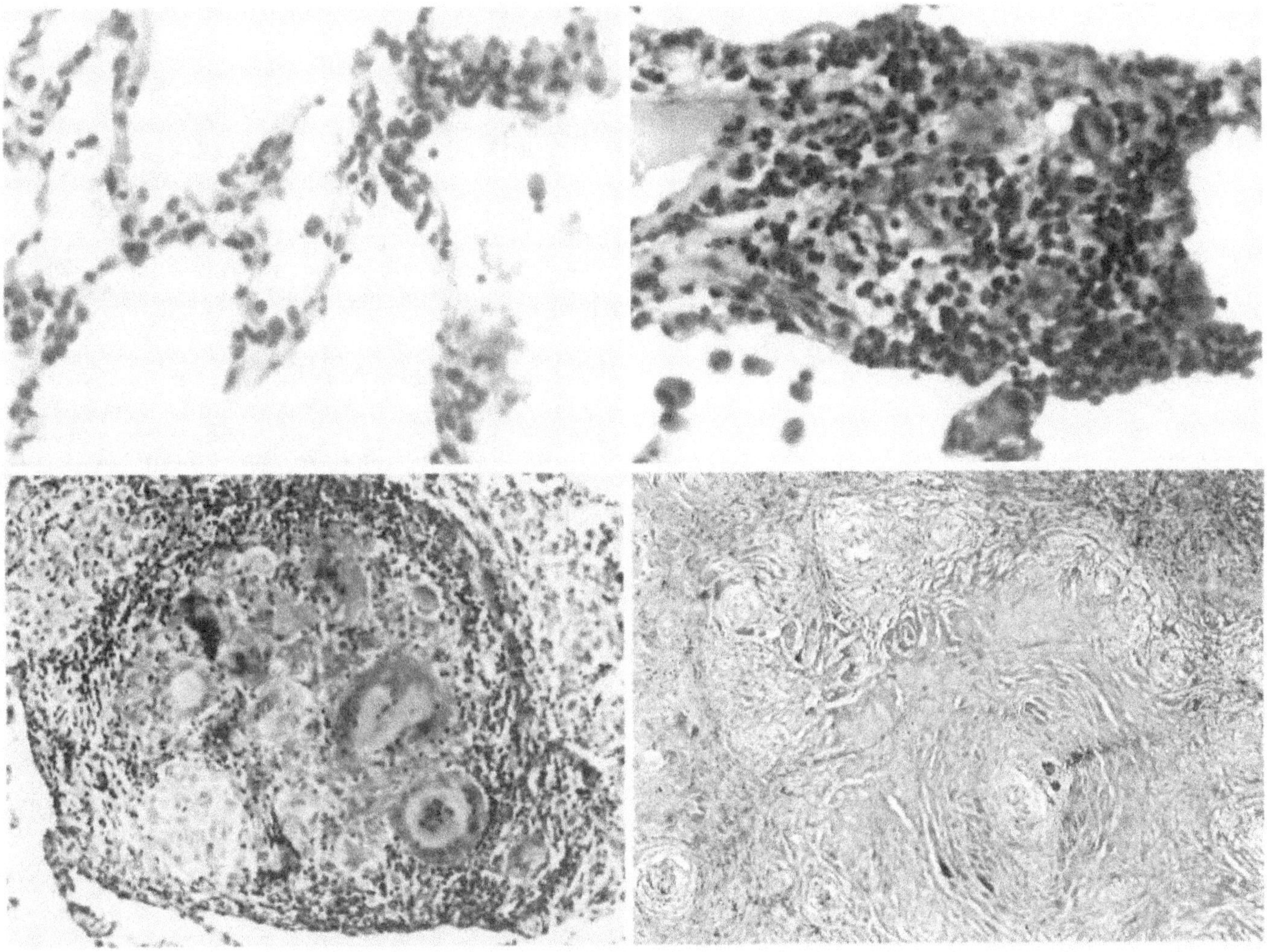

Figure 2. Stages of pulmonary sarcoidosis. **Upper Left.** Alveolar septae with increased numbers of mononuclear cells ("sarcoid alveolitis") Hematoxylin and eosin; original magnification, × 500.) **Upper Right.** Larger collection of mononuclear cells with few epithelioid cells and one giant cell in an alveolar septum. (Hematoxylin and eosin; original magnification, × 500.) **Lower Left.** A well-developed sarcoid granuloma with many giant cells and mononuclear cells only in the periphery. (Hematoxylin and eosin; original magnification, × 220.) **Lower Right.** The final stage in the organization of a sarcoid granuloma. The granulomas now consist mainly of relatively dense fibrous tissue, and only an occasional giant or epithelioid cell remains. (Hematoxylin and eosin; original magnification, × 55.)

lymphocyte and contain an irregular nucleus, often with centrioles; the cytoplasm contains large numbers of mitochrondria, dense granules, ribosomes, and rough endoplasmic reticulum.

The extracellular material within and surrounding the central follicle is classically described as *amorphous hyaline material* or *reticulin* (2). Although it has been suggested that some of this material was "para-amyloid" (47), electron microscopy has shown that it is mostly ground substance with interspersed fibers of various diameters (48). The exact nature of the latter is unknown. It has been described as amyloid or fibrin-like, but is more likely one or more types of collagen.

When involving alveolar septa, the sarcoid granuloma distorts the interstitium by its physical bulk and, thus, probably causes derangements in air-blood relations (37, 49). The presence of granulomas, however, does not seem to affect structures composing the so-called alveolar-capillary membrane; measurements of the pathway between air and blood in the sarcoid lung have shown it to be normal or, at most, slightly increased (50).

ALVEOLITIS OF SARCOIDOSIS; EVOLUTION OF DISEASE

Whereas early reports described the granuloma of sarcoid as being monotonously uniform (suggesting they begin at the same time) (51), it is now clear that the lesions of pulmonary sarcoidosis can originate at different times (5, 6). Moreover, although the granulomas are the morphologic hallmarks of pulmonary sarcoidosis, the alveolar structures in this disease also are characterized by accumulations of inflammatory and immune-effector cells within the interstitium and alveolus (5, 36, 52). Commonly referred to as the *alveolitis* of sarcoidosis, these inflammatory and immune effector cell accumulations consist of monocytes, macrophages, and lymphocytes that are present in approximately equal numbers. In most patients, the majority of effector cells are found within the interstitium rather than the alveolar air spaces (36, 52).

Although the diagnosis of sarcoidosis cannot be made without the presence of granulomas, there is increasing evidence that the alveolitis of sarcoidosis precedes the formation of the granulomas (Figure 2) (34, 36, 52-55). The extensive studies by Rosen and associates (52) have shown that early, developing granulomas are composed of a loose collection of inflammatory and immune effector cells in which monocytes, macrophages, and lymphocytes predominate over epithelioid cells. As the granuloma matures, numbers of epithelioid cells increase and numbers of monocytes, macrophages, and lymphocytes decrease (37, 52, 56). In patients with extensive alveolitis, few granulomas are present, but in patients with numerous granulomas, the alveolitis is minimal or absent, further supporting the concept that the alveolitis precedes the granulomas (52). At least part of the alveolitis of sarcoidosis is derived from circulating inflammatory and immune effector cells; Soler and Bassett (37) have presented morphologic evidence that blood monocytes pass from capillaries to the interstitium in this disease.

The fate of the sarcoid granuloma has been well documented morphologically. Although it can appear *fresh* from months to years, the granuloma ultimately either resolves leaving few or no morphologic changes or it undergoes progressive fibrosis (1, 5, 6, 57). The fibrosis begins as a rim of collagen around the granuloma and proceeds in a centripetal fashion until the entire structure is replaced by fibrous tissue (1, 2, 37, 53, 56). It is likely, although unproven, that the collagen composing the fibrous tissue originates from the fibroblasts in the periphery of the granuloma (37). As the lesion "matures," fibroblasts proliferate in the periphery of the granuloma (56). In older granulomas, peripheral fibroblasts are extensive, and the inflammatory and immune effector cells in the periphery of the granuloma disappear (56). As the fibrosis proceeds inward, capillaries in the region are trapped and disappear (37, 55).

In about 20% of patients with sarcoidosis, there is progression to interstitial fibrosis, distortion, and replacement of the pulmonary architecture (58, 59). These progressive lesions are associated with increased amounts of collagen fibers within the interstitium, obliteration of capillaries, and destruction of architecture by inflammatory and immune effector cells, granulomas, and fibroblasts (37). Eventually, the normal alveolar architecture disappears, resulting in cystic spaces interspersed with bands of connective tissue producing the so-called *end-stage*.

Thus, on morphologic grounds, pulmonary sarcoidosis appears to begin as a mononuclear alveolitis that proceeds to a multinucleated, giant cell granulomatous disease. Thereafter, two alternatives are available: The granulomas resolve leaving relatively normal lung (80% of patients), or progressive fibrosis ensues producing end-stage lung. In either case, the process takes place in various alveolar structures at different times and progresses at different rates.

Characterization of the Alveolitis of Sarcoidosis

Dr. Gary W. Hunninghake (Senior Investigator, Pulmonary Branch, National Heart, Lung, and Blood Institute): Pulmonary sarcoidosis is characterized by the presence of granulomas in the lung parenchyma (5, 6, 60). However, as we have just seen, the earliest lesion of this disease is an alveolitis, a diffuse infiltration of the lung parenchyma by mononuclear cells (36, 52-54). We may conceive, therefore, of the sequence of events in the development of pulmonary sarcoidosis as follows. A stimulus, at present not defined, results in an accumulation of mononuclear cells in the lung parenchyma (that is, the alveolitis). The alveolitis either resolves spontaneously or leads to the formation of granulomas. The presence of granulomas is usually associated with at least some degree of alteration of interstitial connective tissue and epithelial, endothelial, and mesenchymal cells that compose the normal alveolar structures. Although whether it is the alveolitis or granulomas, or both, that mediate these alterations is unclear, it is evident that in some cases the derangement of the alveolar structure is progressive, leading to interstitial fibrosis and the eventual end-stage of alveolar-capillary units.

The sequence of events outlined above does not take place in all of the alveolar structures at the same time or at the same rate. Rather, small groups of units are affected at different times and progress through the phases of alveolitis to granulomas, fibrosis, and cellular derangement to end-stage at different rates. Also, the disease within each group of alveoli may halt, resolve, or progress, making the overall picture a montage of alveolar-capillary units in various stages of inflammation and derangement. Thus, a patient with sarcoidosis will have some alveoli that are normal, some with alveolitis, and others with various mixtures of alveolitis, granuloma, fibrosis, and alterations of parenchymal cells. Over a time, the number of units in each phase will probably change, giving an overall picture of either no lung disease, stable lung disease, or progressive lung disease.

On the basis of these observations, it is clear that characterization and quantification of the alveolitis of sarcoidosis is an important means of defining the pathogenesis as well as the activity and prognosis of the disease.

TECHNIQUE

The inflammatory and immune effector cells forming the alveolitis of sarcoidosis can be recovered from the alveolar structures by a technique termed *bronchoalveolar lavage* (28, 32-34, 61-64). With this method, the effector cells within the lower respiratory tract are obtained by placing a fiberoptic bronchoscope in a distal airway, instilling 1 dL of sterile saline in five 20-mL aliquots, and recovering the lavage fluid by suction. With this technique, from 10 to 30 $\times$ 10^6 effector cells can be recovered; with the immunologic methods now available, this is sufficient to permit detailed characterization of the type, number, and state of activation of the cells that are present. Also, because bronchoalveolar lavage is rapid and safe, the procedure can be used to contrast the effector cell populations of the lungs of sarcoidosis patients with those of normal persons and of persons with other lung disorders and can be used to evaluate the effector cell populations of the same patient over a period of time.

One area of concern in using bronchoalveolar lavage to evaluate the inflammatory and immune effector cell populations in the lower respiratory tract is the possibility that the cells recovered by lavage do not accurately reflect the true alveolitis of the disease. However, studies comparing the effector cells in open lung biopsies of patients to the effector cells recovered by lavage have shown that the cells recovered by lavage accurately reflect the ongoing inflammatory and immune processes within the lower respiratory tract (31, 33, 65). In addition, the inflammatory and immune effector cells obtained by lavage of one segment of the lung appear to be representative of the alveolitis of the sarcoid lung as a whole (66). Although it is not known how many alveolar-capillary units are washed out during the lavage procedure, it is apparent that enough alveoli are sampled so that the local differences from one group of alveolar-capillary units to another are averaged out in the lavage specimen.

The current methods of handling the lavage fluid and characterizing and quantifying the recovered cells have been detailed in a recent review (33). The cell populations are usually quantified as a percentage of the total bronchoalveolar cells. Quantifying the absolute numbers of these cells is not very meaningful, because the yield of cells may be influenced by multiple factors such as the placement of the bronchoscope or the relative "stickiness" of the cells to the alveolar epithelial surface.

GENERAL CHARACTERISTICS OF THE ALVEOLITIS OF SARCOIDOSIS

Evaluation of the inflammatory and immune effector cell populations recovered from the lungs of patients with sarcoidosis shows that the alveolitis of this disease contrasts sharply with the effector cell populations of normal lung and is markedly different than the alveolitis of most other interstitial disorders (28, 32-34, 63-71).

The effector cells present in the alveolar structures of normal nonsmokers consist of more than 90% alveolar macrophages, less than 10% lymphocytes, and less than 1% polymorphonuclear leukocytes (28, 32, 33, 64). In contrast, sarcoidosis is characterized by a marked increase in the proportions of lymphocytes in the lower respiratory tract (28, 31-34, 63-71). On the average, our study population had 33% ± 6% lymphocytes in their lavage fluid compared to less than 10% for normal nonsmokers and smokers. In our sarcoidosis patients with clinical criteria associated with active disease (such as fever, weight loss, erythema nodosum, progressive deterioration of lung function) the proportion of lung lymphocytes was 55% ± 8%, almost twofold higher than that of the group average.

Most other interstitial disorders are associated with normal proportions of lymphocytes in the alveolar structures. Other than sarcoidosis, the only lung disorders know to be associated with increased proportions of lymphocytes in lavage fluid are hypersensitivity pneumonitis (62), tuberculosis (33, 72), and lymphoma involving the lung parenchyma (33). As more lung disorders are evaluated by bronchoalveolar lavage, this list is likely to grow; from the pattern emerging, it will probably include most granulomatous lung diseases in addition to lymphocyte-derived malignancies involving lung parenchyma (33).

In addition to lymphocytes, the remainder of the effector cells characterizing the alveolitis of sarcoidosis are monocytes and macrophages (5, 6, 28, 31-34, 36, 52-54, 61-71); as in normal persons, nonsmoking patients with sarcoidosis have less than 1% neutrophils in their lower respiratory tract (28-34, 64, 65). With the technology presently available, it is not possible to distinguish between the small young macrophage and the blood monocyte that has recently migrated to the alveolar structures; hence the terms *macrophages* or *mononuclear phagocytes* are used interchangeably when this population of cells in bronchoalveolar lavage fluid analyses is discussed. Although the proportions of these cells are lower in lavage fluid recovered from patients with sarcoidosis as compared to those in normal persons, it is important to emphasize that the total number of inflammatory and immune effector cells in the sarcoid lung is many times that in the normal lung. Thus, in terms of total numbers, the alveolitis of sarcoidosis is characterized not only by increased numbers of lymphocytes but also by increased numbers of mononuclear phagocytes.

From these studies, it is apparent that bronchoalveolar lavage analysis yields a picture of the alveolitis of pulmonary sarcoidosis similar to that of the open lung biopsy: Sarcoidosis is a disease characterized by the accumulation of large numbers of lymphocytes, monocytes, and macrophages within the alveolar structures.

CHARACTERIZATION AND QUANTIFICATION OF LYMPHOCYTE SUBTYPES

Estimates of the relative numbers of lymphocyte subtypes in the lower respiratory tract can be expressed either as a percentage of the total lymphocytes present or as a percentage of total inflammatory and immune effector cells present. Both methods are valuable, as they give somewhat different insights into the importance of the various cells as components of the inflammatory and immune effector cell populations of the lower respiratory tract. Whereas expressing the numbers of lymphocyte subtypes as a percentage of total lymphocytes present gives an estimate of relative shifts in lymphocyte subpopulations, expressing the numbers of lymphocyte subtypes as a percentage of total alveolar effector cells gives an estimate of the overall intensity of each lymphocyte component of the pulmonary inflammatory and immune process.

In normal persons, the percentage of lung lymphocytes that is T-lymphocytes varies from 65% to 80%; this is also the case for interstitial disorders such as idiopathic pulmonary fibrosis, the collagen-vascular disorders, and histiocytosis-X (28, 32, 33, 64). In marked contrast, our study population with sarcoidosis, unselected for disease activity, had an average of 90% ± 4% of all lung lymphocytes as T-lymphocytes. In fact, T-lymphocytes represented more than 80% (the high normal value) of all lung lymphocytes in 91% of the persons in the study population, in spite of the fact that these patients were unselected in terms of any clinical, roentgenographic, or physiologic criteria. Of the patients with less than 80% T-lymphocytes, none had any evidence of lung disease at

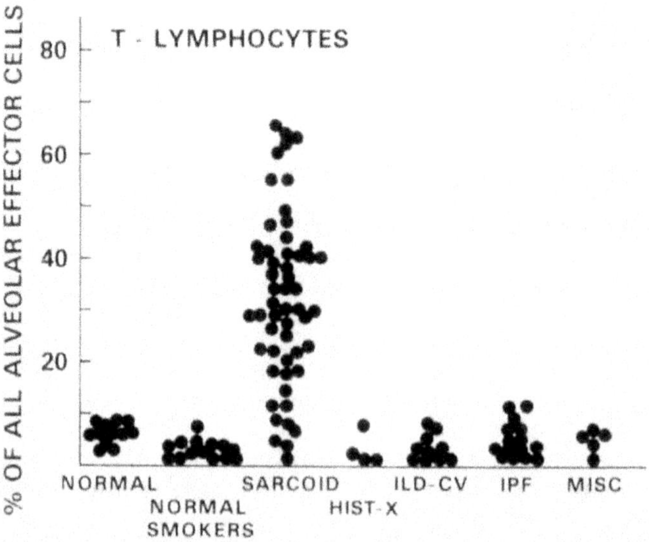

Figure 3. Proportion of all inflammatory and immune effector cells in the alveolar structures that are T-lymphocytes in normal persons and in persons with various chronic lung disorders, including untreated patients with sarcoidosis. The lung effector cells were recovered by bronchoalveolar lavage. For normal persons (nonsmokers and smokers), T-lymphocytes represent less than 8% of all effector cells present. Hist-X = histiocytosis-X; ILD-CV = interstitial lung disease associated with collagen vascular disease (included are patients with rheumatoid arthritis, progressive systemic sclerosis, systemic lupus erythematosus, and mixed connective tissue disease); IPF = idiopathic pulmonary fibrosis; Misc = various miscellaneous lung disorders (included are patients with familial pulmonary fibrosis, Kartagener's syndrome, inorganic dust disease, squamous cell carcinoma, and cystic fibrosis).

the time of evaluation. Thus, pulmonary sarcoidosis is a disease characterized by shifts in the proportions of lung lymphocytes toward more T-lymphocytes (28-34, 65).

That patients with pulmonary sarcoidosis have increased proportions of T-lymphocytes in their alveolar structures is even more remarkable when compared to the findings in their peripheral blood. Although these persons have large amounts of T-lymphocytes in lung, they simultaneously have peripheral blood T-lymphocytopenia (23-34), suggesting that observations of cellular immune processes in blood may give a false view of what is actually occurring in lung. In comparison to persons with sarcoidosis, normal persons have the same proportions of T-lymphocytes in lung and blood as do patients with idiopathic pulmonary fibrosis, interstitial lung disease associated with collagen-vascular disease, and histiocytosis-X (28, 32, 33).

When the numbers of T-lymphocytes in the sarcoid lung are expressed as a proportion of the total inflammatory and immune effector cells present, it becomes apparent that this disease is characterized not only by shifts in the proportions of lung lymphocytes that are T-lymphocytes but also by an intense T-lymphocyte alveolitis. Whereas in normal persons, T-lymphocytes account for less than 8% of all inflammatory and immune effector cells within the alveolar structures, in persons with sarcoidosis, T-lymphocytes represent 31% ± 8% of the effector cells present (Figure 3). By comparison, in most other interstitial disorders, less than 8% of all effector cells present in the lower respiratory tract are T-lymphocytes (28-33). This increased proportion of T-lymphocytes in the sarcoid lung becomes even more impressive when one considers that although normal persons have approximately 25×10^9 effector cells in their lower respiratory tract (73), morphologic observations of biopsies of patients with sarcoidosis with active alveolitis suggest that there are probably five to 20 times more effector cells within their alveolar structures (5, 6, 36, 52-54, 60). It is apparent, therefore, that in absolute numbers T-lymphocytes are tremendously increased within the alveolar structures of the sarcoid lung.

Although the proportions of lung lymphocytes that are T-lymphocytes are increased in the sarcoid lung, the proportions of lung lymphocytes that are B-lymphocytes are significantly reduced (28, 32, 33). In contrast, the proportions of lymphocytes that are B-lymphocytes are increased in the blood of sarcoid patients compared to their own lungs and to the blood of normal persons. Because the sarcoid lung is characterized by an overall increase in total lymphocytes, it is likely that the total number of B-lymphocytes is increased within the sarcoid lung even though the proportion of these cells is reduced. Even so, the total number of T-lymphocytes is still far in excess; on the average, the sarcoid lung has 20 to 25 times more T-lymphocytes than B-lymphocytes (28-33). In comparison, the normal lung has only seven to 10 times more T-lymphocytes than B-lymphocytes (28-33).

If, as suggested above, lung T-lymphocytes are actively involved in the pathogenesis of pulmonary sarcoidosis, many of these lung T-lymphocytes are probably in a state of relative activation and thus function as effector T-lymphocytes. In support of this concept are the findings that in parallel with the marked increase in the numbers of T-lymphocytes in the sarcoid lung, there are also increases in numbers of various subtypes of T-lymphocytes in the alveolar structures of these patients (28-34). Most importantly, persons with sarcoidosis have increased proportions of lung T-lymphocytes that form rosettes with sheep erythrocytes at 37 °C, a subset of T-lymphocytes well known to be in a relative state of activation (Figure 4) (28, 32, 33, 74, 75). Additional evidence of increased numbers of activated T-lymphocytes in the lungs of sarcoid patients comes from the observation that these patients have increased numbers of T-lymphocytes that have receptors for the crystallizable fragment (Fc) portion of IgG (so-called Tγ cells) (28, 32, 33). Although the exact role of Tγ cells in the pathogenesis of sarcoidosis is unknown, several studies have shown that increased numbers of this subset of T-lymphocytes are present when a population of T-lymphocytes has been activated in some manner (76-78).

As pointed out by other investigators, there are increased proportions of T-lymphocytes forming rosettes with sheep erythrocytes at 37 °C (79) and Tγ cells (80) in the blood of patients with sarcoid compared to blood of normals. Although this was also true in our study population, the proportion and total numbers of these T-lymphocyte subtypes in blood were far less than those found in lung, further suggesting that analysis of blood does not give a true picture of the character and magnitude of the immune processes within the lung.

Further evidence of the presence of increased numbers of activated T-lymphocytes in the sarcoid lung comes from studies of the relative proportions of these cells undergoing spontaneous transformation. In this regard, unstimulated, highly purified T-lymphocytes isolated from the lungs of patients with sarcoidosis spontaneously incorporate three- to fourfold greater amounts of [^{3}H]thymidine than do equal numbers of lung T-lymphocytes from normal persons (HUNNINGHAKE GW, CRYSTAL RG. Unpublished observations). In addition, as will be discussed by Dr. Gadek, lung T-lymphocytes from patients with sarcoidosis spontaneously release a variety of lymphokines whereas lung T-lymphocytes from normal persons do not (28, 33, 34).

Thus, it is clear that the alveolitis of sarcoidosis is characterized by increased numbers of lymphocytes, monocytes, and macrophages. Whereas the effector role of the monocytes and macrophages in the sarcoid lung has not been evaluated, it is apparent that this disease is distinguished by large numbers of activated T-lymphocytes within the alveolar structures. Furthermore, these activated T-lymphocytes probably play a major role in the pathogenesis of the disease. Because the activity of the alveolitis can be accurately gauged by analysis of the cell populations in bronchoalveolar lavage fluid, this technique should prove useful in staging patients with sarcoidosis and following their response to therapy.

Maintenance of the Alveolitis of Sarcoidosis

Dr. James E. Gadek (Senior Investigator, Pulmonary Branch, National Heart, Lung, and Blood Institute): Although the initiating stimulus for sarcoidosis is unknown, increasingly there are clues as to how the sarcoid granuloma is formed and maintained. As discussed by Drs. Roberts and Hunninghake, the appearance of granuloma is preceded by an accumulation of monocytes, macrophages, and lymphocytes, particularly T-lymphocytes, within the alveolar structures. I will outline the importance of all these cell types in forming and maintaining granuloma within the lower respiratory tract.

IMPORTANCE OF MONONUCLEAR PHAGOCYTES

Monocytes and alveolar macrophages are part of the *mononuclear phagocyte* system, a term applied to a specific class of phagocytic cells derived from monoblasts within the bone marrow (39, 81-83). The mononuclear phagocyte system forms a continuum of cells that progressively mature from precursor marrow cells to blood monocytes and finally to macrophages. In addition, the evidence is overwhelming that epithelioid cells and giant cells are derived from monocytes and macrophages (53, 54, 83-88). Thus, in pulmonary sarcoidosis, granuloma formation is conceived as a coalescence and maturation of mononuclear phagocytes that are in the alveolar structures. Consequently, although mononuclear phagocytes have a variety of effector functions that may be relevant to the pathogenesis of sarcoidosis (64, 68, 83, 89-98), one critical role of these cells in this disease is to serve as a building block for granuloma formation.

Because granulomas are dynamic structures, there is a need for the constant replenishment of mononuclear phagocytes as epithelioid cells and giant cells either die or move out of granuloma (85, 88). This constant requirement for a monocyte and macrophage pool in the formation of new granuloma and maintenance of established granuloma suggests processes that maintain the mononuclear phagocyte series of cells within the alveolar structures are relevant to the pathogenesis of sarcoidosis.

There are two mechanisms that could serve to replenish the monocyte and macrophage pool within the lung: Monocytes and macrophages within the alveolar structures could proliferate locally, or monocytes could be recruited to the lung from the blood monocyte pool, or both could occur. There are several reasons to think that the second mechanism is more important in pulmonary sarcoidosis. First, although monocytes and macrophages in the lower respiratory tract have the capacity to proliferate (99, 100), large numbers of monocytes and macrophages would have to be constantly dividing to maintain the monocyte series within the sarcoid lung (82). However, evaluation of biopsies of sarcoid lung rarely shows these cells in mitosis (2, 3, 36, 37). Second, studies with experimental models of granuloma formation have shown that most cells composing granuloma are derived from the circulating pool of blood monocytes (45, 53, 68, 83-88). Consistent with this concept, biopsies of patients with sarcoidosis show monocytes migrating from capillaries to the alveolar interstitium (37).

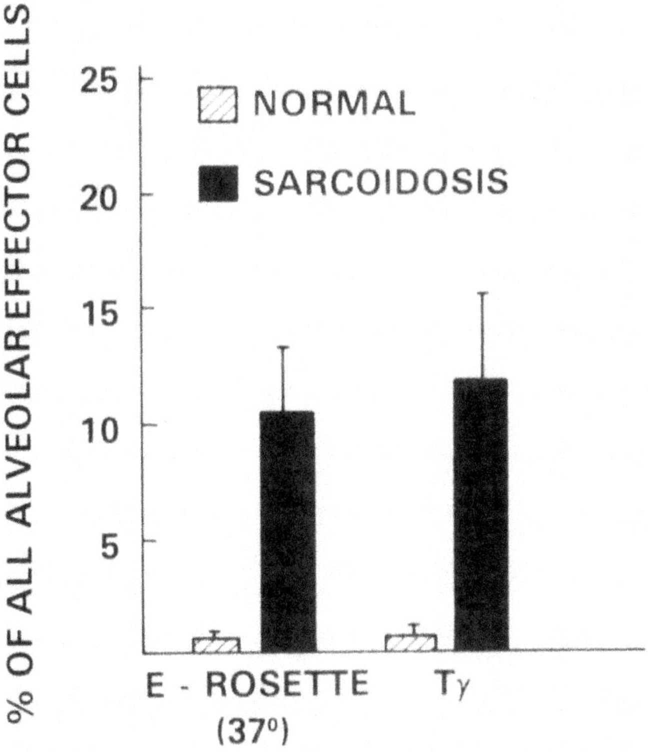

Figure 4. Subtypes of T-lymphocytes in the lungs of patients with sarcoidosis. Two subtypes of T-lymphocytes were evaluated, those forming rosettes with sheep erythrocytes at 37 °C (*E-Rosette, 37°*) and those with receptors for the Fc portion of IgG (*Tγ*). The data are presented as the proportions of all inflammatory and immune effector cells represented as each T-lymphocyte subtype. The normal study population consisted of eight persons and the sarcoid population, of nine. The error bars represent SEM.

Table 1. Role of Lung T-Lymphocytes in Recruiting Blood Monocytes to the Lung in Patients With Pulmonary Sarcoidosis*

Mediator	Function	Normal Persons†		Patients with Sarcoid†	
		Blood	Lung	Blood	Lung
Monocyte chemotactic factor‡	Recruitment of circulating monocytes to the site of mediator release	0	0	1+	4+
Leukocyte inhibitory factor§	Inhibition of polymorphonuclear leukocyte migration	0	0	1+	4+

* Production of soluble mediators of inflammatory cell migration by lung and blood T-lymphocytes of normal persons and patients with pulmonary sarcoidosis.
† Lung and blood T-lymphocytes were incubated for 48 h. at 37 °C and the supernatants evaluated for the production of monocyte chemotactic factor and leukocyte inhibitory factor. The relative amounts of the factors produced are expressed on an arbitrary scale of 0 (none) to 4+ (maximum, equivalent to mitogen-stimulated T-lymphocytes) (28, 34).
‡ Quantified using purified blood monocytes as target cells in a modified Boyden chemotaxis assay (34).
§ Quantified using unfractionated blood leukocytes as target cells in a chemotaxis under agarose assay (28).

MONOCYTE RECRUITMENT TO THE SARCOID LUNG: ROLE OF T-LYMPHOCYTES

The process of recruitment of leukocytes from one compartment to another is known as chemotaxis (101). Chemotactic stimuli are generally protein or lipid and are referred to as "chemotactic factors." A vast array of such factors has been described, some derived from serum and others produced directly by cells (102-115). In addition, a number of chemotactic inhibitors have been characterized (116-121), and thus the process of chemotaxis must be considered as a balance between the attractive nature of chemotactic factors and the restraining influence of chemotactic inhibitors. Whereas some of these processes are directed toward all leukocytes, others affect one cell type more than others allowing for the expression of specificity in cell migrations. This concept is important because neutrophils are rarely found in the sarcoid lung, suggesting that blood monocytes are recruited to the sarcoid lung, and blood neutrophils are excluded.

Chemotactic factors are conventionally evaluated in vitro by the use of chemotactic chambers in which the target cells and putative chemotactic stimuli are separated by a membrane of calibrated pore size. In such a system, chemotactic activity is usually quantitated as the number of target cells moving through the membrane toward the stimulus per unit time (122). To evaluate the role played by lung inflammatory and immune effector cells in recruiting blood monocytes, unstimulated lung T-lymphocytes obtained from sarcoid patients by bronchoalveolar lavage were cultured for 48 hours, after which the supernatants of these cells were evaluated for chemotactic activity using blood monocytes as target cells (34).

Such studies convincingly demonstrate that T-lymphocytes comprising the alveolitis of sarcoidosis are spontaneously elaborating a specific factor (monocyte chemotactic factor) that attracts blood monocytes (34) (Table 1). In contrast, T-lymphocytes present in normal alveolar structures have no influence on the migration of blood monocytes. Monocyte chemotactic factor has a molecular mass of 10 to 15 000 daltons and is probably a protein (110). Whereas T-lymphocytes from the normal lung can be induced to elaborate monocyte chemotactic factor (for example, by stimulation with a mitogen such as concanavalin A), the T-lymphocytes obtained from the lungs of sarcoid patients are spontaneously secreting it (34). This finding is consistent with the concept that increased numbers of T-lymphocytes found in the sarcoid lung are activated.

In addition, comparison of T-lymphocytes from lung and blood of sarcoid patients demonstrates that lung T-lymphocytes spontaneously secrete larger amounts of monocyte chemotactic factor than blood T-lymphocytes of the same person (Table 1). The difference between lung and blood is striking; sarcoid lung T-lymphocytes produce an average of 25 times more of this chemotactic factor per cell than do sarcoid blood T-lymphocytes (34). This observation, together with the finding that the sarcoid lung contains large numbers of T-lymphocytes, suggests that concentrations of this chemotactic factor are higher in lung than in blood. Thus, a gradient of monocyte chemotactic factor between lung and blood of these patients is likely, resulting in the chronic accumulation of blood monocytes within the alveolar structures. In light of this observation, it is not difficult to understand how the pool of mononuclear phagocytes may be maintained within the sarcoid lung, providing a continuous source of basic building blocks for granuloma formation.

Although the elaboration of monocyte chemotactic factor by sarcoid lung T-lymphocytes explains the attraction of blood monocytes to the lung in this disease, it does not explain why monocytes, and not polymorphonuclear leukocytes, are recruited. When neutrophils are used as the target cell, chemotactic chamber studies show that monocyte chemotactic factor attracts neutrophils as well as monocytes (123). Thus, we have to look elsewhere to explain the specificity of the recruitment of monocytes in this disease.

One clue comes from analysis of other products elaborated by activated T-lymphocytes. Along with monocyte chemotactic factor, lung T-lymphocytes from sarcoid patients also spontaneously produced leukocyte inhibitory factor (28), a 68 000-dalton product that prevents the migration of polymorphonuclear leukocytes, but not monocytes (119) (Table 1). In addition, patients with sarcoidosis have elevated levels of serum lysozyme (68), an enzyme that inhibits the migration of neutrophils (124). In sarcoidosis, therefore, blood leukocytes are probably under a number of attractive and inhibitory stimuli, the net result of which is to recruit monocytes, but no neutrophils, to the alveolar structures.

Various studies have shown that blood monocytes of sarcoid patients are in a relative state of activation compared to blood monocytes of normal persons. Monocytes of sarcoid patients have increased numbers of IgG-Fc and C3 receptors (125), show increased spreading (126), and contain more lysozyme (68, 127), β-galactosidase (128), and angiotensin-converting enzyme (68, 129-131), all of which are considered criteria for mononuclear phagocyte activation (68). Although the mechanism of monocyte activation in sarcoidosis is undoubtedly complex and involves a variety of processes, T-lymphocytes probably play a role. In this regard, products elaborated by activated T-lymphocytes are known to be able to stimulate blood monocytes as well as attract them (132). The results of monocyte activation are probably important in helping the monocyte negotiate tissue barriers in its migration from capillary lumen to alveolar interstitium and in preparing the monocyte for its role in granuloma formation. In addition, that lung T-lymphocytes from sarcoid patients also spontaneously elaborate macrophage migration inhibitory factor (HUNNINGHAKE GW, GADEK JE, CRYSTAL RG. Unpublished observations) may provide a mechanism for the immobilization of the monocyte once it arrives within the alveolar structures. Although the relative state of cells composing sarcoid granuloma has not yet been studied, evidence from other forms of granuloma, such as that found in tuberculosis and schistosomasis, suggests that monocytes, macrophages, and epithelioid cells forming granuloma are in a relative state of activation (68, 83-88).

In addition to locally produced T-lymphocyte products, numerous inhibitory factors have been found in serum of patients with sarcoidosis. Although these circulating inhibitory factors probably play an important role in the cutaneous anergy of sarcoidosis, their presence does not seem to be related to disease activity in the lung (133-141). Thus, their role, if any, in the recruitment of blood monocytes to the sarcoid lung is unclear.

In summary, quantitative analysis of the alveolitis of sarcoidosis has shown that it is made up of monocytes, macrophages, and lymphocytes, including large numbers of activated T-lymphocytes. Analysis of the products elaborated by T-lymphocytes composing the alveolitis of sarcoidosis shows that these cells produce factors whose net effect is to attract blood monocytes specifically. Although these observations are relevant only to a part of the pathogenesis of sarcoidosis, they explain how one important cellular constituent of the sarcoid alveolitis is maintained.

Skin Testing, Blood Studies, and Bronchoalveolar Lavage to Assess Activity

Dr. Ronald G. Crystal: Traditionally, the activity of pulmonary sarcoidosis has been assessed with a number of loosely defined clinical criteria such as the presence or absence of weight loss, fatigue, weakness, malaise, fever, erythema nodosum, dry cough, progressive dyspnea, and worsening exercise intolerance (1, 3-5, 7, 12-16, 35). However, true activity of pulmonary sarcoid can be defined only in terms of the actual disease process in the lung. Because the alveolitis of sarcoidosis clearly precedes, and probably causes, the anatomic derangements of the alveolar structures that are characteristic of this disease, assessments of disease activity must take into account the number, type, and functional state of the inflammatory and immune effector cells in the lower respiratory tract. Thus, in view of our previous discussions, monitors of disease activity should assess the status of lung T-lymphocytes, lung mononuclear phagocytes, or both.

Table 2. Skin Test and Blood Studies Suggested in the Literature as Means to Assess the Activity of Pulmonary Sarcoidosis

Test	References
Skin testing	
Evaluation of anergy to a variety of antigens	1, 3-5, 12, 19-23, 143-149
Rebuck skin window	170
Evaluation of circulating mononuclear cells	
Number of lymphocytes	24, 25, 146, 150-151
Number of T-lymphocytes	24-27, 145, 149, 151, 152
Number of activated T-lymphocytes	70, 79, 80, 153
Response of lymphocytes to mitogens and antigens	21-23, 35, 145, 146, 154, 155
Response of lymphocytes to mixed lymphocyte cultures	143
Generation of killer cells	143
Spontaneous production of migration inhibition factor	146
Mediation of antibody dependent cellular cytotoxicity	152
Quantitation of serologic variables	
Immune complexes	156-159
Antibodies against infectious agents	160
Serum inhibitors of sheep erythrocyte binding to normal T-lymphocytes	137-139
IgG levels	149
Presence of autoantibodies	149
Anti T-lymphocyte antibodies	161
Lysozyme	7, 162-166, 180
Angiotensin-converting enzyme	7, 11, 131, 166-178, 180

SKIN TESTS AND BLOOD STUDIES

The mechanisms causing the anergic state in sarcoidosis are not well understood but probably involve circulating "factor(s)" that suppress the normal response of circulating inflammatory and immune effector cells to intradermal antigens (*see* Table 2). However, although anergy is a classic finding in pulmonary sarcoidosis (1, 3-5, 12, 19, 20, 133-143), there is no evidence that the anergic state reflects a concomitant high-intensity alveolitis or that normal skin test responses are characteristic of patients with low-intensity alveolitis (143-149). Likewise, although the numbers and function of blood mononuclear cells may have a broad correlation with disease activity, there is little evidence suggesting that such measurements accurately gauge the quantity and activity of the alveolitis of the sarcoid lung (23-29, 150-155).

The same reservations exist for most serologic tests proposed as monitors of disease activity. For example,

Table 3. Comparison of Proportions of T-Lymphocytes in Lavage Cell Differential with Biopsy Assessment of the Intensity of Alveolitis of Sarcoidosis Patients

Biopsy Assessment*	Percentages of T-Lymphocytes in the Lavage Cell Differential†	
	(≤ 28)	(> 28)
Low-intensity alveolitis	6‡	0
High-intensity alveolitis	2	12‡

* Lung biopsies (approximately 1 cm by 1 cm, hemotoxylin and eosin stain), divided in a blinded fashion, were placed into a low- or high-intensity alveolitis group using criteria based on the number of mononuclear cells infiltrating the gas exchange exchange units (36).

† Patients were divided into two groups: those in whom lavage T-lymphocytes represented $\leq 28\%$ of all inflammatory and immune effector cells present (low-intensity alveolitis) and those in whom T-lymphocutes represented $>28\%$ effector cells present (high-intensity alveolitis).

‡ The groupings of low-intensity alveolitis with $\leq 28\%$ lavage T-lympnocytes and the high-intensity alveolitis with $>28\%$ lavage T-lymphocytes was significant at the $p < 0.01$ level.

there is no evidence that circulating immune complexes or various types of antibodies found in the serum of sarcoid patients are related to the inflammatory and immune processes within their lungs (156-161). However, two serologic variables, lysozyme and angiotensin-converting enzyme, should be considered because in theory, serum levels of these enzymes are linked to the class of phagocytic cells composing the alveolitis of sarcoidosis (11, 68, 162-180).

Lysozyme is an enzyme produced and secreted by many different cell types including cells of the mononuclear phagocytic series. In vitro, activated mononuclear phagocytes have an increased content of lysozyme and secrete more lysozyme into the culture medium (179). Thus, when the observation was made that patients with sarcoidosis frequently had increased levels of serum lysozyme, it was suggested that such measurements might reflect the activity of mononuclear phagocytes in these persons (68, 127, 163, 180). Several studies seem to support this concept. Blood monocytes of sarcoid patients secrete increased amounts of lysozyme compared to controls, monocyte lysozyme secretory rates correlate with the patient's lysozyme levels, and alveolar macrophages of these patients have more lysozyme activity than normal macrophages (68, 127).

Angiotensin-converting enzyme is generally regarded as a product of endothelial cells, where it acts to convert serum angiotensin I to angiotensin II and metabolizes bradykinin (181). However, when it was discovered that patients with sarcoidosis had increased serum levels of angiotensin-converting enzymes (168, 170), attention was directed toward the mechanism of this finding. Alveolar capillary endothelial cells seemed unlikely to be the source, because many chronic lung diseases are associated with injury to the alveolar capillary bed, yet increased angiotensin-converting enzyme levels are much commoner in sarcoidosis (11, 171). It was soon ascertained, however, that angiotensin-converting enzyme was present in lymph nodes, higher levels were present in nodes containing sarcoid granuloma (165), cells of the mononuclear phagocyte series contained and secreted angiotensin-converting enzyme (68, 128), and alveolar macrophages from sarcoid patients contained increased levels of this enzyme (68, 131). Thus, the concept evolved that cells of the mononuclear phagocyte series were the source of increased angiotensin-converting enzyme levels in sarcoidosis, and it was proposed that serum angiotensin-converting enzyme levels might reflect the inflammatory and immune processes in the lung parenchyma.

Unfortunately, in spite of the strong theoretical basis for the use of serum lysozyme and angiotensin-converting enzyme levels to gauge the activity of pulmonary sarcoidosis, there is conflicting evidence on the use of these variables in actually staging patients. Wheras some investigators have found that serum lysozyme and angiotensin-converting enzyme levels roughly correlate with disease activity (defined by symptoms or chest film) (11, 68, 131, 164, 166, 167, 169, 171-174), others have found either little or no correlation (168, 177) or have found that more patients with chronic disease than with acute disease have elevated levels (175). In addition, there have been no clinical studies showing a correlation of serum angiotensin-converting enzyme or lysozyme levels with the intensity of the alveolitis of sarcoidosis. In fact, there is direct evidence suggesting there is no correlation; quantitation of angiotensin-converting enzyme levels in lung parenchyma of sarcoid patients has shown them to be no different from those in normal persons (130, 131). Further confusing the picture is the observation that elevated serum angiotensin-converting enzyme levels also have been found in persons with disorders not involving the lungs, such as degenerative arthritis (171), cirrhosis (171), and granulomatous hepatitis (68, 169), suggesting that the quantity of this enzyme in the serum reflects a contribution from many organs. Because sarcoidosis is a systemic disease, the serum angiotensin-converting enzyme level probably reflects disease activity in many organs and has no specificity for disease activity within the alveolar structures.

In view of the above considerations, although it is clear that activated mononuclear phagocytes produce increased amounts of lysozyme and angiotensin converting enzyme, and that these cells are important components of the alveolitis of sarcoidosis, there is little evidence at present that these serum enzyme levels reflect the intensity of the alveolitis.

BRONCHOALVEOLAR LAVAGE

In contrast to the variables listed in Table 2, several lines of evidence support the concept that bronchoalveolar lavage is a useful clinical tool to sequentially measure the intensity of the inflammatory and immune processes within the alveolar structures of patients with pulmonary sarcoidosis.

1. As Dr. Hunninghake has discussed, bronchoalveolar lavage can be used to characterize the type and state of activation of the cells present within the alveolar structures (33). Although this method samples only cells on the epithelial surface of the lower respiratory tract, comparisons with analyses of effector cells in open lung biop-

sy specimens have shown that lavage analyses yield a representative average of the relative proportions of the various inflammatory and immune effector cells present throughout the alveolar structures (33, 65).

2. Even though lavage analyses are usually expressed in proportional terms (for example, proportion of all inflammatory and immune effector cells that are T-lymphocytes), comparison of lavage data with histologic data showed that for patients with pulmonary sarcoidosis, lavage analyses not only characterize the type of cells present but also estimate the overall intensity of the alveolitis (Table 3). To show this, we compared the proportions of T-lymphocytes recovered by lavage of a group of patients with sarcoidosis with a histologic estimate of the intensity of the alveolitis made by open lung biopsy. The biopsies, taken within 1 month of the lavage, were divided into two groups: those showing a high-intensity alveolitis (that is large numbers of mononuclear cells with the alveolar structures) and those showing a low-intensity alveolitis (that is, small numbers of mononuclear cells

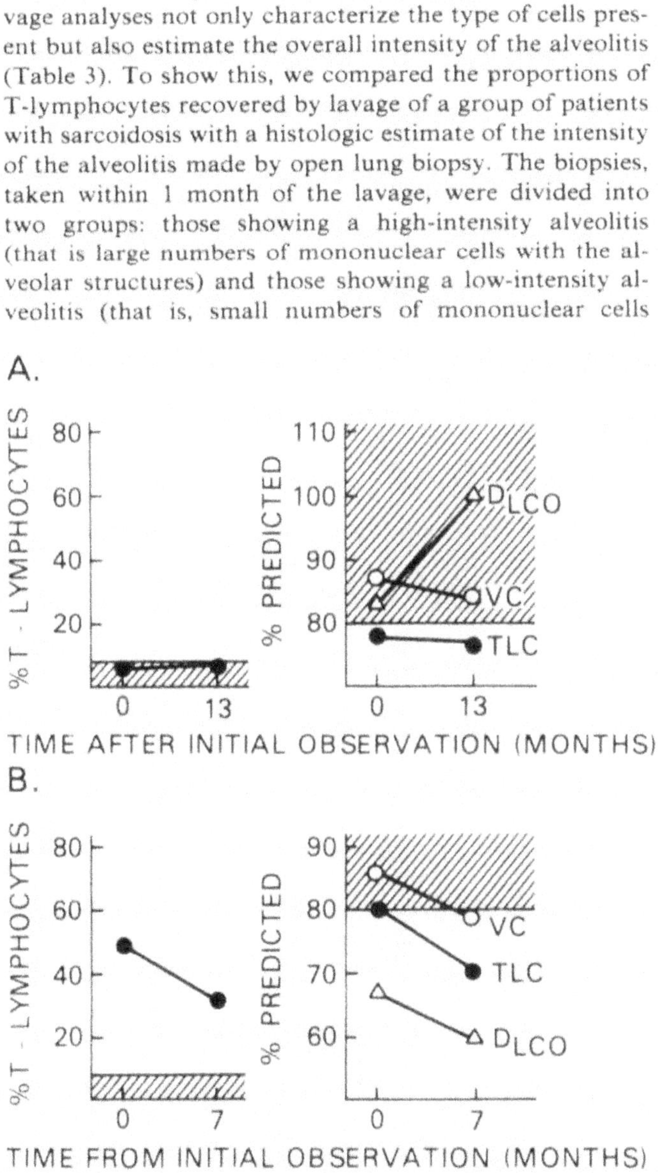

Figure 5. Prognostic use of bronchoalveolar lavage to evaluate the T-lymphocyte component of the alveolitis of pulmonary sarcoidosis. **A.** An untreated 22-year-old woman with pulmonary sarcoidosis seen over 13 months. During this period the alveolitis remained at a low level, and the pulmonary function variables remained stable or improved. **B.** An untreated 25-year-old woman with pulmonary sarcoidosis had a high-intensity alveolitis when first evaluated. After 7 months the alveolitis remained active, and all lung function variables had deteriorated. In both examples, the T-lymphocyte data are presented as the proportion of all lung effector cells that were T-lymphocytes, whereas the pulmonary function data are given in percent of predicted values. Shaded areas represent normal ranges. VC = vital capacity; TLC = total lung capacity; and D_{LCO} = single breath diffusing capacity (predicted based on alveolar volume and hemoglobin).

within the alveolar structures). Likewise, the lavage analyses were divided into two groups: those in which T-lymphocytes accounted for more than 28% of all cells recovered and those in which T-lymphocytes made up less than 28% of the effector cells present. Comparisons of these groupings showed a significant correlation between large numbers of mononuclear cells present in the biopsies and large proportions of T-lymphocytes recovered by lavage (65).

3. In our laboratories, bronchoalveolar lavage has been carried out in over 500 persons; it is associated with minimal discomfort, little morbidity, and no mortality (33). To ensure patient safety, however, it is important not to do lavage in patients with a forced expiratory volume in 1 s of less than 0.8 L. In addition, if inflammatory airway disease is present, lavage analyses must be interpreted cautiously, as it is difficult to estimate the relative contributions of bronchi and alveoli to the recovered cells.

4. Repeat lavage analyses over time show that in persons with pulmonary sarcoidosis in whom the proportion of T-lymphocytes remains low, there is little if any change in lung function over the same period (Figure 5A) (71). In contrast, for untreated patients in whom the proportion of lung T-lymphocytes remains high, lung function deteriorates (Figure 5B).

Such data support the concept that the alveolitis of sarcoidosis is a predecessor and cause of the anatomical derangements characteristic of sarcoidosis and that lavage is a useful monitor of the activity of the sarcoid alveolitis.

Roentgenograms and Physiologic Studies to Assess Activity

Dr. Jack D. Fulmer (Chief, Clinical Service, Pulmonary Branch, National Heart, Lung, and Blood Institute): The most commonly used monitors of pulmonary sarcoidosis are the chest roentgenogram and pulmonary function studies. Inherent in the use of these tests is the assumption that they help to stage the patient, that is, establish the extent and activity of the disease process, the prognosis, and the need for and efficacy of therapy. We will describe, therefore, the roentgenographic and physiologic findings in sarcoidosis and examine the available data concerning the sensitivity and specificity of these tests as monitors of disease activity. Also, because active pulmonary sarcoidosis is characterized by increased numbers of activated T-lymphocytes within the alveolar structures, we will evaluate the usefulness of the chest roentgenogram and common pulmonary function tests as detectors of the T-lymphocyte component of the alveolitis of this disease.

CHEST ROENTGENOGRAMS

The roentgenographic findings in pulmonary sarcoidosis have been well defined, and various classifications have been developed (12, 182-194). However, by international convention, the chest roentgenograms of patients with sarcoidosis are grouped according to the following scheme (12, 186): stage O, normal; stage I, bilateral hilar adenopathy; stage II, hilar adenopathy and diffuse parenchymal changes; and stage III, diffuse pulmonary infiltrates without hilar adenopathy. In this classification, the parenchymal changes most commonly described are fine or coarse nodules or a fluffy, cottonwood appearance; films with fibrotic changes, cysts, and bullae are usually assigned to stage III (12, 186). The proponents of this classification scheme view stages I through III as the roentgenographic manifestations of disease progression (186, 188). A worldwide review of 3676 patients with sarcoidosis showed that at the initial presentation to a physician, 8% had stage O roentgenograms, 51% had stage I, 29% had stage II, and 12% had stage III (186).

Although this international staging scheme is widely used in epidemiologic studies, most investigators believe that it often gives a false impression of the extent and activity of the disease process. Importantly, comparative morphologic-radiographic studies have shown that alveolitis and granulomas are present in the lung parenchyma of persons with stage I roentgenograms (5, 36, 195-198), even though the lung fields appear normal on the roentgenogram. In addition, although stage III roentgenograms are usually found only in those persons with progressive disease, it cannot be assumed that roentgenographic stages I and II always precede stage III (5).

To evaluate the usefulness of the classic roentgenographic staging in detecting the alveolitis in sarcoidosis, we categorized our study population into roentgenographic stages O to III and compared theses stages to estimates of the intensity of the alveolitis made from the lung biopsy. Consistent with the concept that the classic roentgenogram does not yield specific information concerning the activity of pulmonary sarcoidosis, no association was found between the roentgenographic stage and the quantitation of inflammatory and immune effector cells seen in the biopsy (33, 65). Further, comparison of the classic roentgenographic stages to the proportion of the T-lymphocytes recovered by bronchoalveolar lavage also showed no correlation.

In an attempt to escape the rigidity of the classic roentgenographic staging system, many investigators choose to simply describe the pattern seen; the most commonly described parenchymal patterns are reticulonodular, acinar, and fibrotic (189-192). Occasional patients also have large nodular lesions that simulate pulmonary metastasis, and cavitary lesions are sometimes found (184, 189, 193, 194). Although reticulonodular, acinar, and fibrotic patterns are widely recognized as manifestations of sarcoidosis, like the classic roentgenographic stages, their usefulness in staging the disease is unclear. It is generally accepted that the acinar and reticulonodular patterns precede the fibrotic pattern (189, 199, 200), but most evidence suggests that the chest film cannot be used to predict the morphologic findings (5, 36, 195, 201). Closely packed mononuclear cells within the alveolar air spaces have been suggested as the cause of the acinar pattern in sarcoidosis (191, 192), but there is also evidence that it is brought about by interstitial granulomas compressing the air spaces (190, 191). Attempts to correlate the alveolitis of sarcoidosis with these various roentgenographic presentations of sarcoidosis have failed. Evaluation of our study population also shows that there is little relation between the reticulonodular, acinar, and fibrotic patterns and the extent of alveolitis estimated by lung biopsy. Patients with acinar or nodular patterns generally had alveolitis and those with a coarse reticular pattern generally did not, but there was a great deal of overlap between groups. Likewise, no relationship could be found between the roentgenographic pattern and the proportion of bronchoalveolar lavage cells that were T-lymphocytes (33).

PHYSIOLOGIC TESTING

The usual physiologic findings in a patient with pulmonary sarcoidosis are characteristic of those of other patients with interstitial lung disease (3, 8, 189, 202-207). Lung volumes are reduced as are the diffusing capacity and lung compliance (202, 208-215). In addition, airway obstruction is a frequent physiologic finding in patients with sarcoidosis and seems to be unrelated to smoking history or the presence of bronchitis (8, 205, 206, 211, 215-223). Although many patients with sarcoidosis have a normal resting arterial oxygen tension, the resting alveolar-arterial oxygen gradient is often widened. In mild sarcoidosis, the arterial Po_2 may not change with exercise, but in persons with moderate and severe disease, increasing workloads cause the arterial oxygen tension to fall and the alveolar-arterial oxygen gradient to widen (8, 224-226).

Part of the problem in defining the functional consequences of sarcoidosis is that instead of using morphologic data as the standard for classifying patients, most investigators analyze the functional derangements from the perspective of the patient's roentgenographic stage (224). However, even though those with extensive roentgenographic changes usually have severe functional disturbances and those with minimal radiographic findings usually have few functional abnormalities (214), chest film and pulmonary function tests clearly have only a rough correlation to each other. A few studies have suggested that there is progressive impairment of pulmonary function with progressive roentgenographic changes (that is, stage I to III) (207), but for the majority of patients with sarcoidosis, most investigators have found little association between the chest film and physiologic tests (205, 211, 224, 227).

Functional testing is clearly more sensitive, however, to the disease process than the chest film. Many studies have shown examples of patients with stage I sarcoidosis who have abnormal diffusing capacity (189, 202, 207, 211, 224, 226). However, pulmonary function testing can be normal in the presence of parenchymal involvement (226, 227). Likewise, pulmonary function tests can be markedly abnormal but with the patient having little awareness of the functional derangement (228, 229).

As might be expected, some pulmonary function tests are more sensitive than others to this disease process. Measurements of lung volume are generally less sensitive than diffusing capacity, which in turn is less sensitive than gas exchange studies (particularly with exercise) (226, 227).

In our study population, comparison of the lung biopsy to the vital capacity, total lung capacity, diffusing capaci-

Figure 6. Evaluation of the ability of various pulmonary function variables to monitor the extent of the T-lymphocyte component of the alveolitis of sarcoidosis. The proportion of all lung effector cells that were T-lymphocytes (*% T-lymphocytes*) are compared to the percent predicted values for the following: **A.** Vital capacity. **B.** Total lung capacity. **C.** Single breath diffusing capacity (predicted based on alveolar volume and hemoglobin). **D.** Resting arterial oxygen tension. **E.** Change in arterial oxygen tension with exercise (PaO_2 [exercise]; PaO_2 [rest]).

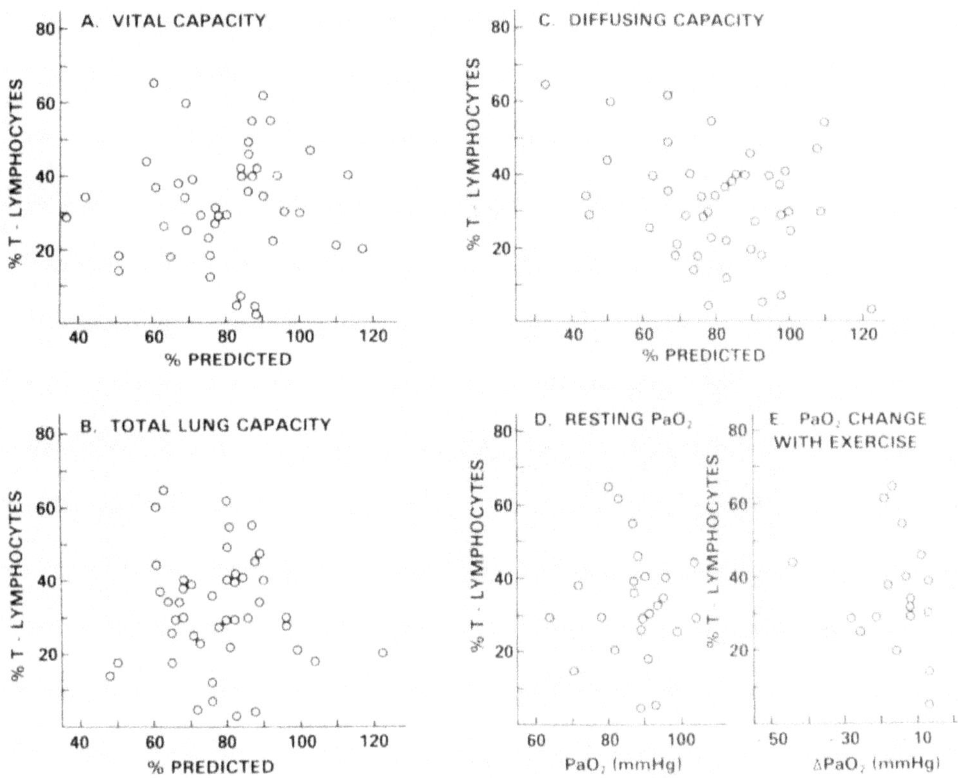

ty, and resting exercising gas exchange data suggests that those studies are abnormal in the presence of alveolitis but cannot predict the extent of parenchymal inflammation. In addition, comparison of the proportion of T-lymphocytes in the lower respiratory tract to these variables showed that the magnitude of the functional abnormality has no relationship to the magnitude of the T-lymphocyte component of the alveolitis (Figure 6).

In summary, although radiographic and functional tests are useful to estimate the extent of disease within the alveolar structures, they cannot distinguish between alveolitis and anatomic derangement. Because the pathogenesis of the disease appears to be closely associated with the magnitude and characteristics of the alveolitis, we do not rely on roentgenographic and pulmonary function tests alone to make prognostic and therapeutic decisions in this disease (71).

Gallium Scanning to Assess Activity

Dr. Bruce R. Line (Senior Investigator, Department of Nuclear Medicine, Clinical Center and Laboratory of Applied Studies, Division of Computer Research and Technology): Gallium-67 (^{67}Ga) is a cyclotron-produced radionuclide with a half-life of 78 hours. This isotope was first used clinically to detect neoplastic disease (230-235). Soon thereafter, it was recognized that ^{67}Ga would also concentrate in sites of acute and chronic inflammation (231, 232, 235, 236). This property of ^{67}Ga is now widely used in the scintigraphic assessment of occult inflammation (237-245). It is thus natural to consider ^{67}Ga scanning as a noninvasive means of assessing the intensity of the alveolitis of sarcoidosis.

Gallium-67 scans are technically simple to do, cause no patient discomfort, and are associated with low radiation exposures (246, 247). The localization of ^{67}Ga in the region from the head to the pelvis is assessed from anterior and posterior rectilinear scans obtained 48 to 72 hours after intravenous administration of ^{67}Ga citrate (35 to 50 μCi/kg). Normal lung tissue does not exceed the uptake of the nonspecific body background. Tissues that show significant physiologic uptake include the skeleton (spine, sternum, pelvis), the liver, and the spleen (Figure 7A) (248). To estimate the quality of ^{67}Ga taken up by lung alveolar tissues and minimize the effects of body structure and interpretive subjectivity, a semiquantitative "^{67}Ga-index" was devised (Figure 7) (249).

Abnormal gallium uptake in the lung is found in various pulmonary disorders with different pathogenesis and by itself is not diagnostic for any particular disease. Most categories of active interstitial lung disease have been associated with positive gallium scans (8). In some of these disorders, such as untreated idiopathic pulmonary fibrosis (249) and sarcoidosis (236, 242, 250, 251), positive gallium scans are the rule. In others, such as histiocytosis-X (LINE BR, FULMER JD, CRYSTAL RG. Unpublished observations), pulmonary uptake of ^{67}Ga is only occasionally observed. The reason for this wide range in sensitivity of the gallium scan is not clear but is probably associated with the type, intensity, and duration of the alveolitis of each disease.

GALLIUM SCANNING IN PULMONARY SARCOIDOSIS

A spectrum of ^{67}Ga uptake patterns can be found in the lungs of patients with sarcoidosis (Figure 7B to D). Diffuse mid- and lower lung zone parenchymal uptake are frequent, but focal or patchy localizations may be

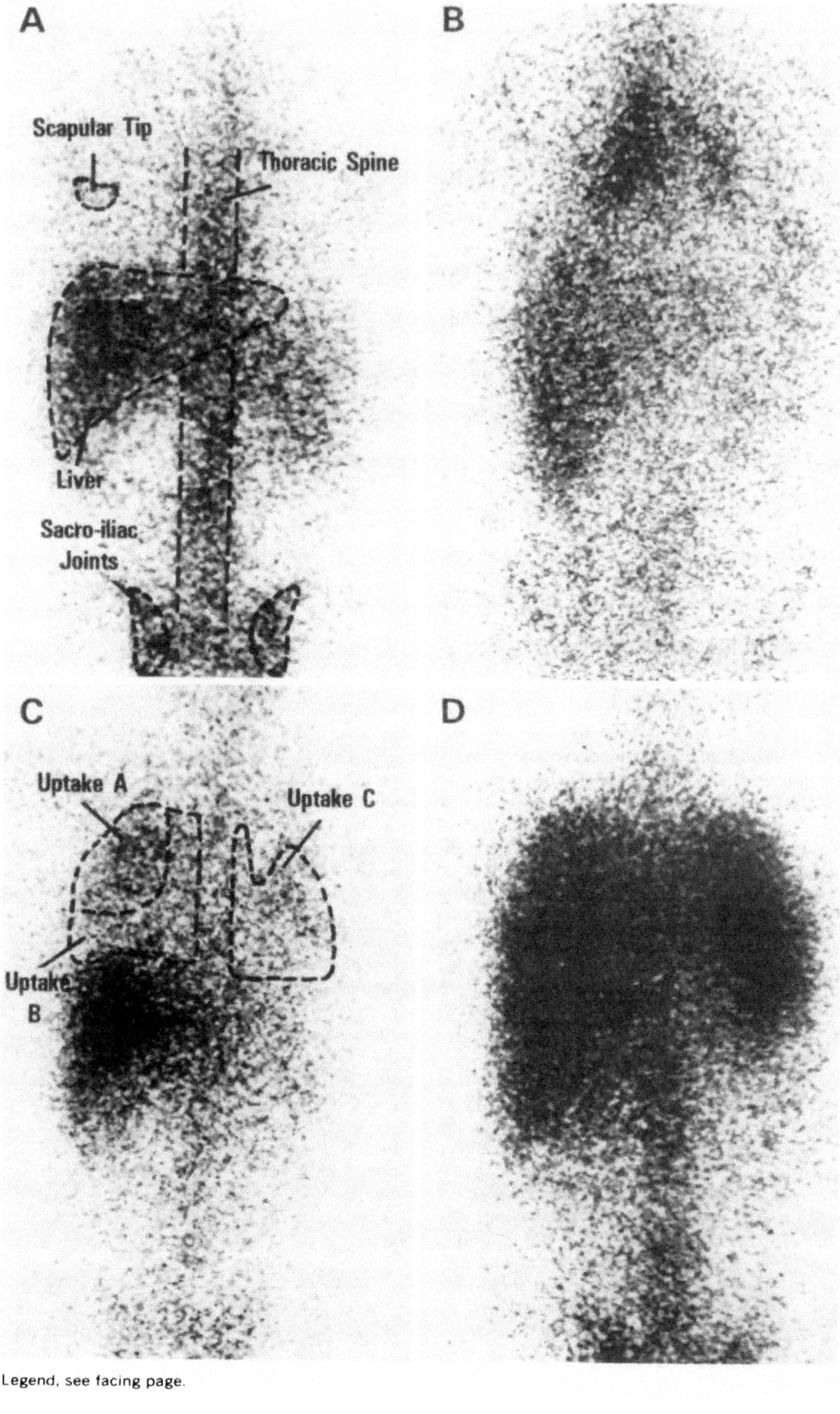

Figure 7. For Legend, see facing page.

present in any lung zone.

Although ^{67}Ga uptake is seen in other thoracic structures other than the lung parenchyma (such as hilar and paratracheal nodes), such uptake is not indicative of alveolitis and therefore not included in the computation of the parenchymal gallium uptake (249).

SIGNIFICANCE OF POSITIVE GALLIUM SCANS

The uptake of gallium in the lungs of patients with sarcoidosis is not associated with age, sex, smoking history, or duration of symptoms. In addition, there is no relation between the level of ^{67}Ga uptake and the functional status of the lung as assessed by lung volumes, by diffusing capacity, or by arterial blood gases at rest or with exercise.

To evaluate the usefulness of ^{67}Ga scans as an indicator of the alveolitis of sarcoidosis, we correlated ^{67}Ga-index estimates of pulmonary ^{67}Ga uptake with assessments of parenchymal inflammation by bronchoalveolar lavage. In the studies to date, there is a significant association of gallium uptake and the proportion of lung effector cells that are lymphocytes but an even stronger association of gallium uptake with the proportion of effector cells that were T-lymphocytes (unpublished observations). Because T-lymphocytes are important in the alveolitis of sarcoidosis, this evidence suggests that gallium uptake reflects the intensity of the T-lymphocyte component of the alveolitis. Consistent with the concept that T-lymphocytes may be responsible for ^{67}Ga uptake in sarcoidosis, Mertz and associates (252) showed in vitro that ^{67}Ga binds to the plasma membrane of lymphocytes. Further, the uptake was doubled when the lymphocytes were activated with phytohemagglutinin.

Further evidence for the usefulness of ^{67}Ga scans in assessing the alveolitis of sarcoidosis comes from the studies in Niden and associates (253) who showed good agreement between ^{67}Ga uptake and the presence of active inflammation in lung tissue obtained by biopsy. In addition, several studies have shown that parenchymal ^{67}Ga uptake is reduced when there is clinical remission of the disease (242, 250-252).

The spectrum of ^{67}Ga index in untreated patients with sarcoidosis (Figure 8) shows uptake scored from 10 to 340 units with indexes in more than two/thirds of patients above the normal limit of 50 units. Scans of untreated patients with sarcoid, compared to untreated patients with idiopathic pulmonary fibrosis, are generally more intense (Figure 8).

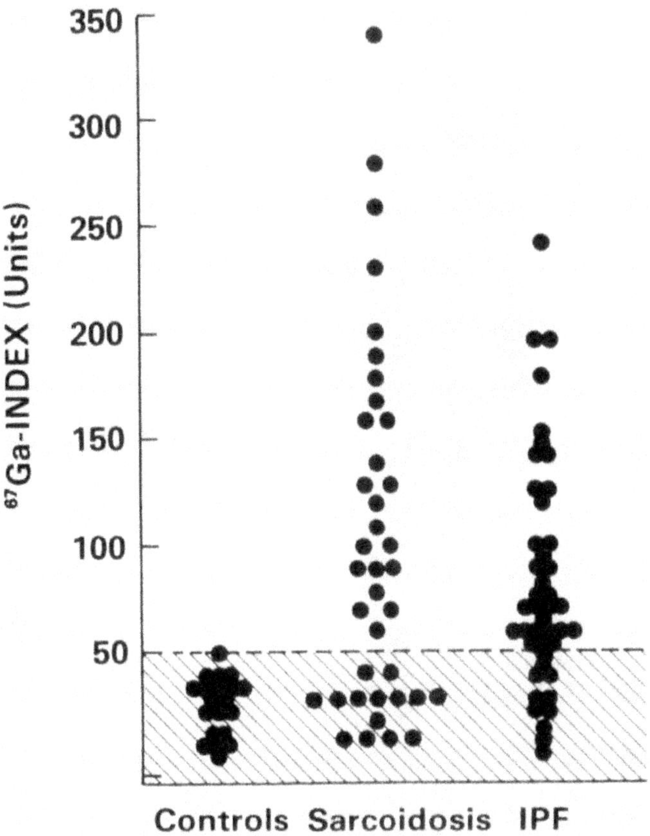

Figure 8. Distribution of ^{67}Ga index in control patients and in untreated patients with sarcoidosis and idiopathic pulmonary fibrosis (*IPF*). All control scans show ^{67}Ga index values below 50 ^{67}Ga index units. Sixty-three percent of the untreated patients with sarcoidosis show ^{67}Ga index values greater than 50 index units. In contrast, 74% of the untreated patients with idiopathic pulmonary fibrosis have ^{67}Ga index values greater than 50 index units (249). As a group, untreated patients with sarcoidosis show greater gallium lung uptake than do untreated patients with idiopathic pulmonary fibrosis. Shaded area represents normal range.

EXTRATHORACIC GALLIUM SCANNING

Although most interest in ^{67}Ga scanning in sarcoidosis has centered on the ^{67}Ga uptake by thoracic structures, gallium often localizes in extrathoracic tissues in this disease (Figures 9 and 10). As in the lung, ^{67}Ga uptake in extrathoracic structures is probably associated with increased proportions of T-lymphocytes. For example, the left iliac crest localization in the patient shown in Figure 10 was associated with larger than normal numbers of T-lymphocytes in the bone marrow of that region. In comparison, the iliac crest on the right did not take up gallium and has normal proportions of T-lymphocytes (28).

In summary, although not diagnostically specific, the ^{67}Ga scan can be used to repetitively characterize the severity and anatomic location of regions of alveolitis and can provide a longitudinal assessment of the degree of inflammation in the whole parenchyma. Gallium-67 scanning is available, noninvasive, and involves low radi-

Figure 7. Examples of ^{67}Ga index computation in a normal person and in three patients with pulmonary sarcoidosis; the method used to quantitate the ^{67}Ga index is as outlined in reference 249. **A.** Normal scan in a 36-year-old man showing physiologic ^{67}Ga uptake in skeletal tissues (scapular tips, spine, pelvis, sacroiliac joints), liver, and spleen. Localization in the pulmonary parenchyma is similar to background (estimated from uptake in abdominal region below kidneys). Gallium-67 index = 10 index units. **B.** Scan of 45-year-old woman with pulmonary sarcoidosis showing right paratracheal and bilateral hilar nodal uptake and mild lower lung zone ^{67}Ga uptake (intensity = 1, area = 30%, equivalent to a ^{67}Ga index of 30 units. **C.** Scan of a 42-year-old man with pulmonary sarcoidosis. Three regions show uptake greater than the background area. Region A (intensity = 2, area = 20%, index = 40 units), region B (intensity = 1 area = 20%, index = 20 units), and region C (intensity = 1, area = 30%, index = 30 units) are summed to give a total ^{67}Ga index of 90 units. **D.** Diffuse high intensity ^{67}Ga uptake in a 36-year-old man with pulmonary sarcoidosis. The ^{67}Ga index is equivalent to 340 units.

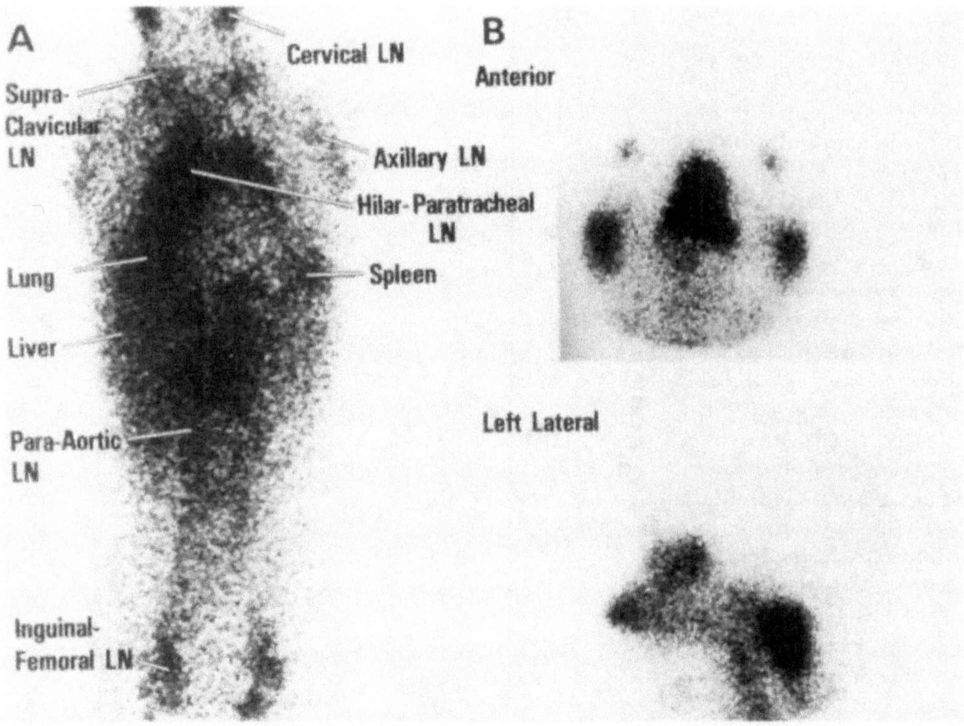

Figure 9. Extrathoracic ^{67}Ga localization in sarcoidosis. **A.** Sarcoidosis in 32-year-old woman. Gallium localization is noted in cervical, supraclavicular, axillary, mediastinal, para-aortic, inguinal, and femoral lymph nodes (*LN*) and in pulmonary parenchyma at base of right lung. **B.** Nasopharyngeal and parotid gland uptake of ^{67}Ga in 24-year-old man with sarcoidosis. There was clinical evidence of sarcoidosis of the nasopharynx but not of the parotids.

ation exposures. It should prove useful in staging patients with sarcoidosis and in following their response to therapy.

Treatment of Pulmonary Sarcoidosis

Dr. Ronald G. Crystal: Although the cause of pulmonary sarcoidosis is unknown, the disease clearly is characterized and perpetuated by activated T-lymphocytes within the alveolar structures. This is probably only part of the picture. For example, an important effector role will probably be found for mononuclear phagocytes in the lung other than simply as building blocks for granuloma formation. However, the knowledge that activated lung T-lymphocytes play a central role in the pathogenesis of this disease permits a rational assessment of therapeutic strategies.

CORTICOSTEROID THERAPY

Corticosteroids are the principal therapy against sarcoidosis. During the past 25 years, the following concepts have emerged (1, 3, 5, 7, 13, 15, 16, 35, 215, 254-261): [1] Corticosteroids generally improve symptoms, may or may not improve roentgenographic abnormalities, and variably improve lung function. [2] To be effective, corticosteroids must be given early and for at least 3 to 6 months. When they are withdrawn, relapses are frequent. Although long-term corticosteroid therapy seems to benefit most patients, the conditions of a small proportion will still deteriorate. [3] If low doses are used for maintenance therapy (for example, prednisone $\leq$ 0.25 mg/kg of body weight a day), complications are infrequent and mild.

Most of these observations are consistent with the concept that corticosteroids suppress the alveolitis of sarcoidosis but have little direct influence on the anatomic derangements of the alveolar structures that occurred before the institution of therapy. In humans, corticosteroids impair T-lymphocyte proliferation (262-264) and T-cell effector functions (265-266). They may affect the distribution of immune effector cells, including the proportioning of T-lymphocytes between blood and various organs (267, 268). These agents also have a profound effect on the capacity of mononuclear phagocytes to respond to mediators produced by T-lymphocytes (269). Thus it is reasonable to hypothesize that when corticosteroids are given in appropriate doses to patients with pulmonary sarcoidosis, they should prevent T-lymphocyte-mediated recruitment of blood monocytes to the lung and thus inhibit granuloma formation. Also, because granulomas are dynamic structures (85, 88), the reduction in recruitment of blood monocytes probably will cause a reduction in the number and size of existing granulomas.

Because both the alveolitis and granulomas impair lung function, therapy with corticosteroids should improve lung function by reducing the intensity of the alveolitis and reducing the lung burden of granuloma. In addition, by suppressing the alveolitis, corticosteroids prevent future derangements of the alveolar structures. However, there is no evidence that corticosteroids can improve interstitial fibrosis or alterations in lung parenchymal cells once present, that is, a deranged alveolus cannot be rebuilt and is lost forever as a gas-exchanging unit (270, 271).

Generally, studies evaluating the efficacy of corticosteriods in pulmonary sarcoidosis have relied on one or more of the following criteria as evidence for a beneficial therapeutic effect: a reduction in symptoms related to the lungs, particularly dyspnea; improvement in the chest roentgenogram; and improvement in functional tests such as lung volumes, diffusing capacity, and arterial

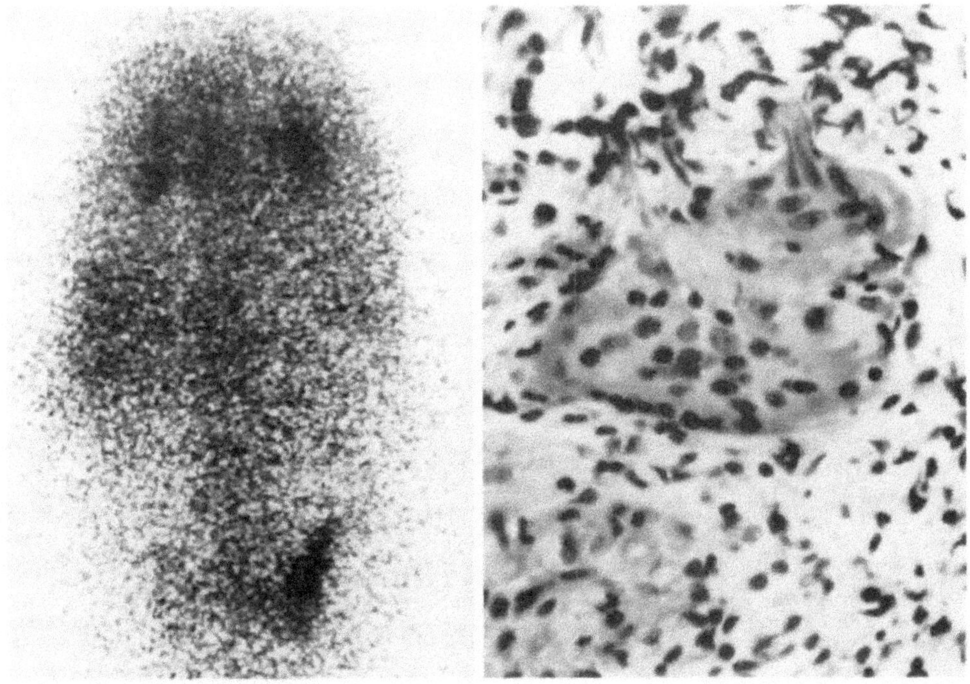

Figure 10 Left. Extrathoracic uptake in left posterior iliac crest of a 63-year-old man. There is also diffuse parenchymal ^{67}Ga uptake with right apical prominence and mediastinal-bilateral hilar node involvement. **Right.** Biopsy of left posterior iliac crest of the patient in left-hand panel showing noncaseating granulomas consistent with sarcoidosis.

blood gases at rest and during exercise. However, in view of our previous discussions, the difficulty assessing the efficacy of corticosteroids using these variables is understandable. Corticosteroids act on the alveolitis, not the derangements of the alveolar structures, yet there have been no studies comparing pulmonary symptoms to the intensity of the alveolitis or the anatomic derangements of the alveolar structures; the chest roentgenogram cannot clearly distinguish between alveolitis and anatomic derangement and is relatively insensitive to the presence of alveolitis; and because functional tests probably detect alveolitis as well as granulomas, fibrosis, and other derangements of the alveolar structures, they cannot be used to follow change in the alveolitis. Thus, even if corticosteroids were to effectively reduce the proportion of T-lymphocytes within the lung of a person with sarcoidosis, this beneficial effect may not be detected by the conventional monitors of the disease process. Because both alveolitis and anatomic derangements seem to influence radiographic and functional tests, an improvement in the alveolitis may be masked by a stabilized, but abnormal, anatomic arrangement of the alveolar structures.

THERAPY OF SARCOIDOSIS: OTHER AGENTS

Besides corticosteroids, chloroquine (272), D-penacillamine (273), spironolactone (274), allopurinol (275), levamisole (276), heparin (277), and phenylbutazone (278) have also been used in the therapy of sarcoidosis. Except for chloroquine, none have been evaluated by controlled trials, and the results with chloroquine are equivocal (272). In view of the current concepts of the disease, there is little theoretical basis for the use of any of these agents. Cytotoxic agents such as chlorambucil (279), azathioprine (280), and methotrexate (279) have also been used, but only in a few patients. No controls were used, the patients were mostly those with advanced disease, and the effect of these drugs on the alveolitis was not evaluated. Thus, although such drugs might suppress lung T-lymphocytes, at this time they cannot be considered as tested therapies for this disease.

FUTURE APPROACHES

The observations that T-lymphocytes play an important role in the pathogenesis of pulmonary sarcoidosis and that the alveolitis of this disease precedes anatomic derangements in the alveolar structures suggest that monitors of lung T-lymphocyte number may provide a convenient and logical guide to therapy decisions and the assessment of new treatment protocols.

ACKNOWLEDGMENTS: The authors thank Drs. Gordon Head and Andrew Dwyer of the Radiology Department, Clinical Center, National Institutes of Health, for assistance in classifying the chest radiographs; Charlotte Kenton of the National Library of Medicine for invaluable help in searching the extensive sarcoidosis literature; and Mrs. Lou West and Mrs. Ellen Wright for excellent editorial assistance.

▶ Requests for reprints should be addressed to Ronald G. Crystal, M.D.; Building 10, Room 6D06, National Institutes of Health; Bethesda, MD 20205.

References

1. Scadding JG. *Sarcoidosis.* London: Eyre and Spottiswoode Ltd.; 1967.
2. Spencer H. *Pathology of the Lung.* New York: Pergammon Press; 1977.
3. Crofton J, Douglas A. *Respiratory Disease.* Oxford: Blackwell Scientific Publications; 1975.
4. Fraser RG, Pare JAP. *Diagnosis of Diseases of the Chest.* Philadelphia: W. B. Saunders Co.; 1979.
5. Mitchell DN, Scadding JG. Sarcoidosis. *Am Rev Respir Dis.* 1974;**110:**774-802.
6. Mitchell DN, Scadding JG, Heard BE, et al. Sarcoidosis: histopathological definition and clinical diagnosis. *J Clin Pathol.* 1977;**30:**395-408.
7. Israel H. Sarcoidosis. In: Simmons DH, ed. *Current Pulmonology.* Vol. 1. Boston: Houghton Mifflin; 1979:163-82.
8. Fulmer JD, Crystal RG. Interstitial lung disease. In: Simmons DH, ed. *Current Pulmonology.* Vol. 1. Boston: Houghton Mifflin; 1979:1-65.
9. Kent DC, Houk VN, Elliott RC, Sokolowski JW Jr, Baker JH,

Sorensen K. The definitive evaluation of sarcoidosis. *Am Rev Respir Dis.* 1970;**101**:721-7.

10. Koerner SK, Sakowitz AJ, Appelman RI, Becker NH, Schoenbaum SW. Transbronchial lung biopsy for the diagnosis of sarcoidosis. *N Engl J Med.* 1975;**293**:268-70.
11. Lieberman J, Nosal A, Schlessner L, Sastre-Foken A. Serum angiotensin-converting enzyme for diagnosis and therapeutic evaluation of sarcoidosis. *Am Rev Respir Dis.* 1979;**120**:329-35.
12. Siltzbach LE, James DG, Neville E, et al. Course and prognosis of sarcoidosis around the world. *Am J Med.* 1974;**57**:847-52.
13. James DG, Neville E, Siltzbach LE, et al. A worldwide survey of sarcoid. In: Siltzbach LE, ed. Seventh International Conference on Sarcoidosis. *Ann NY Acad Sci.* 1976;**278**:321-34.
14. Mayock RL, Bertrand P, Morrison CE, Scott JH. Manifestations of sarcoidosis: analysis of 145 patients with a review of 9 series selected from the literature. *Am J Med.* 1963;**35**:67-89.
15. Israel HL. Prognosis of sarcoidosis. *Ann Intern Med.* 1970;**73**:1038-9.
16. Sones M, Israel HL. Course and prognosis of sarcoidosis. *Am J Med.* 1960;**28**:84-93.
17. Bacharach T. Sarcoidosis: a clinical review of 111 cases. *Am Rev Respir Dis.* 1961;**84**:12-6.
18. Longcope WT, Freiman DG. A study of sarcoidosis. *Medicine (Baltimore).* 1952;**31**:1-132.
19. Geraint-James D. Immunology of sarcoidosis. *Lancet.* 1966;**2**:633-4.
20. Sones M, Israel HC. Altered immunologic reactions in sarcoidosis.
21. Hirschhorn K, Schreibman RR, Bach FH et al. *In vitro* studies of lymphocytes from patients with sarcoidosis and lymphoproliferative diseases. *Lancet.* 1964;**2**:842-3.
22. Sharma OP, James DG, Fox RA. A correlation of *in vitro* delayed type hypersensitivity and *in vitro* lymphocyte transformation in sarcoidosis. *Chest.* 1971;**60**:35-7.
23. Kataria YP, Sagone AL, LoBuglio AF, et al. *In vitro* observations on sarcoid lymphocytes and their correlation with cutaneous anergy and clinical severity of disease. *Am Rev Respir Dis.* 1973;**108**:767-76.
24. Hedfors E, Holm G, Petterson E. Lymphocyte subpopulations in sarcoidosis. *Clin Exp Immunol.* 1974;**17**:219-26.
25. Daniele RP, Rowlands DT Jr. Lymphocyte subpopulations in sarcoidosis: correlation with disease activity and duration. *Ann Intern Med.* 1976;**85**:593-600.
26. Ramachandar K, Douglas SD, Siltzbach LE, et al. Peripheral blood lymphocyte subpopulations in sarcoidosis. *Cell Immunol.* 1975;**16**:422-6.
27. Sorensen SF, Hardt F, Veien NF. Estimation of lymphocyte subpopulations in peripheral blood of patients with sarcoidosis. *Scand J Immunol.* 1976;**5**:117-22.
28. Hunninghake GW, Fulmer JD, Young RC Jr, Gadek JE, Crystal RG. Localization of the immune response in sarcoidosis. *Am Rev Respir Dis.* 1979;**120**:49-57.
29. Hunninghake G, Kelman J, Weinberger S, Young R, Fulmer J, Crystal RG. Lung lymphocyte subpopulations in sarcoidosis. *Clin Res.* 1978;**26**:448A. Abstract.
30. Hunninghake GW, Kelman JA, Gadek JE, Elson NA, Fulmer JD, Crystal RG. Comparison of inflammatory and immune effector cell populations in lavage fluid and lung biopsies of patients with pulmonary fibrosis. *Am Rev Respir Dis.* 1978;**177** (suppl): 68. Abstract.
31. Hunninghake G, Gadek J, Weinberger S, et al. Comparison of the alveolitis of sarcoidosis and idiopathic pulmonary fibrosis. *Chest.* 1979;**75S**:266S-67S.
32. Hunninghake GW, Fulmer JD, Young RC, Crystal RG. Comparison of lung and blood lymphocyte subpopulations in pulmonary sarcoidosis. In: Williams, WJ, Davies, BH, eds. *Proceedings of the 8th International Conference on Sarcoidosis and Other Granulomatous Disease.* London: Alpha Omega Publishing, Ltd.; 1980:426-35.
33. Hunninghake GW, Gadek JE, Kawanami O, Ferrans VJ, Crystal RG. Inflammatory and immune processes in the human lung in health and disease: evaluation by bronchoalveolar lavage. *Am J Pathol.* 1979;**97**:149-206.
34. Hunninghake GW, Gadek JE, Young RC Jr, Kawanami O, Ferrans VJ, Crystal RG. Mechanisms of granuloma formation in pulmonary sarcoidosis by T-lymphocytes within the lung. *N Engl J Med.* 1980;**302**:594-8.
35. Siltzbach LE. Sarcoidosis. In: Fishman AP, ed. *Pulmonary Diseases and Disorders.* New York: McGraw-Hill; 1980:899-908.
36. Carrington CB, Gaensler EA, Mitsus JP, et al. Structure and function in sarcoidosis. *Ann NY Acad Sci.* 1976;**278**:265-82.
37. Soler P, Basset F. Morphology and distribution of the cells of a sarcoid granuloma: ultrastructural study of serial sections. *Ann NY Acad Sci.* 1976;**278**:147-60.
38. Soler P, Bernaudin JF, Basset F, Basset G. Epithelioid cell and sarcoid-like granuloma: a review of human and experimental material. *Mt Sinai J Med.* 1977;**44**:767-71.
39. Van Furth R. Origin and kinetics of monocytes and macrophages. *Semin Hematol.* 1970;**7**:125-41.
40. James EM, Williams WJ. Fine structure and histochemistry of epithelioid cells in sarcoidosis. *Thorax.* 1974;**29**:115-20.
41. Wanstrup J, Christensen HE. Sarcoidosis: I. Ultrastructural investigations on epithelioid cell granulomas. *Acta Pathol Microbiol Scand.* 1966;**66**:169-85.
42. Jones-Williams W, Erazmus DA, Valerie-James EM, Davies T. The fine structure of sarcoid and tuberculous granulomas. *Postgrad Med J.* 1970;**46**:496-500.
43. Fuse Y, Hiragi Y. The fine structures of sarcoidal and Kveim granulomas. In: Iwai K, Hasodo Y, eds. *Proceedings of the VI International Conference on Sarcoidosis.* Baltimore: University Park Press; 1974;269-75.
44. Fukushiro R, Hirone T, Eryn Y. Ultrastructural and cytochemical observations on sarcoid granulomas. In: Levinsky L, Macholda F, eds. *Fifth International Conference on Sarcoidosis.* Prague: Universita Karlova; 1971:276-9.
45. Carr I, Norris P. The fine structure of human machrophage granules in sarcoidosis. *J Pathol.* 1977;**122**:29-32.
46. Biberfield P. Morphogenesis in blood lymphocytes stimulated with phytohaemagglutinin (PITA): a light and electron microscopic study. *Acta Pathol Microbiol Scand [A].* **223** (suppl):1-70.
47. Teilum G. Allergic hyperglobulinosis and hyalinosis (paraamyloidosis) in the reticulo-endothelial system in Boecks sarcoid and other conditions: a morphologic immunity reaction. *Am J Pathol.* 1948;**24**:389-407.
48. Kalifat SR, Bouteille M, Belarue J. Changes in connective tissue in sarcoid granuloma: hyalin, paraamyloid and fibrinoid: electron microscopic study of 11 cases. *Virchows Arch Abt B Zellpath.* 1969;**3**:348-58.
49. Weinberger SE, Crystal RG. Reactions of the interstitial space to injury. In: Fishman AP, ed. *Pulmonary Diseases and Disorders.* New York: McGraw-Hill; 1980;640-7.
50. Divertie MB, Cassan SM, Brown AL. Ultrastructural morphometry of blood-air barrier in pulmonary sarcoidosis. *Chest.* 1976;**69**:154-7.
51. Pinner M. Noncaseating tuberculosis. *Am Rev Tuberc.* 1938;**37**:690-728.
52. Rosen Y, Athanassiades TJ, Moon S, et al. Nongranulomatous interstitial pneumonitis in sarcoidosis: relationship to the development of epithelioid granulomas. *Chest.* 1978;**74**:122-5.
53. Takahashi M. Histopathology of sarcoidosis and its immunological basis. *Acta Pathol Jpn.* 1970;**20**:171-82.
54. Teilum G. Morphogenesis and development of sarcoid lesions: similarities to the group of collagenosis. *Acta Med Scand.* 1964;**425** (suppl):14-8.
55. Judd PA, Finnegan P, Curran RC. Pulmonary sarcoidosis: a clinicopathologic study. *J Pathol.* 1975;**115**:191-8.
56. Cain H, Kraus B. Asteroid bodies: derivatives of the cytosphere. *Virchows Arch [Cell Pathol].* 1977;**26**:119-32.
57. Obel AL, Löfgren S. Pathogenesis of hyaline formation in sarcoidosis lymph nodes. *Acta Med Scand.* 1964;**425**(suppl):27-30.
58. DiBenedetto RJ, Ribaudo C. Bronchopulmonary sarcoidosis. *Am Rev Respir Dis.* 1966;**94**:952-5.
59. Scadding JG. The late stages of pulmonary sarcoidosis. *Postgrad Med J.* 1970;**46**:530-6.
60. Boros OL. Granulomatous inflammations. *Prog Allergy.* 1978;**24**:183-267.
61. Reynolds HY, Newball HH. Analysis of proteins and respiratory cells obtained from human lungs by bronchial lavage. *J Lab Clin Med.* 1974;**84**:559-73.
62. Reynolds HY, Fulmer JD Kazmierowski JA, Roberts WC, Frank MM, Crystal RG. Analysis of bronchoalveolar lavage fluid from patients with idiopathic pulmonary fibrosis and chronic hypersensitivity pneumonitis. *J Clin Invest.* 1977;**59**:165-75.
63. Weinberger SE, Kelman JA, Elson NA, et al. Bronchoalveolar lavage in interstitial lung disease. *Ann Intern Med.* 1978;**89**:459-66.
64. Hunninghake GW, Gadek JE, Szapiel SV, et al. The human alveolar macrophage. In: Harris CC, Trump BF, Stoner GD, eds. *Cultured Human Cells and Tissues in Bio-Medical Research.* New York: Academic Press; 1980. *(Methods and Perspectives in Cell Biology*, Vol. 1).
65. Hunninghake GW, Kawanami O, Ferrans VI, et al. Characterization of the inflammatory and immune effector cells in lung parenchyma of patients with interstitial lung disease. *Am Rev Respir Dis.* In press.
66. Yeager J, Williams MC, Beekman JF, Bayly TC, Beaman BL, Hawley RJ. Sarcoidosis: analysis of cells obtained by bronchial lavage. *Am Rev Respir Dis.* 1977;**116**:951-5.
67. Reynolds HY. The importance of lymphocytes in pulmonary health and disease. *Lung.* 1978;**155**:225-42.
68. Gee JB, Godel PT, Zorn SK, et al. Sarcoidosis and mononuclear

phagocytes. *Lung.* 1978;**155:**243-53.

69. Danel C, Arnoux A, Marsac J, et al. Cellular data from bronchoalveolar lavages in various interstitial diseases. *Bull Europ Physiopath Respir.* 1979;**15:**42P-43P.
70. Rossman MD, Daniele RP, Dauber JH. Bronchoalveolar lymphocytes in sarcoidosis. *Am Rev Respir Dis.* 1979;**119:**795.
71. Keogh B, Hunninghake G, Line B, et al. Therapeutic decisions in sarcoidosis: prospective evaluation of the effect of corticosteroids on lavage lymphocytes and [67] gallium scans. *Clin Res.* 1979;**27:**400A. Abstract.
72. Clot J, Andary M, Bonsequet J, Godart P, Michel FB. Lous populations lymphocytaires des iquides de lavage bronchoalveolaire. *Bull Europ Physiopath Respir.* 1979;**15:**27P-28P.
73. Barry BE, Crapo JD, Gehr P, Bachofen M, Weibel ER. Population characteristics of the cells in normal human lung. *Am Rev Respir Dis.* 1979;**119:**287A. Abstract.
74. Wybran JM, Carr C, Fudenbert HH. The human-rosette forming cell as a marker of a population of thymus-derived cells. *J Clin Invest.* 1972;**51:**2537-43.
75. Katoh AK, Charoensiri S. The formation of stable E-rosettes by human T-lymphocytes activated by phytohemagglutinin. *J Immunol.* 1977;**118:**2291-2.
76. Ferranrini M, Morretta L, Abile R, Durante ML. Receptors for IgG molecules on human lymphocytes forming spontaneous rosettes with sheep red cells. *Eur J Immunol.* 1975;**5:**70-2.
77. Krammer PH, Hudson C, Sprent J. Fc receptor, Ia-antigens, and immuno-globulin on normal and activated mouse T-lymphocytes. *J Exp Med.* 1975;**142:**1403-14.
78. Fridman WH, Fradelizi D, Guimezanes A, Plates C, Leclerc JC. The role of the Fc receptor (FcR) on thymus-derived lymphocytes. II. Presence of FcR on suppressor cells and direct involvement in suppression. *Eur J Immunol.* 1977;**8:**549-54.
79. Rossman MD, Dauber JH, Daniele RP. Elevation of stable (37°) E-rosettes in sarcoidosis. *Am Rev Respir Dis.* (suppl:73)1977:111.
80. Katz P, Haynes BF, Fauci AS. Alteration of T-lymphocyte subpopulations in sarcoidosis. *Clin Immunol Immunopathol.* 1978;**10:**350-4.
81. Hocking WG, Golde DW. The pulmonary-alveolar macrophage. *N Engl J Med.* 1979;**301:**580-7.
82. Blusse van Oud Alblas A, van Furth R. Origin, kinetics, and characteristics of pulmonary macrophages in the normal steady state. *J Exp Med.* 1979;**149:**1504-18.
83. Carr I. *The Macrophage.* London: Academic Press, Inc.; 1973:80-5.
84. Adams DO. The structure of mononuclear phagocytes differentiating *in vivo.* *Am J Pathol.* 1974;**76:**17-39.
85. Spector WG. The dynamics of granulomas and the significance of epithelioid cells. *Pathologie-Biologie.* 1975;**6:**437-9.
86. Black MM, Epstein WL. Formation of multinucleate giant cells in organized epithelioid cell granulomas. *Am J Pathol.* 1974;**74:**262-74.
87. Sutton JS, Weiss L. Transformation of monocytes in tissue culture into macrophages, epithelioid cells, and multinucleated giant cells: an electron microscope study. *J Cell Biol.* 1966;**28:**303-32.
88. Mariano M, Spector WG. The formation and properties of macrophage polykaryous (inflammatory giant cells). *J Pathol.* 1974;**113:**1-19.
89. Johnston RB Jr, Godzik CA, Cohn ZA. Increased superoxide anion production by immunologically activated and chemically elicited macrophages. *J Exp Med.* 1978;**148:**115-27.
90. Drath DB, Karnovsky ML, Huber GL. Hydroxyl radical formation in phagocytic cells of the rat. *Am J Physiol.* 1979;**46:**136-40.
91. Werb Z, Gordon S. Secretion of a specific collagenase by stimulated macrophages. *J Exp Med.* 1975;**142:**346-60.
92. Horowitz AL, Kelman JA, Crystal RG. Activation of alveolar macrophage collagenase by a neutral protease secreted by the same cell. *Nature.* 1976;**264:**772-4.
93. Janoff A, Rosenberg R, Gladston M. Elastase-like esteroprotease activity in human and rabbit alveolar macrophage granules. *Proc Soc Exp Biol Med.* 1971;**136:**1054-8.
94. Polverini PF, Cotran RS, Gimbrome MA, Unanue ER. Activated macrophages induce vascular proliferation. *Nature.* 1977;**269:**804-6.
95. Rosenthal AS, Lipsky PE, Shevach EM. Macrophage-lymphocyte interaction and antigen recognition. *Fed Proc.* 1975;**34:**1743-8.
96. Unanue ER. Secretory function of mononuclear phagocytes. *Am J Pathol.* 1976;**83:**396-417.
97. Evans R, Alexander P. Mechanisms of extracellular killing of nucleated mammalian cells by macrophages. In: Nelson DS, ed. *Immunobiology of the Macrophage.* New York: Academic Press; 1976:535-76.
98. Ward PA, Unanue ER, Goralnick SJ, Schreiner GF. Chemotaxis of rat lymphocytes. *J Immunol.* 1977;**119:**416-421.
99. Golde DW, Byers LD, Finley TN. Proliferative capacity of the human alveolar macrophage. *Nature.* 1974;**247:**373-5.
100. Adamson IYR, Bowden DH. Role of monocytes and interstitial cells in the generation of alveolar macrophages. *Fed Proc.* 1979;**38:**1205.
101. Boyden S. The chemotactic effect of mixtures of antibody and antigen on polymorphonuclear leukocytes. *J Exp Med.* 1962;**115:**453-66.
102. Kazmierowski JA, Gallin JI, Reynolds HY. Mechanisms for the inflammatory response in primate lungs: demonstration and partial characterization of an alveolar macrophage-derived chemotactic factor with preferential activity for polymorphonuclear leukocytes. *J Clin Invest.* 1977;**59:**273-81.
103. Hunninghake GW, Gallin JI, Fauci AS. Immunologic reactivity of the lung. The *in vivo* and *in vitro* generation of a neutrophil chemotactic factor by alveolar macrophages. *Am Rev Respir Dis.* 1978;**117:**15-23.
104. Hunninghake GW, Gadek JE, Crystal RG. Human alveolar macrophage chemotactic factor for neutrophils: stimuli and partial characterization. *J Clin Invest.* In press.
105. Merrill WW, Naegel GP, Matthay RA, Reynolds HY. Alveolar macrophage-derived chemotactic factor: kinetics of *in vitro* production and partial characterization. *J Clin Invest.* 1980;**65:**268-76.
106. Gadek JE, Hunninghake GW, Zimmerman RL, Crystal RG. Regulation of release of the alveolar macrophage-derived chemotactic factor. *Am Rev Respir Dis.* 1980;**121:**823-33.
107. Gallin JI, Quie PG. *Leukocyte Chemotaxis: Methods, Physiology, and Clinical Implications.* New York: Raven Press; 1978:1-429.
108. Ward PA, Remold HG, David JR. Leukotactic factor produced by sensitized lymphocytes. *Science.* 1969;**163:**1079-81.
109. Snyderman R, Altman LC, Hausman MS, et al. Human mononuclear leukocyte chemotaxis: a quantitative assay for humoral and cellular chemotactic factors. *J Immunol.* 1972;**108:**857-60.
110. Altman LC, Snyderman R, Oppenheim JJ, et al. A human mononuclear leukocyte chemotactic factor: characterization, specificity and kinetics of production by homologous leukocytes. *J Immunol.* 1973;**110:**801-10.
111. Kay AB, Stechschulte DJ, Austen KF. An eosinophilic leukocyte chemotactic factor of anaphylaxis. *J Exp Med.* 1971;**133:**602-19.
112. Zigmond SH, Hirsch JG. Leukocyte locomotion and chemotaxis: new methods for evaluation and demonstration of cell-derived chemotactic factor. *J Exp Med.* 1973;**137:**387-410.
113. Goetzl EJ, Woods JM, Gorman RR. Stimulation of human eosinophil and neutrophil polymorphonuclear leukocyte chemotaxis and random migration by 12-L-hydroxy-5,8,10,14-eicosatetraenoic acid. *J Clin Invest.* 1977;**59:**179-83.
114. Sobel JD, Gallin JI. Polymorphonuclear leukocyte and monocyte chemoattractants produced by human fibroblasts. *J Clin Invest.* 1979;**63:**609-18.
115. Kaplan AP, Goetzl EJ, Austen KF. The fibrinolytic pathway of human plasma. II. The generation of chemotactic activity by activation of plasminogen proactivator. *J Clin Invest.* 1973;**52:**2591-5.
116. Berenberg JL, Ward PA. Chemotactic factor inactivator in normal human serum. *J Clin Invest.* 1973;**52:**1200-6.
117. Goetzl EJ, Rocklin RE. Amplification of the activity of human leukocyte inhibitory factor (LIF) by the generatipn of a low molecular weight inhibitor of PMN leukocyte chemotaxis. *J Immuno.* 1978;**121:**891-6.
118. Till G, Ward PA. Two distinct chemotactic factor inactivators in human serum. *J Immunol.* 1975;**114:**843-7.
119. Rocklin RE. Products of activated lymphocytes: leukocyte inhibitory factor (LIF) distinct from migration inhibitory factor (MIF). *J Immunol.* 1974;**112:**1461-6.
120. Goetzl EJ. Plasma and cell-derived inhibitors of human neutrophil chemotaxis. *Ann NY Acad Sci.* 1975;**256:**210-21.
121. Wright DG, Gallin JI. Modulation of the inflammatory response by products released from human polymorphonuclear leukocytes during phagocytosis: generation and inactivation of the chemotactic factor C5a. *Inflammation.* 1975;**1:**23-39.
122. Cates KL, Ray CA Quie PG. Modified Boyden chamber method of measuring polymorphonuclear leukocyte chemotaxis. In: Gallin JI, Quie PG, eds. *Leukocyte Chemotaxis: Methods, Physiology, and Clinical Applications.* New York: Raven Press; 1978:67-72.
123. Altman LC. Chemotactic lymphokines. In: Gallin JI, Quie PG, eds. *Leukocyte Chemotaxis: Methods, Physiology, and Clinical Implications.* New York: Raven Press; 1978:267-88.
124. Gordon LI, Douglas SD, Kay NE, Yamada O, Osserman EF, Jacob HS. Modulation of neutrophil function by lysozyme: potential feedback system of inflammation. *J Clin Invest.* 1979;**64:**226-32.
125. Douglas SE, Doughaday CC, Schmidt ME, Siltzbach LE. Kinetics of monocyte receptor activity for immunoproteins in patients with sarcoidosis. *Ann NY Acad Sci.* 1976;**278:**190-6.
126. Douglas SE. Human monocyte spreading *in vitro*: inducers and effects on Fc and C3 receptors. *Cell Immunol.* 1976;**21:**344-9.
127. Himan LM, Stevens CA, Matthay RA, Reynolds HY, Gee JBL. Lysozyme and angiotensin convertase activity in human alveolar macrophages: the effects of cigarette smoking and pulmonary sarcoidosis.

Am Rev Respir Dis. 1978;**117**(Part 2):67. Abstract.

128. SHIMA K, TAMIYA J, TSUDA T, TOKUOMI H. Lysosomal enzyme activation of monocytes in sarcoid patients and activation factor in their sera. In: *Proceedings of the 8th International Conference on Sarcoidosis.* Cardiff, Wales, UK. 1978:9.
129. FRIEDLAND J, SETTON C, SILVERSTEIN E. Induction of angiotensin converting enzyme in human monocytes in culture. *Biochem Biophys Res Comm.* 1979;**83**:843-9.
130. SILVERSTEIN E, FRIEDLAND J, LYONS HA, et al. Markedly elevated angiotensin converting enzyme in lymph nodes containing non-necrotizing granulomas in sarcoidosis. *Proc Nat Acad Sci USA.* 1976;**73**:2137-41.
131. SILVERSTEIN E, FRIEDLAND J, LYONS HA, et al. Elevation of angiotensin-converting enzyme in granulomatous lymph nodes and serum in sarcoidosis: clinical and possible pathogenic significance. *Ann NY Acad Sci.* 1976;**278**:498-513.
132. DAVID JR, REMOLD HG. Macrophage activation by lymphocyte mediators and studies on the interaction of macrophages and lymphocytes. In: NELSON DS, ed. *Immunobiology of the Macrophage.* New York: Academic Press, 1976;401-27.
133. GORDON LI, DOUGLAS SE, KAY NE, OSSERMAN EF, JACOB HD. Modulation of neutrophil function by lysozyme: a macrophage secretory product. In: WILLIAMS WJ, DAVIES BH, eds. *Proceedings of the 8th International Conference on Sarcoidosis and Other Granulomatous Disease.* London: Alpha Omega Publishing, Ltd; 1980:76-83.
134. MADERAZO EG, WARD PA, WORONICK CL, KUBIK J, DEGRAFF AC JR. Leukotactic dysfunction in sarcoidosis. *Ann Intern Med.* 1976;**84**:414-9.
135. CAMPBELL PB. Defective monocyte leukotaxis in sarcoidosis: possible relationship to a plasma factor. *Am Rev Respir Dis.* 1977;**116**:251-9.
136. YOSHIDA T, SILTZBACK LE, MASIH N, COHEN S. Serum-migration inhibitory activity in patients with sarcoidosis. *Clin Immunol Immunopathol.* 1979;**13**:39-46.
137. SHIMA K, IKEDA S, HORIUCHI S, TOKUOMO H. Lysosomal enzyme activity of monocytes and activation factors in the sera of sarcoidosis patients. In: WILLIAMS WJ, DAVIES BH, eds. *Proceedings of the 8th International Conference on Sarcoidosis and Other Granulomatous Disease,* London: Alpha Omega Publishing, Ltd; 1980:89-98.
138. SEMENZATO G, CIORANI A, COLOMBATTI M, AMADORI G, GASPAROTTO G. Inhibitors of T-cell immune function in sarcoidosis. In: WILLIAMS WJ, DAVIES BH, eds. *Proceedings of the 8th International Conference on Sarcoidosis and Other Granulomatous Disease.* London: Alpha Omega Publishing, Ltd.; 1980:466-71.
139. DAVIES BH, JONES KP, EVANS P, JONES-WILLIAMS W. Thymic lymphocyte responses in sarcoidosis: effect of sera and levamisole. In: WILLIAMS WJ, DAVIES BH, eds. *Proceedings of the 8th International Conference on Sarcoidosis and Other Granulomatous Disease.* London: Alpha Omega Publishing, Ltd.; 1980:477-84.
140. HORSMANHEIMO A, HORSMANHEIMO M, FUDENBERG HH, SILTZBACK LE, MCKEE KT. Kveins test reactivity with leukocyte migration in agarose and lymphocyte transformation tests. In: WILLIAMS WJ, DAVIES BH, eds. *Proceedings of the 8th International Conference on Sarcoidosis and Other Granulomatous Disease.* London: Alpha Omega Publishing, Ltd.; 1980:186-90.
141. MANGI RJ, DWYER JM, KANTOR FS. The effect of plasma upon lymphocyte responses *in vitro*: demonstration of a humoral inhibitor in patients with sarcoidosis. *Clin Exp Immunol.* 1974;**18**:519-28.
142. DRUTZ DJ, CLINE MJ. Intermittent neutrophil-monocyte bactericidal defects in a patient with sarcoidosis. *Am Rev Respir Dis.* 1975;**112**:387-92.
143. BROOM BC, MACLAURIN BP. Sarcoidosis: correlation of delayed hypersensitivity, MLC reactivity and lymphocytotoxicity with disease activity. *Clin Exp Immunol.* 1973;**15**:355-64.
144. FRIOU GJ. Delayed cutaneous hypersensitivity in sarcoidosis. *J Clin Invest.* 1952;**31**:630.
145. HORSMANHEIMO M. Correlation of tuberculin-induced lymphocyte transformation with skin test reactivity and with clinical manifestations of sarcoidosis. *Cell Immunol.* 1974;**10**:329-37.
146. KATARIA YP, LOBUGLIO AF, BROMBERG PA. Sarcoid lymphocytes: spontaneous transformation and release of macrophage migration inhibition activity. *Am Rev Respir Dis.* 1976;**113**:315-23.
147. SELROOS O, NIEMISTO M. Tuberculin sensitivity in active and cured sarcoidosis in Finland. In: IWAI K, HOSODA Y, eds. *Proceedings of the VI International Conference on Sarcoidosis,* Baltimore: University Park Press; 1974;248-52.
148. SONES M, ISRAEL HL. Altered immunologic reactions in sarcoidosis. *Ann Intern Med.* 1954;**40**:260-8.
149. VEIEN NK, HARDT F, BENDIXEN G, et al. Immunological studies in sarcoidosis: a comparison of disease activity and various immunologic parameters. *Ann NY Acad Sci.* 1976;**278**:47-51.
150. HOFFBRAND BI. Occurrence and significance of lymphopenia in sarcoidosis. *Am Rev Respir Dis.* 1968;**98**:107-10.
151. SORENSEN SF, HARDT F, VEIEN NK. Estimation of lymphocyte subpopulations in the peripheral blood of patients with sarcoidosis. *Scand J Immunol.* 1976;**5**:1117-22.
152. KALDEN JR, PETER HH, LOHMANN E, SCHEDEL J, DIEHL V, VALKE D. Estimation of T- and K-cell activity in the peripheral blood of sarcoidosis patients. *Ann NY Acad Sci.* 1976;**278**:52-68.
153. HSU CCS, WU SJY, CELIC L, WEAVER LJ, SOLLIDAY N. Increased proportion of active sheep erythrocyte rosette-forming lymphocytes and plasma rosette enhancement in sarcoidosis. *Am Rev Respir Dis.* 1979;**119**:383-9.
154. GOLDSTEIN RA, JANICKI BW, MIRRO J, FOELLMER JW. Cell-mediated immune responses in sarcoidosis. *Am Rev Respir Dis.* 1978;**117**:55-62.
155. SILTZBACH LE, GLADE PR, HIRSHANT Y, VIEIRA LOBD, CELIKOGLU IS, HIRSCHHORN K. In vitro stimulation of peripheral lymphocytes in sarcoidosis. In: LEVINSKY L, MACHOLDA F. *Fifth International Conference on Sarcoidosis.* Prague: University Karlova; 1971:217-20.
156. DANIELE RP, MCMILLAN LJ, DAUBER JH, ROSSMAN MD. Immune complexes in sarcoidosis: a correlation with activity and duration of disease. *Chest.* 1978;**74**:261-4.
157. GUPTA RC, KUEPPERS F, DEREMEE RA, et al. Pulmonary and extrapulmonary sarcoidosis in relation to circulating immune complexes: a quantification of immune complexes by two radioimmunoassays. *Am Rev Respir Dis.* 1977;**116**:261-6.
158. HEDFORS E, NORBERG R. Evidence for circulating immune complexes in sarcoidosis. *Clin Exp Immunol.* 1974;**16**:493-6.
159. VERRIER-JONES J, CUMMING RH, ASPLIN CM. Evidence for circulating immune complexes in erythema nodosum and early sarcoidosis. *Ann NY Acad Sci.* 1976;**278**:212-9.
160. KUEPPERS F, DEREMEE RE. Search for a specific antibody in sera from patients with sarcoidosis. *Ann NY Acad Sci.* 1976;**278**:220-4.
161. DANIELE RP, ROWLANDS DT. Antibodies to T cells in sarcoidosis. *Ann NY Acad Sci.* 1976;**278**:88-100.
162. KLOCKARS M, SELROOS O. Immunohistochemical demonstration of lysozyme in the lymph nodes and Kveim reaction papules in sarcoidosis. *Acta Pathol Microbiol Scand.* 1977;**85A**:169-73.
163. PASCUAL RS, GEE JBL, FINCH SC. Usefulness of serum lysozyme measurement in diagnosis and evaluation of sarcoidosis. *N Engl J Med.* 1973;**289**:1074-6.
164. SELROOS O, KLOCKARS M. Serum lysozyme in sarcoidosis. Evaluation of its usefulness in determination of disease activity. *Scand J Respir Dis.* 1977;**58**:110-6.
165. SILVERSTEIN E, FRIEDLAND J, ACKERMAN T. Elevation of granulomatous lymph node and serum lysozyme in sarcoidosis and correlation with angiotensin-converting enzyme. *Am J Clin Pathol.* 1977;**68**:219-24.
166. SILTZBACK LE, KRAKOFF L, DORPH D, TIERSTEIN AS. Elevated levels of serum angiotensin-converting enzyme (ACE) and lysozyme (L) levels in sarcoidosis. In: WILLIAMS WJ, DAVIES BH, eds. *Proceedings of the 8th International Conference on Sarcoidosis and Other Granulomatous Disease.* London: Alpha Omega Publishing, Ltd.; 1980:298-302.
167. ASHUTOSH K, KEIGHLEY JFH. Diagnostic value of serum angiotensin converting enzyme activity in lung disease. *Thorax.* 1976;**31**:552-7.
168. FANBURG BL, SCHOENBERGER MD, BACHUS B, SNIDER GL. Elevated serum angiotensin I converting enzyme in sarcoidosis. *Am Rev Respir Dis.* 1976;**114**:525-8.
169. FERLITSCH A, KOHOUT J, KUMMER F, LEGENSTEIN E, MULLER MM. Angiotensin converting enzyme in the diagnosis of sarcoidosis. In: WILLIAMS WJ, DAVIES BH, eds. *Proceedings of the 8th International Conference on Sarcoidosis and Other Granulomatous Disease.* London: Alpha Omega Publishing, Ltd.; 1980:22.
170. LIEBERMAN J. Elevation of serum angiotensin-converting-enzyme (ACE) level in sarcoidosis. *Am J Med.* 1975;**59**:365-72.
171. LIEBERMAN J. The specificity and nature of serum angiotensin-converting-enzyme (serum ACE) elevations in sarcoidosis. *Ann NY Acad Sci.* 1976;**278**:488-97.
172. LIEBERMAN J, KANESHIRO W, WEISSER K, et al. Update on serum ACE: angiotensin converting enzyme assays for diagnosis and therapeutic evaluation in sarcoidosis. In: WILLIAMS WJ, DAVIES BH, eds. *Proceedings of the 8th International Conference on Sarcoidosis and Other Granulomatous Disease.* London: Alpha Omega Publishing, Ltd.; 1980:320-7.
173. ROHRBACH MS, DEREME RA. Serum angiotensin converting enzyme activity in sarcoidosis as measured by a simple radiochemical assay. *Am Rev Respir Dis.* 1979;**119**:761-7.
174. SANDRON D, LECOSSIER D, MOREUN F, BASSET G, BATTESTI JP. Comparison between two methods of determining serum angiotensin converting enzyme in sarcoidosis and other pulmonary diseases. In: WILLIAMS WJ, DAVIES BH, eds. *Proceedings of the 8th International Conference on Sarcoidosis and Other Granulomatous Disease.* London: Alpha Omega Publishing, Ltd.; 1980; 317-9.
175. ABBOY R, KANADA DJ, SHARMA OP. Serum angiotensin converting

enzyme in sarcoidosis. In: Williams WJ, Davies BH, eds. *Proceedings of the 8th International Conference on Sarcoidosis and Other Granulomatous Disease.* London: Alpha Omega Publishing; 1980:273-6.

176. Simonowitz LJ, Solliday N, Celic L, Cugell E. Serial measurements of angiotensin converting enzyme and diffusing capacity in sarcoidosis. *Am Rev Respir Dis.* 1977;**115**(suppl):164. Abstract.
177. Studdy P, Bird R, Geraint JD, Sherberb S. Serum angiotensin converting enzyme (SACE) in sarcoidosis and other granulomatous disorders. In: Williams WJ, Davies BH, eds. *Proceedings of the 8th International Conference on Sarcoidosis and Other Granulomatous Disease.* London: Alpha Omega Publishing, Ltd.; 1980:259-65.
178. Ueda E, Hishimurak, Hawada K, et al. Serum angiotensin-converting enzyme activity in patients with sarcoidosis. *Jpn J Thorac Dis.* 1976;**14**:736-42.
179. Nelson DS. *Immunobiology of the Macrophage.* New York: Academic Press; 1976.
180. Pascual RS, Perille PE, Gee JBL, Finch SC. Serum and urine lysozyme in sarcoidosis. In: Osserman E, Cenfield R, Beychok S, eds. *Lysozyme.* New York: Academic Press; 1974:391.
181. Ng KKF, Vane JR. Fate of angiotensin I in the circulation. *Nature (London).* 1968;**218**:144-50.
182. Renzi G, Dutton RE. Pulmonary function in diffuse sarcoidosis. *Respiration.* 1973;**31**:124-31.
183. James DG, Carstairs LS, Trowell J, Sharma OP. Treatment of sarcoidosis: report of a controlled therapeutic trial. *Lancet.* 1967;**2**:526-8.
184. Kirks DR, McCormick VD, Greenspan RH. Pulmonary sarcoidosis: roentgenologic analysis of 150 patients. *Am J Roentgenol Radium Therap Nucl Med.* 1973;**117**:777-8.
185. James DG. Diagnosis and treatment of sarcoidosis. *Br Med J.* 1956;**2**:900-04.
186. James DG, Neville E, Siltzbach LE, et al. A worldwide view of sarcoidosis. *Ann NY Acad Sci.* 1976;**278**:321-34.
187. DeRemee RA, Andersen HA. Sarcoidosis: a correlation of dyspnea with roentgenographic stage and pulmonary function changes. *Mayo Clin Proc.* 1974;**49**:742-5.
188. Freundlich IM, Libshitz HI, Glassman LM, Israel HL. Sarcoidosis: typical and atypical thoracic manifestations and complications. *Clin Radiol.* 1970;**21**:376-83.
189. Fraser RG, Pare JAP. *Diagnosis of Diseases of the Chest.* Philadelphia: W.B. Saunders; 1979:1659-90.
190. Felson B. *Chest Roentgenology.* Philadelphia: W.B. Saunders; 1973:302.
191. Rabinowitz JG, Ulreich S, Soriano C. The usual unusual manifestations of sarcoidosis and the "hilar haze"—a new diagnostic aid. *Am J Roentgenol Rad Therap Nucl Med.* 1974;**120**:821-39.
192. Shigematsu N, Emori K, Matsuba K, Harada S, Takahahi T. Clinico-pathologic characteristics of pulmonary acinar sarcoidosis. *Chest.* 1978;**73**:186-8.
193. Felson B. Uncommon roentgen patterns of pulmonary sarcoidosis. *Dis Chest.* 1958;**34**:357-67.
194. Sharma OP, Hewlett R, Gordonson J. Nodular sarcoidosis: an unusual radiographic appearance. *Chest.* 1973;**64**:189-92.
195. Kirks DR, McCormick VD, Greenspan RH. Pulmonary sarcoidosis: roentgenologic analysis of 150 patients. *Am J Roentgenol.* 1973;**117**:777-86.
196. Young RC, Titus-Dillon PY, Schneider ML, Shelton TG, Hackney RL, Harden KA. Sarcoidosis in Washington, D.C.: clinical observations in 105 black patients. In: Levinsky DL, Macholda F, eds. *Fifth International Conference on Sarcoidosis.* Prague: Universita Karlova; 1971:513-20.
197. Rosen Y, Amorosa JK, Moon S, Cohen J, Lyons HA. Occurrence of lung granulomas in patients with stage I sarcoidosis. *Am J Roentgenol.* 1977;**129**:1083-85.
198. Epler GR, McLoud TC, Gaensler ER, Mickus JP, Carrington CB. Normal chest roentgenograms in chronic diffuse infiltrative lung disease. *N Engl J Med.* 1978;**298**:934-9.
199. McCort JJ, Pare JAP. Pulmonary fibrosis and cor pulmonale in sarcoidosis. *Radiology.* 1954;**62**:496-504.
200. Scadding JG. Prognosis of intrathoracic sarcoidosis. *Br Med J.* 1961;**2**:1165-72.
201. Mikhail JR, Drury RA, Mitchell DN. Evaluation of the clinical and histological features of paratracheal and hilar gland enlargement. *Postgrad Med J.* 1970;**46**:515-8.
202. Boushy SF, Kurtzman RS, Martin ND, Lewis BM. The course of pulmonary function in sarcoidosis. *Ann Intern Med.* 1965;**62**:939-55.
203. Berg GR. Pulmonary function in sarcoidosis. *N Engl J Med.* 1968;**278**:1019. Letter.
204. O'Brien LE, Forsman PJ, Wiltse HE. Early onset sarcoidosis with pulmonary function abnormalities. *Chest.* 1974;**65**:472-4.
205. Renzi G, Dutton RE. Pulmonary function in diffuse sarcoidosis. *Respiration.* 1974;**31**:124-36.
206. Colp C, Park SS, Williams MH Jr. Pulmonary function follow-up to 120 patients with sarcoidosis. *Ann NY Acad Sci.* 1976;**278**:301-07.
207. Miller A, Chuang M, Teirstein AS, Siltzbach LE. Pulmonary function in stage I and II pulmonary sarcoidosis. *Ann NY Acad Sci.* 1976;**278**:292-300.
208. Hamer NA. Changes in the components of the diffusing capacity in pulmonary sarcoidosis. *Thorax.* 1963;**18**:275-87.
209. Saumon G, Georges R, Loiseau A, Turiaf J. Membrane diffusing capacity and pulmonary capillary blood volume in pulmonary sarcoidosis. *Ann NY Acad Sci.* 1976;**278**:284-91.
210. Sellers RD, Siebens AA. The effects of sarcoidosis on pulmonary function with particular reference to changes in pulmonary compliance. *Am Rev Respir Dis.* 1965;**91**:660-4.
211. Ting GY, Williams MH Jr. Mechanics of breathing in sarcoidosis of the lung. *JAMA.* 1965;**192**:619-24.
212. Harden KA, Young RC Jr, Carr C, Laurey JR. Oxygen cost of breathing. II. Studies in patients with sarcoidosis. *Am Rev Respir Dis.* 1968;**97**:1127-30.
213. Snider GL, Doctor LR. The mechanics of ventilation in sarcoidosis. *Am Rev Respir Dis.* 1964;**89**:897-908.
214. Tabiri G, Arndt H, Behrend H, Dombrowski H. Lung volumes, compliance and diffusing capacity in advanced pulmonary sarcoidosis. In: Levinsky DL, Macholda F, eds. *Fifth International Conference on Sarcoidosis.* Prague: Universita Karlova; 1971:442-6.
215. Young RL, Harkleroad CE, Lordon RE, Weg JG. Pulmonary sarcoidosis: a prospective evaluation of glucocorticoid therapy. *Ann Intern Med.* 1970;**73**:207-12.
216. Kaneko K, Sharma OP. Airway obstruction in pulmonary sarcoidosis. *Bull Eur Physiopathol Respir.* 1977;**13**:231-40.
217. Rizzato G, Brambilla I, Bertoli L, Conti F, Merlin R, Mantaro O. Impaired airway function and pulmonary hemodynamics in sarcoidosis. In: Williams WJ, Davies BH, eds. *Proceedings of the 8th International Conference on Sarcoidosis and Other Granulomatous Disease.* London: Alpha Omega Publishing, Ltd.; 1980:349-60.
218. Sahetya GK, Covy WB, Facen HK, Hassan S, Kumar B, Young RC. Pulmonary sarcoidosis: a significant cause of chronic airway obstruction. In: Williams WJ, Davies, BH, eds. *Proceedings of the 8th International Conference on Sarcoidosis and Other Granulomatous Disease.* London: Alpha Omega Publishing, Ltd.; 1980:361-7.
219. Miller A, Teirstein AS, Jackler I, Chuang M, Siltzbach LE. Airway function in chronic pulmonary sarcoidosis with fibrosis. *Am Rev Respir Dis.* 1974;**109**:179-89.
220. Tammeling GJ, de Vries K, Sluiter HJ, et al. Obstructive lung disease in pulmonary sarcoidosis. *Acta Med Scand.* 1964;**176**(suppl):275-77.
221. Levinson RS, Metzger LF, Stanley NN, et al. Airway function in sarcoidosis. *Am J Med.* 1977;**62**:51-9.
222. Radwan L, Grebska E, Koziorowski A. Small airway function in pulmonary sarcoidosis. *Scand J Respir Dis.* 1978;**59**:37-43.
223. Sharma OP. Airway obstruction in sarcoidosis. *Chest.* 1978;**73**:6-7. Editorial.
224. Bates DV, Macklem PT, Christie RV. Pulmonary sarcoidosis. In: *Respiratory Function in Disease.* Philadelphia: W.B. Saunders Co.; 1971:287-9.
225. Staneck V, Widimsky J, Navratil M, Daum S, Levinsky L. The pulmonary gas exchange during exercise in patients with pulmonary fibrosis. *Scand J Respir Dis.* 1967;**48**:11-2.
226. Sears MR. Pulmonary gas transfer and alveolar-oxygen differences in sarcoidosis. In: Williams WJ, Davies BH, eds. *Proceedings of the 8th International Conference on Sarcoidosis and Other Granulomatous Disease.* London: Alpha Omega Publishing, Ltd.; 1980:343-8.
227. Colp C. Sarcoidosis: course and treatment. *Med Clin N Am.* 1977;**61**:1267-78.
228. Young RC Jr, Carr C, Shelton TG, et al. Sarcoidosis: relationship between changes in lung structure and function. *Am Rev Respir Dis.* 1967;**95**:224-38.
229. Young RL, Lordon RE, Krumholz RA, Harkleroad LE, Branam GE, Weg JG. Pulmonary sarcoidosis. I. Pathophysiologic correlations. *Am Rev Respir Dis.* 1968;**97**:997-1008.
230. Edwards CL, Hayes RL. Tumor scanning with ^{67}Ga citrate. *J Nucl Med.* 1969;**10**:103-5.
231. Lavender PJ, Lowe J, Barker JR, Burn JI, Chaudhri MA. Gallium-67 citrate scanning in neoplastic and inflammatory lesions. *Br J Radiol.* 1971;**44**:361-6.
232. Kanno I. Diagnostic evaluation of ^{67}Ga scanning of lung cancer and other diseases. *Radiology.* 1971;**101**:355-62.
233. Hisasi T, Nakayama Y. Clinical evaluation of ^{67}Ga citrate scanning. *J Nucl Med.* 1972;**13**:196-201.
234. van der Schoot JB, Groen AS, de Jons J. Gallium-67 scintigraphy in lung diseases. *Thorax.* 1972;**27**:543-6.
235. Teates CD, Bray ST, Williamson BR. Tumor detection with ^{67}Ga citrate: a literature survey (1970-1978). *Clin Nucl Med.* 1978;**3**:456-60.
236. Dise-Peterson H, Heckscher T, Hertz M. ^{67}Ga-scintigraphy in

nonmalignant lung diseases. *Scand J Respir Dis.* 1972;**53**:314-31.

237. LITTENBERG RL, TAKETA RM, ALAZRAKI NP, HALPERN SE, ASHBURN WL. Gallium-67 for localization of septic lesions. *Ann Intern Med.* 1973;**79**:403-6.
238. ISRAEL HL, ATKINSON GW. Sarcoidosis: basics of respiratory disease. *Am Thoracic Soc.* 1978;**7**:1-6.
239. SILBERSTEIN EB. Gallium detection of inflammation. *Ann Intern Med.* 1974;**80**:774. Letter.
240. TEATES CD, HUNGER JG. Gallium scanning as a screening test for inflammatory lesions. *Radiology.* 1975;**116**:383-7.
241. KUMAR B, COLEMAN RE, ALDERSON PO. Gallium citrate Ga-67 imaging in patients with suspected inflammatory processes. *Arch Surg.* 1975;**110**:1237-42.
242. SIEMSEN JK, GREBE SF, SARGENT EN, WENTZ D. Gallium-67 scintigraphy of pulmonary diseases as a complement to radiography. *Radiology.* 1976;**118**:371-5.
243. VALLIERES BJ, JOHNSTON GS, JONES AE, LINE BR. Gallium-67 citrate scintigraphy: II. Clinical aspects. *Union Med Can.* 1977;**106**:1382-91.
244. STAAB EV, MCCARTNEY WH. Role of gallium-67 in inflammatory disease. *Semin Nucl Med.* 1978;**8**:219-34.
245. MYERSON PJ, MYERSON DA, SPENCER RP. Anatomic correlations in radiogallium imaging of the peritoneum and retroperitoneum. *Semin Nucl Med.* 1979;**9**:66-70.
246. LANSHAMMER H, GLAUBITT G, GREBE SF, et al. Gallium-67 for tumor scanning. *J Nucl Med.* 1972;**13**:25-30.
247. NELSON B, HAYES RL, EDWARDS CL, et al. Distribution of gallium in human tissues after intravenous administration. *J Nucl Med.* 1972;**13**:92-100.
248. LARSON SM, MILDER MS, JOHNSTON GS. Interpretation of the ^{67}Ga photoscan. *J Nucl Med.* 1973;**14**:208-14.
249. LINE BR, FULMER JD, REYNOLDS HY, et al. Gallium-67 citrate scanning in the staging of idiopathic pulmonary fibrosis: correlation with physiologic and morphologic features and bronchoalveolar lavage. *Am Rev Respir Dis.* 1978;**118**:355-65.
250. SIEMSEN JK, GREBE SF, WAXMAN AD. The use of gallium-67 in pulmonary disorders. *Semin Nucl Med.* 1978;**8**:235-49.
251. HESHIKI A, SCHATZ SL, MCKUSICK KA, BOWERSOX DW, SOIN JS, WAGNER HN. Gallium-67 citrate scanning in patients with pulmonary sarcoidosis. *Am J Roentgenol Radium Ther Nucl Med.* 1974;**122**:744-9.
252. MERTZ T, MALMUD L, MCKUSICK KA, WAGNER HN. Mechanisms of ^{67}Ga association with lymphocytes. *Cancer Res.* 1974;**34**:2495-9.
253. NIDEN AH, MISHKIN FS, KHURANA ML. ^{67}Gallium citrate lung scans in interstitial lung disease. *Chest.* 1976;**69**:266-8.
254. STONE DJ, SCHWARTZ A, FELTMAN JA, LOVELOCK FJ. Pulmonary function in sarcoidosis: results with cortisone therapy. *Am J Med.* 1953;**15**:468-78.
255. ISRAEL HL, SONES M, HARRELL D. Cortisone treatment of sarcoidosis: experience with thirty-six cases. *JAMA.* 1954;**156**:461-8.
256. SMELLIE H, APTHORP GH, MARSHALL R. The effect of corticosteroid treatment on pulmonary function in sarcoidosis. *Thorax.* 1960;**16**:87-90.
257. SHARMA OP, COLP C, WILLIAMS MH. Course of pulmonary sarcoidosis with and without corticosteroid therapy as determined by pulmonary function studies. *Am J Med.* 1966;**41**:541-51.
258. SILTZBACH LE. Sarcoidosis: clinical features and management. *Med Clin N Am.* 1967;**51**:483-502.
259. AMERICAN THORACIC SOCIETY MEDICAL SECTION OF THE NATIONAL TUBERCULOSIS AND RESPIRATORY DISEASE ASSOCIATION: Treatment of sarcoidosis. *Am Rev Respir Dis.* 1971;**103**:433-4.
260. ISRAEL HL, FOUTS DW, BEGGS RA. A controlled trial of prednisone treatment of sarcoidosis. *Am Rev Respir Dis.* 1973;**107**:609-14.
261. JOHNS CJ, ZACHARY JB, BALL WC. A ten-year study of corticosteroid treatment of pulmonary sarcoidosis. *Hopkins Med J.* 1974;**134**:271-83.
262. HEDFORS E. Influence of steroid treatment on lymphocyte response in sarcoidosis. *Clin Immunol Immunopathol.* 1975;**4**:96-100.
263. BALOW JE, HURLEY DL, FAUCI AS. Immuno-suppressive effects of glucocorticoids: differential effects of acute vs. chronic administration on cell-mediated immunity. *J Immunol.* 1975;**114**:1072-6.
264. FAUCI AS, DALE DC, BALOW JE. Glucocorticosteroid therapy: mechanisms of action and clinical considerations. *Ann Intern Med.* 1976;**84**:304-15.
265. ROSENAU W, MOON HD. The inhibitory effect of hydrocortisone on lysis of homologous cells by lymphocytes in vitro. *J Immunol.* 1962;**89**:422-6.
266. STAVEY L, COHEN IR, FELDMAN M. The effect of hydrocortisone on lymphocyte-mediated cytolysis. *Cell Immunol.* 1973;**7**:302-12.
267. FAUCI AS. Corticosteroids and circulating lymphocytes. *Transplant Proc.* 1975;**7**:37-40.
268. HAYNES BF, FAUCI AS. The differential effect of in vivo hydrocortisone on the kinetics of subpopulations of human peripheral blood thymus-derived lymphocytes. *J Clin Invest.* 1978;**61**:703-7.
269. BALOW JE, ROSENTHAL AS. Glucocorticoid suppression of macrophage migration inhibitory factor. *J Exp Med.* 1973;**137**:1031-41.
270. CRYSTAL RG, FULMER JD, BAUM B, et al. Cells, collagen and idiopathic pulmonary fibrosis. *Lung.* 1978;**155**:199-224.
271. VRACKO R. Significance of basal lamina for regeneration of injured lung. *Virchows Arch [Pathol Anat].* 1972;**355**:264-74.
272. BRITISH TUBERCULOSIS ASSOCIATION: Chloroquine in the treatment of sarcoidosis. *Tubercle.* 1967;**48**:257-72.
273. BREYNE H. Experiences with immunological therapy of sarcoidosis over 13 years. *Z Erkrank Atm Org.* 1977;**149**:160-3.
274. WANDETT-FREERKSEN E. Aldactone in the treatment of sarcoidosis of the lungs. *Z Erkrank Atm Org.* 1977;**149**:156-9.
275. ROSOF BM. Allopurinol for sarcoid. *N Engl J Med.* 1964;**294**:447. Letter.
276. ROSENTHAL M, TRABERT U, MÜLLER W, MÜLLER S, WURM K. Levamisole in sarcoidosis. *N Engl J Med.* 1974;**294**:112-3.
277. HEDFORS E. Possible role for anticoagulant treatment in sarcoidosis. *Mt Sinai J Med.* 1977;**44**:745-7.
278. GERAINT-JAMES D, CARSTAIRS LS, TROWELL J, SHARMA OP. Treatment of sarcoidosis: report of a controlled therapeutic trial. *Lancet.* 1967:526-8.
279. ISRAEL HL. Effects of chlorambucil and methotrexate in sarcoidosis. In: LEVINSKY L, MACKOLDA F, eds. *Fifth International Conference on Sarcoidosis.* Prague: Universita Karlova; 1971:632-4.
280. SHARMA O, HUGHES DTD, GERAINT-JAMES D, NAISH P. Immunosuppressive therapy with azathioprine in sarcoidosis. In: LEVINSKY L, MACHOLDA F, eds. *Fifth International Conference on Sarcoidosis.* Prague: Universita Karlova; 1971:635-7.

Characterization of the Inflammatory and Immune Effector Cells in the Lung Parenchyma of Patients with Interstitial Lung Disease[1,2]

GARY W. HUNNINGHAKE, OICHI KAWANAMI, VICTOR J. FERRANS, ROSCOE C. YOUNG, JR., WILLIAM C. ROBERTS, and RONALD G. CRYSTAL

SUMMARY The pathogenesis of the interstitial lung disorders is intimately related to the number, type, and state of activation of inflammatory and immune effector cells (the alveolitis) within the alveolar structures. To directly characterize the type and status of the cells comprising the alveolitis of various interstitial lung disorders, a method was developed to isolate inflammatory and immune effector cells from open lung biopsies of patients with idiopathic pulmonary fibrosis (n = 9) and sarcoidosis (n = 6). The cells isolated from these biopsies were compared with effector cells obtained from normal lung (n = 3). The effector cell populations in normal lung contained alveolar macrophages (84 ± 17%), lymphocytes (16 ± 4%), and rare polymorphonuclear leukocytes (<1%); of the lymphocytes present, 73 ± 4% were T-lymphocytes, 7 ± 2% were "activated" T-lymphocytes, and 9 ± 2% were B-lymphocytes. In contrast, a characteristic feature of the alveolitis of idiopathic pulmonary fibrosis was the presence of increased proportions of polymorphonuclear leukocytes, primarily neutrophils (18 ± 4%); the percentages of lymphocytes and various lymphocyte subpopulations were similar to those found in the normal lung. By comparison, the alveolitis of sarcoidosis was characterized by the presence of increased proportions of lymphocytes (57 ± 7%), T-lymphocytes (91 ± 5%), and "activated" T-lymphocytes (19 ± 4%); neutrophils were rarely found in the lung of nonsmoking patients with sarcoidosis. The proportions of various inflammatory and immune effector cells isolated from the lung of normal subjects as well as from biopsies of patients with idiopathic pulmonary fibrosis and sarcoidosis were similar to those cell populations that were present in the respective bronchoalveolar lavage fluids. Thus, the alveolitis of the interstitial lung diseases can be directly characterized by the types of inflammatory and immune effector cells present within the lung parenchyma. In addition, the cells recovered by bronchoalveolar lavage accurately reflect the alveolitis of these disorders.
AM REV RESPIR DIS 1981; 123:407-412

Introduction

The interstitial lung diseases are a heterogeneous group of disorders characterized by a chronic accumulation of increased numbers of inflammatory and immune effector cells within the alveolar structures (the "alveolitis"), a derangement of interstitial collagen (the "fibrosis"), alterations in lung parenchymal cells, and a progressive disordering of alveolar-capillary units (1-13). Although the fibrosis of interstitial disease likely plays an important role in disordering alveolar-capillary units, the current concepts of the pathogenesis of these disorders suggest that the alveolitis occurs early in the disease process and likely mediates both the fibrosis and the alterations in lung parenchymal cells (5, 10-14). Thus, to understand the pathogenesis of the different interstitial diseases, it was first necessary to define the type and function of the cells comprising the alveolitis that is characteristic of each disorder.

The classic approach to evaluate the alveolitis of interstitial disease has been to biopsy the lung parenchyma and, using conventional histologic methods, to describe qualitatively the inflammatory and immune effector cells that have accumulated within the alveolar structures (1-13). However, although such methods are useful to determine the degree of the cellular infiltrate, the integrity of the alveolar structures, and the amount of fibrosis, they yield little information as to the type and function of the cells comprising the alveolitis.

A newer approach to evaluate the alveolitis of interstitial disease has been the use of the fiberoptic bronchoscope to lavage the lower respiratory tract of these patients to obtain inflammatory and immune effector cells that are lining the epithelial surface of the lung parenchyma (5, 11-13, 15-22). This technique holds great promise, because, for the first time, it permits detailed morphologic surface marker, and functional evaluation of the inflammatory and immune effector cells involved in various chronic lung diseases. In addition, bronchoalveolar lavage is a safe, easily repeatable procedure that can be used to follow the status of the alveolitis of interstitial disease and its response to therapy (11-13, 15-21).

Although the formation derived from bronchoalveolar lavage of patient with interstitial disease is consistent with the theoretical concepts of the pathogenesis of these disorders, it has not been demonstrated that the inflammatory and immune effector cells collected by lavage are truly representative of the effector cells within the alveolar structures. The present study, therefore, was designed to study directly the inflammatory and immune effector cells that comprise the alveolitis of these disorders by isolating these cells from biopsies of lung parenchyma of patients with interstitial disease and comparing these cells with the cell populations obtained by bronchoalveolar lavage of the same patients. Two diverse disorders, sarcoidosis and idiopathic pulmonary fibrosis, were chosen for study, because they likely represent diseases whose pathogenesis is me-

(*Received in original form January 31, 1980 and in revised form December 10, 1980*)

[1] From the Pulmonary Branch and Pathology Branch, National Heart, Lung and Blood Institute, National Institutes of Health, Bethesda, MD 20205, and the Pulmonary Division, Department of Medicine, Howard University, Washington, DC 20001.

[2] Requests for reprints should be addressed to Gary W. Hunninghake, M.D., Building 10, Room 6D06 National Heart, Lung and Blood Institute, Bethesda, MD 20205.

diated through markedly different inflammatory and immune effector cells (1–21). For comparison, similar studies were carried out using lung biopsies from normal lung obtained from patients who underwent thoracotomy and biopsy of what turned out to be nonmalignant, noninfectious localized pulmonary lesions.

Methods

Study population: normal control subjects. Fiberoptic bronchoscopy was performed on 6 nonsmoking normal volunteers (2 men and 4 women with a mean ± SE age of 28 ± 6yr). The pulmonary function tests and chest roentgenograms of all 6 subjects were within normal limits, and none of the subjects were taking medication. Open lung biopsies were not performed on these 6 volunteers.

Normal lung parenchyma was obtained from patients who underwent thoracotomy for removal of solitary lung nodules. The nodule and a portion of the surrounding parenchyma were examined histologically and the remaining parenchyma was used for isolation of inflammatory and immune effector cells, as described subsequently. Data were used from only those patients fulfilling he following criteria: (*1*) nonsmoking, (*2*) normal pulmonary function tests and normal chest roentgenograms (except for the solitary nodules), and (*3*) nodules that proved to be noninfectious and nonmalignant and surrounding parenchyma that was normal by histologic examination. Three patients fulfilled all of these criteria. There were 2 men and 1 woman with a mean age of 42 ± 8 yr.

Study population: patients with idiopathic pulmonary fibrosis. A diagnosis of idiopathic pulmonary fibrosis (IPF) was made in 9 nonsmoking patients (5 men and 4 women with a mean age of 46 ± 8 yr) by established criteria (5, 10, 11, 13). All patients were in mid-course of their disease and none were taking medication. As a group, the patients with IPF had the following functional abnormalities: vital capacity, 71 ± 14% predicted; total lung capacity, 65 ± 9% predicted; single breath diffusing capacity, 58 ± 7% predicted, forced expiratory volume in one second/forced vital capacity, 96 ± 8% predicted; resting Pa_{O_2}, 77 ± 7 mm Hg; Pa_{O_2} at maximal steady-state exercise, 56 ± 12 mm Hg. All 9 patients underwent open lung biopsy and fiberoptic bronchoscopy with lavage.

Study population: patients with sarcoidosis. A diagnosis of sarcoidosis was established in 6 patients using the following criteria (10–13, 21): (*1*) an open lung biopsy demonstrating noncaseating epithelioid granulomata with giant cell formation in the lung parenchyma and coexisting morphologic features compatible with sarcoidosis; (*2*) a compatible clinical picture without evidence of mycobacterial, fungal, or parasitic infection; (*3*) no history of exposure to inorganic or organic material known to cause granulomatous lung disease; (*4*) a positive reaction to a Kveim-Siltzbach skin test (materials for the Kveim-Siltzbach skin test were kindly provided by Dr. L. Siltzbach). All patients had active sarcoidosis with lung parenchymal and hilar node involvement. None was taking medication. As a group, these patients had the following functional abnormalities: vital capacity, 74 ± 9% predicted; total lung capacity, 77 ± 7% predicted; single breath diffusing capacity, 62 ± 14% predicted; forced expiratory volume in one second/forced vital capacity, 101 ± 8% predicted; resting Pa_{O_2}, 87 ± 9 mm Hg; Pa_{O_2} at maximal steady-state exercise, 74 ± 12 mm Hg. All 6 patients underwent open lung biopsy and fiberoptic bronchoscopy with lavage.

Bronchoalveolar lavage. Patients and normal subjects were premedicated intravenously with valium (2 to 10 mg) and intramuscularly with atropine (0.8 mg). After local anesthesia with 2% lidocaine spray, examination of the airways was carried out with a flexible fiberoptic bronchoscope (Model BF-B2; Olympus Corporation of America, New Hyde Park, NY). The tip of the bronchoscope was then wedged in B4 or B5 in the left lung. Lavage was carried out with 100 ml of sterile saline in 5 20-ml aliquots with immediate vacuum aspiration after each aliquot. Immediately after lavage, the fluid was filtered through several layers of surgical gauze and the volume was measured. The cells were separated from the lavage fluid by centrifugation (500 *g* for 5 min) and resuspended in Hanks' balanced salt solution (HBSS) without Ca^{++} or Mg^{++}. The cells were then evaluated for total number (Model FN, Coulter Electronics, Hialeah, FL), viability (trypan blue dye exclusion), and differential count (Wright-Giemsa stained cytocentrifuge preparation, Cytospin®, Shandon Southern Instruments, Sewickley, PA). Macrophages were distinguished from lymphocytes by nonspecific esterase stains (11). The bronchoalveolar lavage cells (in HBSS) were then subjected to Hypaque-Ficoll density (1.077 to 1.080 g/ml) centrifugation (23), and the purified mononuclear cells were suspended in HBSS at a concentration of 4 × 10^6 cells/ml.

Lung biopsy. All lung biopsy specimens were immediately placed in sterile heparanized 0.9% saline (100 units/ml) at 4° C and portions removed for histologic examination and culture. The remaining tissue was then used to obtain inflammatory and immune effector cell populations by first teasing the parenchyma in HBSS in a petri dish. The resulting material was filtered through several layers of sterile surgical gauze to obtain a single cell suspension. Mononuclear cells were then isolated from these cell suspensions by Hypaque-Ficoll density centrifugation (23) and resuspended in HBSS at a concentration of 4 × 10^6 cells/ml. A small aliquot of the original cell suspension, the mononuclear cell band from the Hypaque-Ficoll gradient, and the cells going to the bottom of the Hypaque-Ficoll gradient were used to make a cytocentrifuge smear for cell differential, as described previously. Evaluation of these cell differentials demonstrated that, in addition to inflammatory and immune effector cells additional lung cells were also present in the unfractionated biopsy cell suspensions. These cells were distinguished from lymphocytes and alveolar macrophages by their morphologic features, their inability to phagocytize, their lack of cell surface markers and their density on Hypaque-Ficoll (these cells went to the bottom along with polymorphonuclear leukocytes). For these reasons, these cells were not considered to be inflammatory and immune effector cells and they were not considered during subsequent analyses. Only polymorphonuclear leukocytes, macrophages, and lymphocytes were included in the cell differentials; in all biopsies, these cells comprised more than 75% of the cells isolated.

Identification of lymphocyte subpopulations. Identical methods were used to identify lymphocyte subpopulations in the post-Hypaque-Ficoll mononuclear cell suspensions from lavage fluid and the lung biopsies (11, 20). The viability of the cell suspensions was more than 95% in all cases. To exclude phagocytic cells from quantitation of lymphocyte subpopulations, neutral red dye was added to the mononuclear cell suspensions before the rosetting procedure used to identify lymphocyte subpopulations. "Total lymphocytes" were arbitrarily identified as all cells not taking up the red dye. The use of the dye did not affect the percentages of lymphocytes forming rosettes in any of the testing procedures subsequently described.

The T-lymphocytes were identfied by their ability to form spontaneous rosettes at 4° C with neuraminidase-treated sheep red blood cells (SRBC) (24) and B-lymphocytes by the presence of surface immunoglobulin using a fluorescein conjugated $F(ab')_2$ goat antihuman immunoglobulin reagent (Cappel Laboratory, Cochranville, PA) (25). Both tests were performed as previously described (11, 21).

"Activated" T-lymphocytes, defined as subset of T-lymphocytes capable of forming rosettes with SRBC (not neuraminidase treated) at 37° C, were identified by combining 0.25 ml of the mononuclear cell suspension (4 × 10^6 cells/ml in HBSS) with 0.25 ml of 0.5 SRBC and incubating at 37° C for 5 min (26–28). The cells were then pelleted (100 *g* for 5 min at 37° C), incubated (at 37° C for 15 min), and the rosette-forming cells enumerated as previously described (11, 21).

Analysis of data. All data were presented as mean ± SE of the mean; comparison between values were made using the two-tailed t test.

Results

Bronchoalveolar lavage was performed without difficulty in each of the patients and in each of the normal volunteers. Visualization of the tracheobronchial tree prior to lavage demonstrated normal airways in all of the subjects, with no evidence of bronchitis. There was no significant difference in the total fluid recovered from the normal or the patient groups ($p > 0.2$, all comparisons). The recovered fluid was sterile in all cases, except for rare oral flora.

The biopsies of normal lung were characterized by thin alveolar septums and pleura, and the alveolar walls formed a fine, fishnet pattern. Within the interstitium and the alveoli there were a few mononuclear cells, primarily alveolar macrophages. Polymorphonuclear leukocytes were rarely found in the alveolar structures of the normal lung (data not shown).

The biopsies of the IPF lung were characterized by thickened interstitial areas and a derangement of the structure of alveolar-capillary units. In addition to alveolar macrophages/monocytes, increased numbers of polymorphonuclear leukocytes and lymphocytes were also present both within the interstitium and on the epithelial surface of the alveoli. Granulomata were not present within the lung in these patients (data not shown).

The biopsies of sarcoid lung were also characterized by thickened interstitial areas and a derangement of alveolar-capillary units. In contrast to the IPF lung, the inflammatory and immune effector cells present within the interstitium and alveoli of the sarcoid lung were comprised primarily of lymphocytes and monocytes/macrophages. Polymorphonuclear leukocytes were only rarely found in the lung in nonsmoking patients with this disorder. The lung lesions of sarcoidosis were always associated with the presence of granulomata within the lung parenchyma (data not shown).

The unfractionated single cell suspensions isolated from normal lung biopsies contained alveolar macrophages, small numbers of lymphocytes, and a variety of lung parenchymal cells; polymorphonuclear leukocytes were not present. After Hypaque-Ficoll centrifugation, the lung parenchymal cells pelleted to the bottom of the gradient and the macrophages and lymphocytes remained at the top of the gradient (data not shown).

In contrast to normal lung, the unfractionated single cell suspensions from the IPF lung were characterized by the presence of polymorphonuclear leukocytes in addition to macrophages, small numbers of lymphocytes, and lung parenchymal cells. After Hypaque-Ficoll centrifugation, the polymorphonuclear leukocytes and the lung parenchymal cells pelleted to the bottom of the gradient and the macrophages and lymphocytes remained at the top of the gradient (data not shown).

Compared with those from both normal and IPF lung, the unfractionated single cell suspensions from the sarcoid lung were characterized by the presence of large numbers of both lymphocytes and alveolar macrophages together with small numbers of eosinophils, basophils, and lung parenchymal cells; neutrophils were not present in these cell suspensions. After Hypaque-Ficoll centrifugation, the lung parenchymal cells, eosinophils, and basophils pelleted to the bottom of the gradient and the macrophages and lymphocytes remained at the top of the gradient (data not shown).

Comparison of the inflammatory and immune effector cells in lavage fluid and the lung biopsies. The cell yield per standard 100-ml bronchoalveolar lavage was $14 \pm 5 \times 10^6$ cells in normal subjects, $22 \pm 6 \times 10^6$ cells in patients with IPF, and $66 \pm 8 \times 10^6$ cells in patients with sarcoidosis (table 1).

An average of $7 \pm 3 \times 10^6$ inflammatory and immune effector cells/cm^3 of tissue were obtained from normal lung, $11 \pm 5 \times 10^6$ cells/cm^3 of lung tissue from patients with IPF, and $44 \pm 13 \times 10^6$ cells/cm^3 of lung tissue from patients with sarcoidosis (table 1). Sufficient numbers of cells were obtained from all biopsies to characterize the inflammatory and immune effector cells that were present in the lung tissues. This technique appeared to isolate almost all inflammatory and immune effector cells from the biopsies since histologic analysis of the parenchymal tissue that remained after teasing the specimens revealed only a rare macrophage, lymphocyte, or neutrophil (data not shown). Using the total number of red blood cells recovered in the biopsies as a reference, the percentages of blood-derived mononuclear cells were calculated; in all cases it was < 3%.

In the normal lung, the percentages of lymphocytes were $7 \pm 1\%$ in lavage fluid and $16 \pm 4\%$ in the unfractionated cell suspensions from the lung biopsies ($p < 0.01$) (figure 1). Polymorphonuclear leukocytes were rarely present in either lavage fluid or in the cell suspensions from the lung biopsies. Macrophages comprised the rest of the cell differential in both the lavage and biopsy cell suspensions. The other lung cells present in the unfractionated cell suspensions that were not considered inflammatory and immune effector cells were not included in the cell differentials.

In the IPF lung, the percentages of lymphocytes were $5 \pm 3\%$ in lavage fluid and $14 \pm 5\%$ in the unfractionated biopsy cell suspensions (figure 2). The percentages of these cells in lavage fluid and the lung biopsies were not significantly different from those in lavage fluid and lung biopsies of normal lung ($p > 0.2$, each comparison). In contrast to the normal lung, there was a marked increase in the percentages of polymorphonuclear leukocytes, primarily neutrophils but including eosinophils, in both lavage fluid and in

TABLE 1

ABSOLUTE NUMBER OF INFLAMMATORY AND IMMUNE EFFECTOR CELLS RECOVERED FROM OPEN LUNG BIOPSIES AND BRONCHOALVEOLAR LAVAGE FLUID OF PATIENTS WITH SARCOIDOSIS AND IPF AND NORMAL CONTROL SUBJECTS

	Cell Yield ($\times 10^{-6}$)	
Patient Groups	Biopsy*	Lavage Fluid†
Sarcoidosis	44 ± 13‡	66 ± 8
IPF	11 ± 5	22 ± 6
Normal subjects	7 ± 3§	14 ± 5‖

* Cell yield per cm^3 of lung tissue.
† Cell yield per standard 100 ml lavage.
‡ Mean ± SEM.
§ Includes normal lung from 3 patients with solitary lung nodules; *see* Methods.
‖ Includes 6 normal volunteers; *see* Methods.

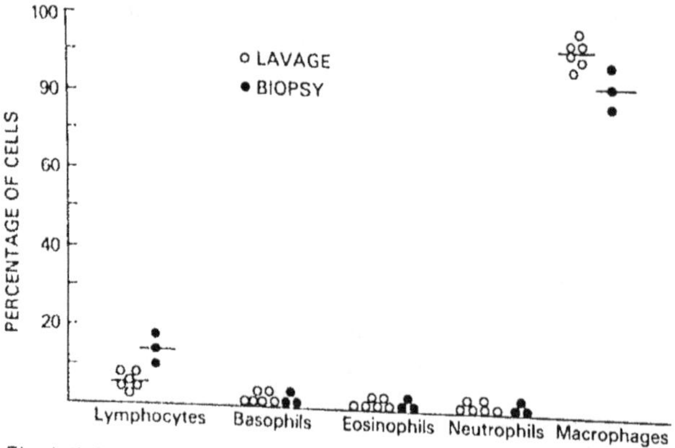

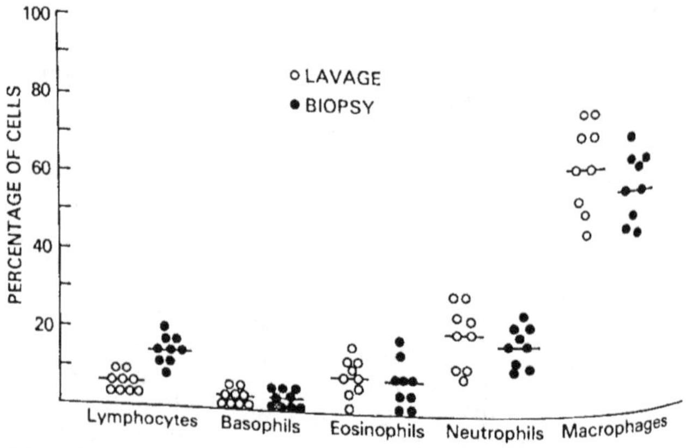

Fig. 1. (*left*) Inflammatory and immune effector cells obtained from bronchoalveolar lavage and open lung biopsies of normal lung. The percentage of cells is on the ordinate, and various cell types including macrophages, lymphocytes, basophils, eosinophils, and neutrophils are indicated on the abscissa. The data represent the mean ± SEM of cells from bronchoalveolar lavage of 6 normal subjects and cells from biopsies of 3 normal subjects. Fig. 2. (*right*) Inflammatory and immune effector cells obtained from bronchoalveolar lavage and open lung biopsies of patients with idiopathic pulmonary fibrosis. The percentage of cells is on the ordinate, and various cell types including macrophages, lymphocytes, basophils, eosinophils, and neutrophils are indicated on the abscissa. The data represent the cells from bronchoalveolar lavage and open lung biopsies of 9 patients with IPF.

the lung biopsies of patients with IPF ($p < 0.01$, each comparison). There was no significant difference in the percentages of either neutrophils or eosinophils in lavage fluid of patients with IPF compared with the IPF biopsy cell suspensions ($p > 0.2$, each comparison). Macrophages comprised the rest of the cell differentials in both the lavage and biopsy cell suspensions.

In the sarcoid lung, there was a marked increase in the percentages of lymphocytes in both lavage fluid and lung biopsies, compared with both control subjects and patients with IPF ($p < 0.01$, all comparisons) (figure 3). There was no significant difference in the percentages of lymphocytes in lavage fluid compared with the biopsy cell suspensions in patients with sarcoidosis (48 ± 12% versus 57 ± 7%, respectively, $p > 0.2$). In addition, there were no significant numbers of neutrophils in the lung of these patients. However, 2 to 3% basophils and eosinophils were routinely present in both lavage fluid and the biopsy cell suspensions. Macrophages comprised the rest of the cell differential in both the lavage and biopsy cell suspensions.

Comparisons of lymphocyte subpopulations in lavage fluid and the biopsy cell suspensions. In normal subjects, the percentages of T-lymphocytes, "activated" T-lymphocytes, and B-lymphocytes were similar in cell suspensions from lavage fluid and from lung parenchyma ($p > 0.2$). In addition, in patients with IPF or with sarcoidosis there also were no differences in the proportions of each of these lymphocyte subpopulations in cell suspensions isolated from lavage fluid compared with those isolated from lung parenchyma ($p > 0.2$, each comparison). Thus, the lymphocytes in lavage fluid reflected those present in the lung parenchyma in normal subjects as well as in patients with IPF or sarcoidosis (figure 4).

There were no significant differences in the percentages of T-lymphocytes, "activated" T-lymphocytes, or B-lymphocytes between control subjects and patients with IPF in either the lavage cell suspensions or the post-Hypaque-Ficoll biopsy cell suspensions ($p > 0.2$, all comparisons). In patients with sarcoidosis, however, the percentages of T-lymphocytes and "activated" T-lymphocytes were significantly increased in both lavage fluid and in the lung biopsies, compared with both the normal and the IPF lung ($p < 0.01$, all comparisons). In contrast, the percentages of B-lymphocytes were significantly decreased in both lavage fluid and lung biopsies of patients with sarcoidosis, compared with the normal and IPF lung ($p < 0.01$, all comparisons). Although the percentages of B-lymphocytes were decreased in the lung of patients with sarcoidosis, it is likely that the absolute numbers of these cells as well as the T-lymphocytes were actually increased because of the marked increase in the total number of lymphocytes that were present in the lungs of these patients.

Discussion

From histologic studies, it has been known for some time that the cell populations of the alveolar structures of the human lung include significant numbers of inflammatory and immune effector cells (1–14). The present study demonstrated that these effector cells can be isolated directly from lung biopsies in numbers adequate to characterize them. By comparing the effector cell populations present in biopsies of normal, IPF, and sarcoid lung, it has become apparent that the inflammatory and immune effector cells present in the IPF and the sarcoid lung are markedly different from those in normal lung and from each other. In addition, these studies have also shown that the proportions of effector cells recovered by bronchoalveolar lavage of patients with IPF or sarcoidosis closely resemble the proportions of effector cells actually present within the alveolar structures of the lungs of these patients. This observation, together with the study which demonstrated that samples of lavage fluid obtained from different sites within the lung contain a similar composition of cell types (18) validates the concept that bronchoalveolar lavage is a useful technique by which to characterize the alveolitis of these disorders.

Effector cells in the normal lung. Consistent with histologic studies, most of the inflammatory and immune effector cells isolated directly from normal lung were alveolar macrophages; a smaller proportion were lymphocytes. The lymphocytes present were primarily T-lymphocytes; most of these cells were not activated. The B-lymphocytes were also present, but in much smaller numbers than the T-lymphocytes. In normal lung, polymorphonuclear leukocytes were rarely found.

Lavage of the normal lung yielded

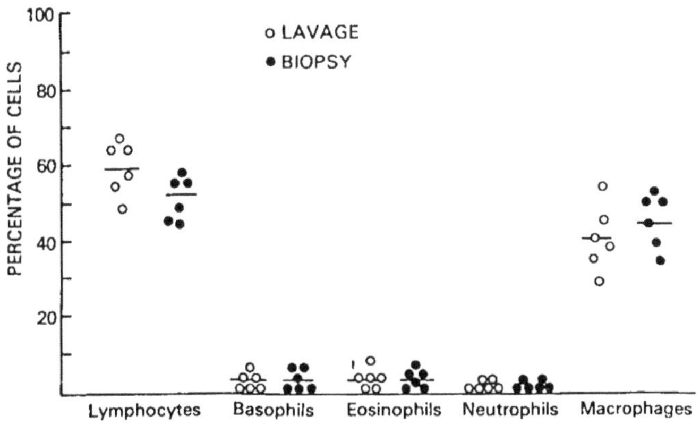

g. 3. Inflammatory and immune effector cells obtained from bronchoalveolar lavage and open lung opsies of patients with pulmonary sarcoidosis. The percentage of cells is on the ordinate, and various ell types including macrophages, lymphocytes, basophils, eosinophils, and neutrophils are indicated n the abscissa. The data represent the cells from bronchoalveolar lavage and open lung biopsies of 6 atients with sarcoidosis.

milar results. The only significant diference between the effector cells reovered from the biopsies of normal ng and the lavage of normal lung was nat a relatively larger proportion of mphocytes were present in the parenyma than was reflected by lavage nalysis. This observation was consisnt with animal studies (29) and histogic observations (30) of human lung nowing that, in normal lung parenyma, the majority of lymphocytes re in the interstitium, not in the alveor air spaces. However, analysis of the mphocytes present in lavage did acurately reflect the distribution of lymhocyte subtypes in the alveolar strucres (figure 4).

Effector cells in the IPF lung. In ontrast to the normal lung, the effecor cells isolated from biopsies of paents with IPF were characterized by e presence of large proportions of eutrophils. The proportions and subpes of lymphocytes, however, closely sembled those of normal lung.

Analysis of effector cells recovered y bronchoalveolar lavage of the same PF patients revealed similar results. his is particularly important in relaon to the neutrophils found in lavage f these patients (10, 11, 13, 17–21). lthough patients with IPF do not as a ile have bronchitis, lavage samples ontaining neutrophils must be interreted in the context that clinically oclt inflammatory airway disease ight be present, and thus the neutrohils might be airway, rather than alcolar, derived. However, the fact that e proportions of neutrophils reovered from IPF parenchymal biopes were similar to those in lavage strongly supported the concept that bronchoalveolar lavage of these patients yields a valid assessment of the character and intensity of the alveolitis that is present.

Effector cells in the sarcoid lung. The inflammatory and immune effector cells associated with the alveolitis of sarcoidosis were characterized by much larger proportions of lymphocytes than were found in either the normal or the IPF lung. Not only were there increased proportions of lymphocytes in the sarcoid lung, but more of

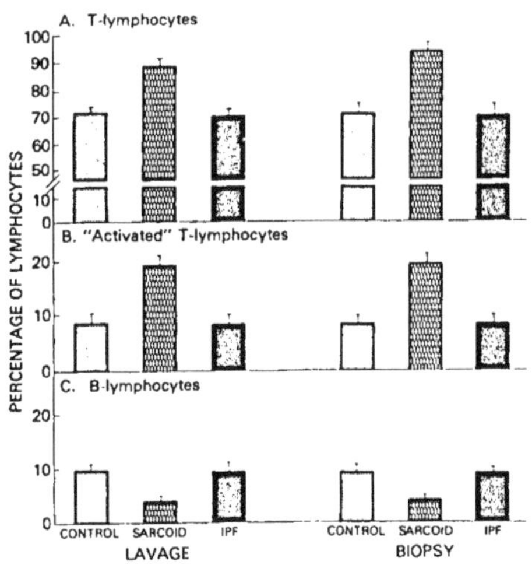

Fig. 4. Lymphocyte subpopulations in bronchoalveolar lavage fluid and open lung biopsies of patients with normal lung and patients with IPF and sarcoidosis. The percentage of lymphocytes is on the ordinate and the source of cells is indicated on the abscissa. A. percentage of T-lymphocytes; B. percentage of "activated" T-lymphocytes; C. percentage of B-lymphocytes. The lavage data represent the mean ± SEM of cells obtained from 6 normal subjects, 9 patients with IPF, and 6 patients with sarcoidosis; and the biopsy data represent cells obtained from 3 normal subjects, 9 patients with IPF, and 6 patients with sarcoidosis.

these lymphocytes were T-lymphocytes and more of these T-lymphocytes were "activated." In addition, the alveolitis of sarcoid lung was further distinguished by the absence of neutrophils from the alveolar structures of these patients.

When the alveolitis of sarcoidosis was characterized by lavage techniques, it was found to consist of increased proportions of activated T-lymphocytes (10–13, 19–21, 31–35), similar to what was found on direct analysis of the biopsy specimens. Thus, as in IPF, lavage is a valid means to assess the alveolitis of sarcoidosis.

The present study demonstrated that adequate numbers of effector cells can be isolated directly from biopsies of normal subjects and patients with common forms of interstitial lung disease. These techniques should be generally applicable to the evaluation of other interstitial disorders and permit a validation of lavage assessments of the alveolitis of each disease. In addition, the numbers of effector cells recovered from the biopsies are sufficient to permit detailed characterizations of the types and functions of various subpopulations of effector cells comprising the alveolitis of these disorders. This should prove useful in helping to understand the pathogenesis of the interstitial lung diseases, and also in staging the intensity of the alveolitis of individual patients. The latter is critical in terms of making rational therapy decisions in these disorders.

References

1. Spencer H. Interstitial pneumonia. Annu Rev Med 1967; 18:423–42.
2. Scadding JG, Hinson KFW. Diffuse fibrosing alveolitis (diffuse interstitial fibrosis of the lungs): correlation with histology at biopsy with prognosis. Thorax 1967; 22:291–304.
3. Hinson KFW. Diffuse pulmonary fibrosis. Hum Pathol 1970; 1:275–88.
4. Scadding JG. Diffuse pulmonary alveolar fibrosis. Thorax 1974; 29:271–81.
5. Crystal RG, Fulmer JD, Roberts WC, Moss ML, Line BR, Reynolds HY. Idiopathic pulmonary fibrosis: clinical, histologic, radiographic, physiologic, scintigraphic, cytologic and biochemical aspects. Ann Intern Med 1976;85:769–88.
6. Fulmer JD, Crystal RG. The biochemical basis of pulmonary function. In: Crystal RG, ed, The Biochemical Basis of Pulmonary Function. New York: Marcel Dekker, 1976:419–66.
7. Weinburger SE, Crystal RG. Reactions of the interstitial space to injury. In: Fishman AP, ed, Textbook of pulmonary diseases. New York: McGraw-Hill, 1979:640–47.
8. Basset F, Soler P, Bernandin JF. Contribu-

tion of electron microscopy to the study of interstitial pneumonias. Prog Respir Dis 1975; 8:45-58.

9. Brody AR, Craighead JE. Interstitial association of cells lining air spaces in human pulmonary fibrosis. Virchows Arch [Pathol Anat] 1976; 372:39-49.

10. Fulmer JD, Crystal RG. Interstitial lung disease. In: Simmons DH, ed, Current pneumonology. Boston: Houghton Mifflin, 1979:1-65.

11. Hunninghake GW, Gadek JE, Kawanami O, Ferrans VJ, Crystal RG. Inflammatory and immune processes in the human lung in health and disease: evaluation by bronchoalveolar lavage. Am J Pathol 1979; 97:149-206.

12. Crystal RG, Roberts WC, Hunninghake GW, Gadek JE, Fulmer JD, Line BR. Pulmonary sarcoidosis: a disease characterized and perpetuated by activated lung T-lymphocytes. Ann Intern Med (in press).

13. Crystal RG, Ferrans VJ, Gadek JE, Fulmer JD, Line BR, Hunninghake GW. Interstitial lung disease: current concepts of pathogenesis, staging, and therapy. Am J Med (in press).

14. Rosen Y, Athanassiades TJ, Moon S, Lyons HA. Nongranulomatous interstitial pneumonitis in sarcoidosis. Relationship to development of epithelioid granulomas. Chest 1978; 74:122-5.

15. Finley TN, Swenson EW, Curran WS, Huber GL, Todman AJ. Bronchopulmonary lavage in normal subjects and patients with obstructive lung disease. Ann Intern Med 1967; 66:651-8.

16. Reynolds HY, Newball HH. Analysis of proteins and respiratory cells obtained from human lungs by bronchial lavage. J Lab Clin Med 1974; 84:559-73.

17. Reynolds HY, Fulmer JD, Kazmierowski JA, Roberts WC, Frank MM, Crystal RG. Analysis of bronchoalveolar lavage fluid from patients with idopathic pulmonary fibrosis and chronic hypersensitivity pneumonitis. J Clin Invest 1977; 59:165-75.

18. Weinberger SE, Kelman JA, Elson NA, *et al.* Broncholalveolar lavage in interstitial lung disease. Ann Intern Med 1978; 89:459-66.

19. Hunninghake GW, Fulmer JD, Young RC, Crystal RG. Comparison of lung and blood lymphocyte subpopulations in pulmonary sarcoidosis. In: Eighth International Congress on Sarcoidosis and Other Granulomatous Diseases 1980 (in press).

20. Hunninghake GW, Gadek JE, Szapiel SV, *et al.* The human alveolar macrophage. In: Harris CC, Trump BF, Stoner GD, eds, Methods and perspectives in cell biology: cultured human cells and tissues in biomedical research. New York: Academic Press, 1980 (in press).

21. Hunninghake GW, Fulmer JD, Young RC, Gadek JE, Crystal RG. Localization of the immune response in sarcoidosis. Am Rev Respir Dis 1979; 120:49-57.

22. Daniele RP, Altrose MD, Rowlands DT. Immunocompetent cells from the lower respiratory tract of normal human lungs. J Clin Invest 1925; 56:986.

23. Boyum A. Isolation of mononuclear cells and granulocytes from human blood. Scand J Clin Invest 1968; 21:77-82.

24. Weiner MS, Bianco C, Nussenzweig V. Enhanced binding of neuraminidase-treated sheep erythrocytes to human T-lymphocytes. Blood 1976; 42:939-44.

25. Papamichail M, Brown JC, Holborow EJ. Immunoglobulins in the surface of human lymphocytes. Lancet 1971; 2:850-52.

26. Wybran JM, Carr C, Fudenberg HH. The human rosette-forming cell as a marker of a population of thymus-derived cells. J Clin Invest 1972; 51:2537-42.

27. Katoh AK, Charoensiri S. The formation of stable E-rosettes by human T-lymphocytes activated by photohemagglutinin. J Immunol 1977 118:2291-94.

28. Yu DTY. Human lymphocyte subpopulations: suspension-sheep-red-blood cell rosettes Clin Immunol Immunopathol 1977; 8:190-6.

29. Hunninghake GW, Fauci AS. Immunological reactivity of the lung. I. A guinea pig model for the study of pulmonary mononuclear cell subpopulations. Cell Immunol 1976; 26:89-97.

30. Bienenstock J, Clancy RL, Percy DY. Bronchus associated lymphoid tissue (BALT), its relationship to mucosal immunity. In: Kirkpatrick CH, Reynolds HY, eds, Immunologic and infectious reactions in the lung. New York: Marcel Dekker, 1976:29-58.

31. Reynolds HY. The importance of lymphocytes in pulmonary health and disease. Lung 1978; 155:225-42.

32. Gee JBL, Bodel PT, Zorn SK, Hinman LM, Stevens CA, Matthay RA. Sarcoidosis and mononuclear phagocytes. Lung 1978; 115:243-53.

33. Danel C, Arnoux A, Marsac J, Basset F, Chretien J. Cellular data from bronchoalveolar lavages in various interstitial disease. Bull Eur Physiopathol Respir 1979; 15:42-3P.

34. Rossman MD, Daniele RP, Dauber JH. Bronchoalveolar lymphocytes in sarcoidosis. J Lab Clin Med 1979; 94:862-71.

35. Yeager H, Williams MC, Beckman JF, Bayly TC, Beaman BL, Hawley RJ. Sarcoidosis: analysis of cells obtained by bronchial lavage. Am Rev Respir Dis 1977; 116:951-5.

Carcinoma of the Lung Causing Pulmonary Arterial Stenosis*

Bruce F. Waller, M.D., F.C.C.P.; Ross D. Fletcher, M.D.; and William C. Roberts, M.D., F.C.C.P.

A patient is described in whom carcinoma of the lung caused compression and obstruction of the left and right main pulmonary arteries and auscultatory features of peripheral pulmonary arterial stenosis.

Herein we describe findings in a man with carcinoma of the lung causing auscultatory features of peripheral pulmonary arterial stenosis. To our knowledge, such a patient has not been described previously.

Case Report

A 55-year-old man was healthy until January 1977 (11 months before death), when left anterior chest pain and dyspnea first appeared. He had smoked a package of cigarettes daily for 30 years. The mean jugular venous pressure was equivalent to about 6 cm of water, and a prominent A wave was visible. The carotid arterial pulse was normal. The breath sounds were decreased, and the percussion note was dull over the left chest. A right ventricular impulse was easily palpable. The second heart sound at the base was widely split on inspiration, and never became single during expiration (Fig 1). The pulmonary component of the second heart sound was increased in intensity. A third heart sound, S_3, was present over the right sternal border. A grade 3/6 systolic ejection murmur was heard over the precordium, both axillae and back, loudest over the second right and left intercostal spaces, and the murmur increased in intensity with inspiration, especially along the right sternal border and in the right axilla. No diastolic murmurs were heard. An ECG showed prominent left ventricular voltage and nonspecific ST segment and T wave changes. His chest roentgenogram (Fig 2) disclosed complete opacification of the left lung field. An echocardiogram was consistent with pulmonary hypertension.

Tissue obtained from the left main stem bronchus showed small-cell carcinoma. At right-sided cardiac catheterization, the pressures (in mm Hg) were as follows: right atrium, a = 8, v = 7); right ventricle, 55/10; pulmonary trunk, 55/10; proximal right pulmonary artery, 55/10, and distal right pulmonary artery, 22/10 (Fig 1). Right atrial angiogram (Fig 2) disclosed normal right atrial and ventricular cavities and pulmonary trunk, but severe narrowing of the left main and moderate narrowing of the right main pulmonary arteries.

The patient received chemotherapy and local irradiation, and a chest roentgenogram four weeks later showed considerable clearing of the left lung field. Moreover, the intensity of the systolic ejection murmur had decreased to grade 1/6.

*From the Pathology Branch, National Heart, Lung, and Blood Institute, National Institutes of Health, Bethesda, Md, and the Division of Cardiology, Department of Medicine, Veterans Administration Hospital, Washington, D.C.
Reprint requests: Dr. Roberts, Building 10A, Room 3E30, National Institutes of Health, Bethesda 20205

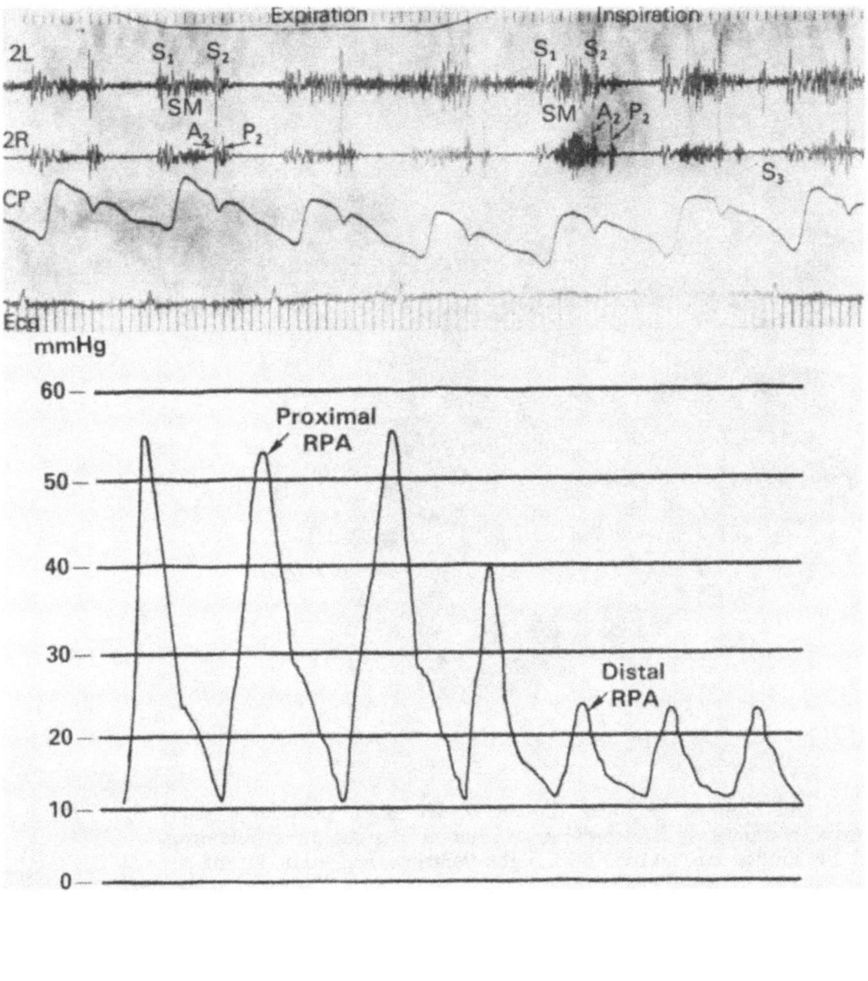

FIGURE 1. Phonocardiogram *(upper)* recorded at second left (2L) and right (2R) intercostal spaces showing systolic murmurs (SM) and a persistently split second heart sound (S_2). A_2= aortic component of S_2, CP=external carotid pulse; P_2=pulmonic component of S_2; S_1=first heart sound; S_3=third heart sound. Pressure tracing *(lower)* with pullback from distal to proximal right main pulmonary artery (RPA).

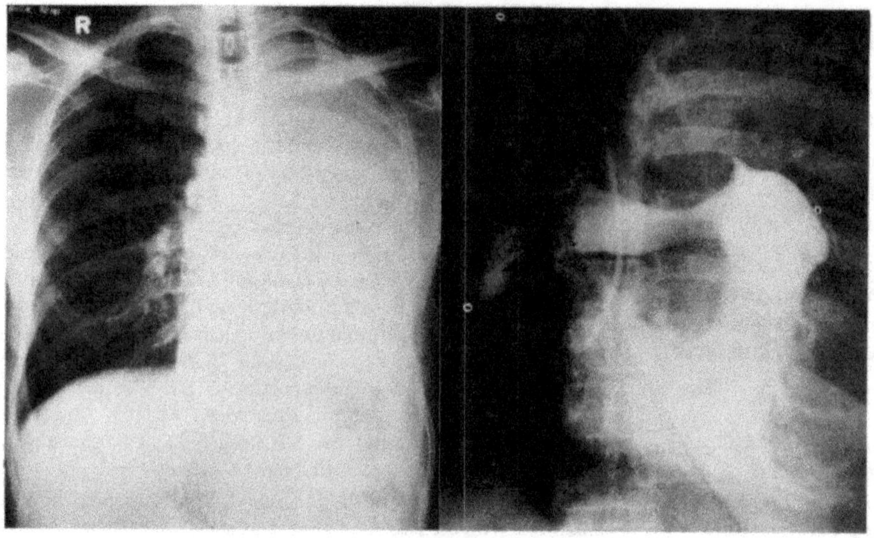

Figure 2. Posteroanterior chest roentgenogram *(left)* showing opacification of left lung field and angiogram *(right)* with injection into right atrium demonstrating severe luminal narrowing of left main and moderate narrowing of right main pulmonary arteries. Roentgenograms done 11 months before death.

He slowly deteriorated, however, and died ten months later (November 1977). His only evidence of right-sided congestive heart failure at any time was the presence of a third heart sound, which varied with respiration.

At necropsy, both right and left lung parenchyma and pleura were extensively replaced by carcinoma (Fig 3). The left main bronchus and pulmonary artery were severely compressed by tumor. The right main pulmonary artery was partially compressed by surrounding tumor. A large cavity filled with necrotic tumor was present in the upper left lobe. Histologic sections showed tumor invasion of the walls of the right and left main pulmonary arteries and intrapulmonary arteries. The heart weighed 420 g, and the right ventricle was dilated.

Discussion

Although many reports have described exterior compression of one or more major extrapulmonary pulmonary arteries by neoplasm, auscultatory evidence of obstruction to one or more major pulmonary arteries has not been documented previously. In our patient, total obstruction to the left main pulmonary artery and partial obstruction to the right main pulmonary artery was documented by both angiography (during life) and

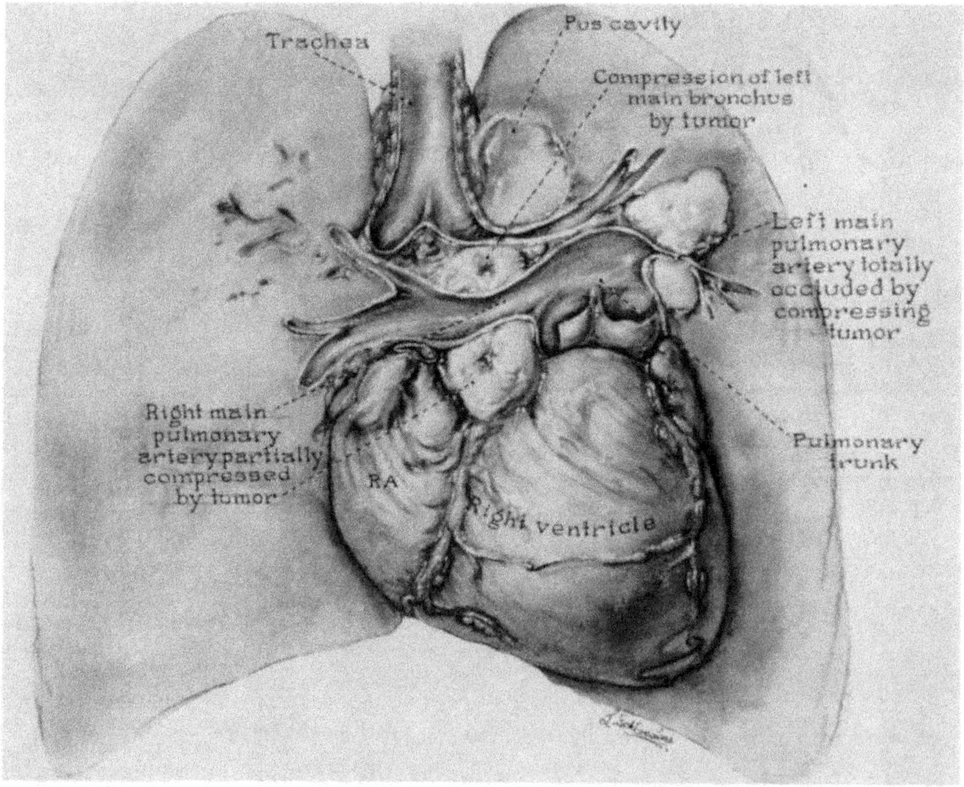

Figure 3. Drawing of heart and lungs at necropsy. Lumen of left main pulmonary artery totally occluded by carcinoma, compressing it externally, and lumen of right main pulmonary artery partially obstructed by similar mechanism. Both right ventricle and right atrium are dilated.

necropsy, and a 33 mm Hg peak systolic pressure gradient between proximal and distal right main pulmonary artery was found at catheterization. The wide splitting of the second heart sound at the cardiac base in our patient can be attributed to the peripheral pulmonary stenosis. There was not enough right ventricular failure (only a third heart sound) in the presence of the pulmonary hypertension in our patient to account for the wide splitting of the second heart sound.

ACKNOWLEDGMENT: The authors thank W. Proctor Harvey, M.D., Chief, Division of Cardiology, Department of Medicine, Georgetown University, Washington, D.C., for reviewing the manuscript and for making useful suggestions.

A Simple Histologic Classification of Pulmonary Arterial Hypertension

For many years students of congenital heart disease were unable to explain the differences in survival patterns in patients with similar-sized isolated communications between systemic and pulmonary circulations. In 1927 Moschcowitz[1] suggested that the explanation may be the presence of pulmonary hypertension in some patients with shunts and its absence in others. In 1935, Brenner[2] described histologic features of the normal pulmonary arteries and veins. In 1936, Parker and Weiss[3] at the Boston City Hospital described changes in the parenchyma and vessels of lungs in patients with mitral stenosis. In the late 1940s, Edwards,[4] who also trained at the Boston City Hospital in the late 1930s, began describing anatomic changes in the pulmonary vasculature in patients with congenital heart disease, and he too attributed the changes to the effects of pulmonary hypertension. In 1958, Heath and Edwards[5] proposed an anatomic classification of hypertensive pulmonary changes (Fig. 1). Their classification was based primarily on observations of necropsy patients with large ventricular septal defect or patent ductus arteriosus having *pulmonary hypertension from birth*, but a few patients had primary pulmonary hypertension.

Although the Heath and Edwards classification brought organization to a complex subject, reevaluation nearly 30 years later indicates that their classification has certain deficiencies. Considerable overlap exists between their grades 2 and 3 and grades 4 and 5. *Alveolar hemosiderosis* (grade 5) does not concern a pulmonary artery and it may occur in patients without pulmonary arterial hypertension. In my view, a classification of pulmonary arterial changes should not include changes in alveolar spaces (hemosiderosis). Their grade 6 category implies that grades 1 through 5 are prerequisites, when, in actuality, necrotizing vasculitis may occur in the absence of grades 1 to 5 and it may occur in the absence of pulmonary hypertension. A classification of hypertensive changes in the pulmonary arteries should be applicable, of course, to all patients with pulmonary hypertension irrespective of its cause and irrespective of whether the hypertension is congenital or acquired in origin.

Basis of Grades of Hypertensive Pulmonary Vascular Disease Found in Association with Large Ventricular Septal Defects and Functionally Related Diseases

<table>
<tr><th rowspan="2"></th><th colspan="6">Grade of hypertensive pulmonary vascular disease</th></tr>
<tr><th>1</th><th>2</th><th>3</th><th>4</th><th>5</th><th>6</th></tr>
<tr><td rowspan="4">Type of intimal reaction</td><td>←None→</td><td colspan="5"></td></tr>
<tr><td></td><td colspan="5">←Cellular→</td></tr>
<tr><td colspan="2"></td><td colspan="4">←Fibrous and fibroelastic→</td></tr>
<tr><td colspan="3"></td><td colspan="3">←Plexiform lesion→</td></tr>
<tr><td rowspan="5">State of media of arteries and arterioles</td><td colspan="6">←Hypertrophied→</td></tr>
<tr><td colspan="2"></td><td colspan="4">←Some generalized dilatation→</td></tr>
<tr><td colspan="3"></td><td colspan="3">←Local "dilatation lesions"*→</td></tr>
<tr><td colspan="4"></td><td colspan="2">←Pulmonary hemosiderosis†→</td></tr>
<tr><td colspan="5"></td><td>←Necrotizing arteritis→</td></tr>
</table>

*Vein-like branches of hypertrophied muscular pulmonary arteries, angiomatoid lesion, and cavernous lesion

†Associated with distended, thin-walled, arterial vessels throughout the lung

FIGURE 1. Classification of hypertensive pulmonary vascular changes by Heath and Edwards in 1958.[5] Reproduced with permission of the publisher.

The classification of pulmonary arterial changes recommended herein consists of only 3 grades, and is based on histologic alterations irrespective of the etiology of or the time of appearance of the pulmonary arterial hypertension. The major changes in the pulmonary arteries include: (1) *medial thickening* (MT), (2) *intimal thickening* (IT), and (3) *plexiform lesion* (PL) (Fig. 2). Grade I includes MT only; grade II, MT plus IT; and grade III, MT plus IT plus PL (Fig. 3). Neither arteritis (vasculitis) nor hemosiderosis are included in the grading system.

Medial thickening: This indicates an increase in the thickness of the media of a pulmonary artery or of a pulmonary arteriole, or both. Whether this occurs entirely from hypertrophy of smooth muscle cells or from both hypertrophy and hyperplasia is unclear. Thus, the reason for the phrase *medial thickening* rather than *medial hypertrophy*.

Intimal thickening: There are 2 types of intimal thickening: the cellular variety, in which the proliferated intima consists primarily of smooth-muscle cells with collagen in between, and the acellular variety, which consists mostly of dense fibrous (collagen) tissue with minimal or no smooth muscle cells.

Plexiform lesion: This is an aneurysmal or glomus-like structure that emerges at more-or-less right angles to a muscular pulmonary artery. Just after origin of the right-angle branch it suddenly bulges into a plexus of channels, the walls of which consist primarily of fibrous tissue covered by endo-

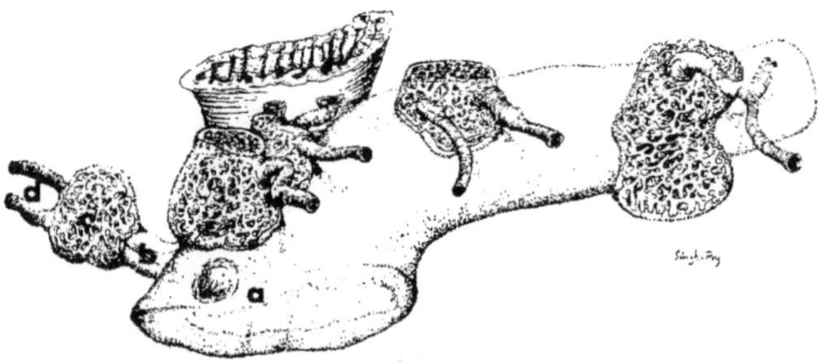

FIGURE 2. Drawing from Moschcowitz et al[10] of plexiform lesions arising from a muscular pulmonary artery. Reproduced with permission of the publisher.

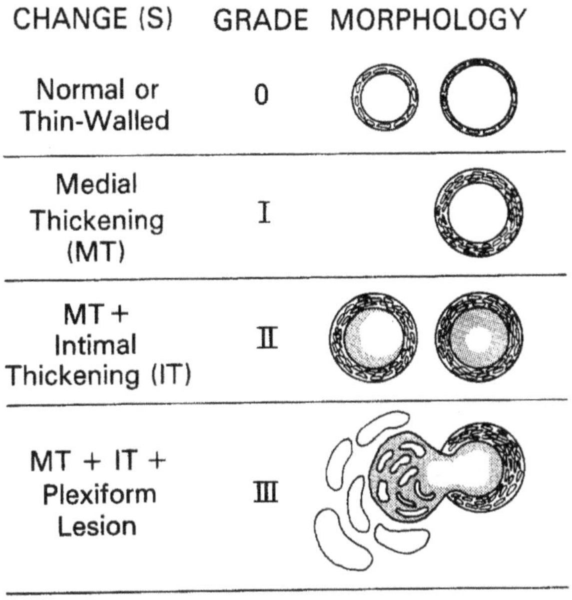

FIGURE 3. Types of grading of the morphologic pulmonary artery changes from Virmani and Roberts.[12] Reproduced with permission of the publisher.

thelial cells. The PL gives rise to thin-walled channels, probably dilated arterioles, which rapidly branch into alveolar septal capillaries. These thin-walled channels when considerably dilated have been called *dilatation lesions.*

Proposed causes: *Medial thickening* is a response of the arterial wall to increased pressure and therefore occurs only in patients with pulmonary arterial hypertension. Medial thickening is never simply a normal consequence of aging. *Intimal thickening* is not necessarily the consequence of pulmonary arterial hypertension, but it is accelerated by elevation of pulmonary arterial pressure. Cellular and acellular IT is frequently observed in older persons, most of whom have normal pulmonary arterial pressures.[6] The occurrence of IT combined with MT, however, is indicative of pulmonary hypertension. *Plexiform lesions* occur only in patients with severe pulmonary hypertension, but most patients with severe pulmonary hypertension do not have them. Plexiform lesions occur in patients with large intravascular shunts or primary pulmonary hypertension or pulmonary embolic or thrombotic disease, but they do not occur in patients in whom the severe pulmonary hypertension is secondary to left-sided cardiac disease (e.g., mitral stenosis). Plexiform lesions do not occur if the cause of the pulmonary hypertension is located distal to the pulmonary capillary level or, stated differently, if the pulmonary arterial hypertension is the consequence of pulmonary venous hypertension. For a PL to occur, the cause of the hypertension must originate at the capillary or recapillary level.[7]

The exact cause of PLs is unknown. Serial sections of lung at sites of a PL generally show extreme narrowing or almost total obstruction of the lumen of the muscular pulmonary artery distal to the origin of the small muscular pulmonary artery or arteriole which is the site of the PL. Kanjuh and colleagues[8] suggested that the PL was a consequence of a *jet lesion* caused by blood rapidly changing its course because of the distal obstruction of the relatively large muscular pulmonary artery distal to the site of the PL. Thus, the PL might act as a dissipator of the extremely high pulmonary arterial pressure. Others have suggested that the PL represents a site of *anastomoses of pulmonary arteries and veins*[9] or it is a *congenital malformation.*[10] PL, however, has never been observed in the lungs at birth; the earliest it has been observed is at 2 months of age.[11] The PL may represent an aneurysm formed at sites of *congenitally underdeveloped or weak media* (analogous to the formation of an intracerebral berry aneurysm in systemic hypertension), the aneurysm later being filled by thrombus, which organizes into multiple minute vascular channels.[12,13] Wagenvoort and Wagenvoort[14] proposed that the PL represents a site of healed necrotizing arteritis. The inflammation weakens the arterial wall, which focally expands, fibrin and platelets are deposited in the aneurysm, and organization of the thrombus produces multiluminal channels lined by endothelial cells.

Whatever its cause, the PL represents irreversible pulmonary hypertension, whereas MT alone or MT plus IT indicates that the pulmonary hypertension is reversible.

William C. Roberts, MD
Editor in Chief

References

1. Moschcowitz E. Hypertension of the pulmonary circulation; its causes, dynamics and relation to other circulatory states. Am J Med Sci 1927;174:388–406.
2. Brenner O. Pathology of the vessels of the pulmonary circulation. Arch Intern Med 1935;56:211–237, 457–497, 724–752, 976–1014, 1189–1241.
3. Parker F, Weiss S. The nature and significance of the structural changes in the lungs in mitral stenosis. Am J Pathol 1936;12:573–598.
4. Edwards JE. Functional pathology of the pulmonary vascular tree in congenital cardiac disease. Circulation 1957;15:164–196.
5. Heath D, Edwards JE. The pathology of hypertensive pulmonary vascular disease. A description of six grades of structural changes in the pulmonary arteries with special reference to congenital cardiac septal defects. Circulation 1958;18:533–547.
6. Wagenvoort CA, Wagenvoort N. Age changes in muscular pulmonary arteries and arterioles. Arch Pathol 1965;79:524–528.
7. Roberts WC, Fredrickson DS. Gaucher's disease of the lung causing severe pulmonary hypertension with associated acute recurrent pericarditis. Circulation 1967;35:783–789.
8. Kanjuh VI, Sellers RD, Edwards JE. Pulmonary vascular plexiform lesion. Arch Pathol 1964;78:513–522.
9. Hufner RF, McNicol CA. The pathologic physiology of microscopic pulmonary vascular shunts. AMA Arch Pathol 1958;65:554–560.
10. Moschcowitz E, Rubin E, Strauss L. Hypertension of the pulmonary circulation due to congenital glomoid obstruction of the pulmonary arteries. Am J Pathol 1961;39:75–93.
11. Hruban Z, Humphreys EM. Congenital anomalies associated with pulmonary hypertension in an infant. Arch Pathol 1960;70:766–779.
12. Virmani R, Roberts WC. Pulmonary arteries in congenital heart disease: a structure-function analysis. In: Roberts WC, ed. Adult Congenital Heart Disease. Philadelphia: FA Davis, 1987:77–131.
13. Naeye RL, Vennart GP. Structure and significance of pulmonary plexiform structures. Am J Pathol 1960;36:593–621.
14. Wagenvoort CA, Wagenvoort N. Pathology of Pulmonary Hypertension. New York: Wiley & Sons, 1977.

Pulmonary Arterial and Venous Hypertension and Left Ventricular Calcification of Undetermined Etiology

DEBORAH J. BARBOUR, MD
THOMAS V. INGLESBY, MD
JOEL A. ROTH, MD
WILLIAM C. ROBERTS, MD

In patients with severe pulmonary hypertension, the cause can nearly always be determined clinically or, if not, by necropsy examination. We recently studied a young woman with severe pulmonary hypertension and, despite cardiac catheterization, echocardiography, radionuclide angiography, pulmonary function studies, and, finally, necropsy, the cause of the severe pulmonary hypertension could not be determined. A description of the findings in this unusual patient is the purpose of this report.

From the Pathology Branch, National Heart, Lung, and Blood Institute, National Institutes of Health, Bethesda, Maryland, and the Departments of Medicine (Cardiology) and Pathology, Overlook Hospital, Summit, New Jersey. Manuscript received and accepted March 6, 1986.

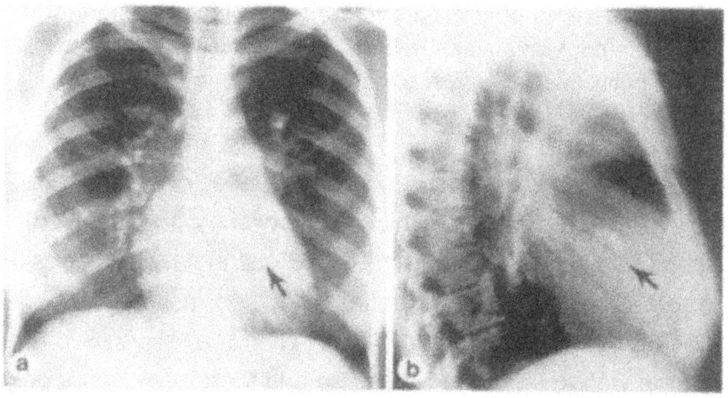

FIGURE 1. Posteroanterior and lateral chest radiographs taken 19 months before the patient's death showing mild cardiomegaly and an intracardiac calcific density (*arrows*) variously interpreted at the time as involving the aortic or mitral valve but which, at necropsy, was present in the ventricular septum.

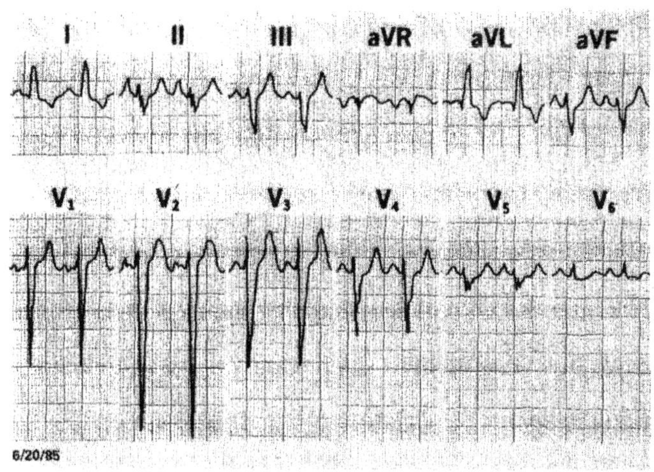

FIGURE 2. Twelve-lead electrocardiogram taken 3 months before death. The QRS axis is leftward (−40°), there is an intraventricular conduction delay and right atrial abnormality.

TABLE I Hemodynamic Data Recorded Two Months Before Death

Pressures (mm Hg) (s/d = peak systole/end diastole)	
Pulmonary artery (PA) (s/d)	145/62
Right ventricle (s/d)	130/16
Right atrium (mean)	9
PA wedge (mean)	22
Left ventricle (s/d)	100/20
Systemic artery (s/d)	100/68
Cardiac index (liters/min/m^2)	1.9
Pulmonary vascular resistance (dynes s cm^{-5})	200

M.B., a 20-year-old white woman, was well until age 14 years, when exertional dyspnea developed and gradually worsened. At age 18, she had several respiratory infections (Fig. 1). She was evaluated 2 months before death and severe pulmonary hypertension was found. Cyanosis was absent and her lungs were clear. Precordial murmurs were absent; S_2 was loud, the interval between A_2 and P_2 did not vary with respiration, and both S_3 and S_4 gallops were present. The electrocardiogram is shown in Figure 2. A radionuclide angiogram revealed right ventricular enlargement and the left ventricular ejection fraction was 52%. On echocardiogram, the left atrial dimension was 42 mm, the left ventricular dimensions were 45 mm in diastole and 22 mm in systole; left ventricular wall thickness and motion and the cardiac valves were normal. Pulmonary function tests showed severe impairment of diffusion capacity, mild obstruction

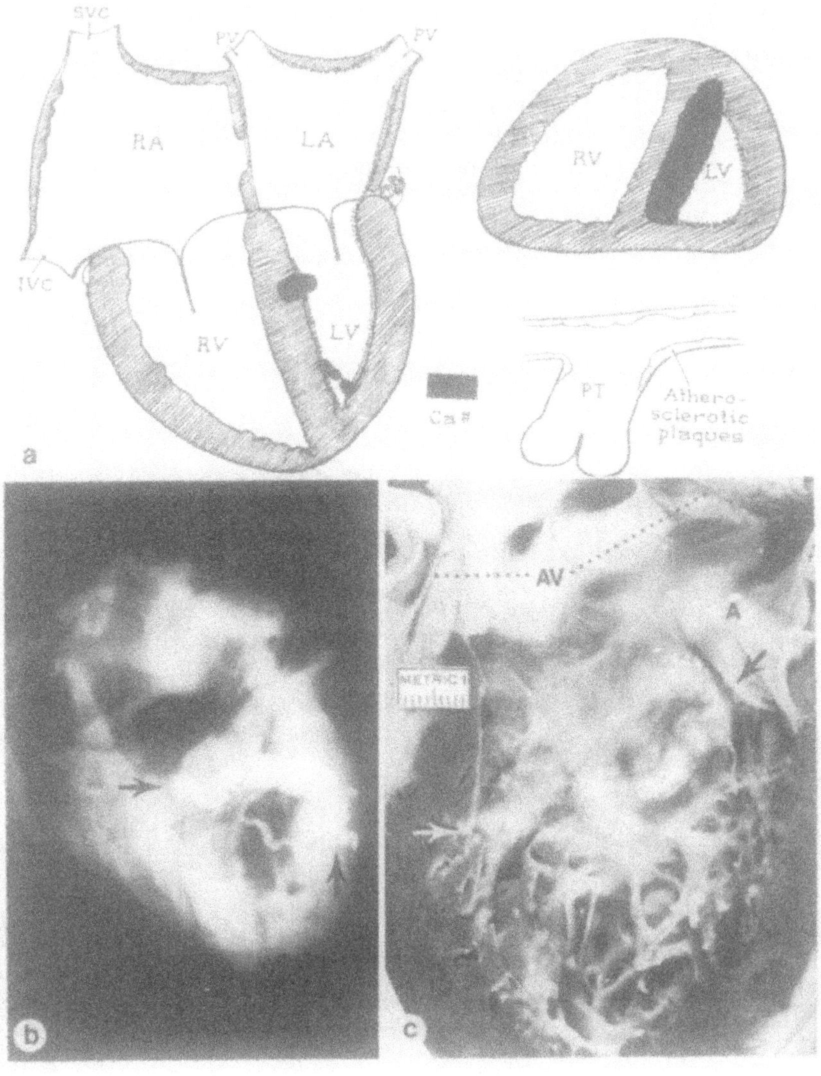

FIGURE 3. Heart. *a* (*left*), schematic representation of longitudinal section through the heart showing calcific bar on ventricular septum and calcified trabeculae within the left ventricular (LV) cavity. *Stippling* indicates thickened endocardium localized to left atrium (LA) and ventricle. The right atrium and ventricle (RA, RV) are dilated. Atherosclerotic plaques are present in the pulmonary trunk (PT) and right and left main pulmonary arteries. *b*, radiograph of the heart at necropsy showing a dense calcific bar (*between arrows*) extending across the ventricular septum and several calcified left ventricular trabeculae. *c*, a long axial cut showing the left ventricular aspect of the ventricular septum, opened aortic valve (AV) and anterior (A) mitral leaflet. The calcific bar (*between arrows*) extends across the ventricular septum. IVC = inferior vena cava; PV = pulmonary valve; SVC = superior vena cava.

and a vital capacity 58% of predicted. Data obtained at cardiac catheterization are summarized in Table I. Plans were made for combined heart and lung transplantation but she died of pneumonia while waiting.

At necropsy, the heart weighed 360 g and the right atrium and ventricle were dilated. The left atrial endocardium was diffusely thickened and the left ventricular endocardium was focally thickened. A dense, calcific bar extended transversely for approximately 4.5 cm in the ventricular septum and protruded approximately 1 cm into the left ventricular cavity (Fig. 3). Several left ventricular trabeculae also were calcified. The valves and coronary arteries were normal. Histologic sections of myocardium disclosed only myocyte hypertrophy.

Atherosclerotic plaques were present in the intima of the pulmonary trunk and in the extraparenchymal pulmonary arteries (Fig. 4). Histologic examination of both ascending aorta and pulmonary trunk (stained for elastic tissue) showed normal configuration of the elastic fibers in the pulmonary trunk (adult pattern).[1] Plexiform lesions were absent in all 16 sections of lung examined. The pulmonary veins were thickened and dilated, the alveolar septae were focally fibrotic and many but not all of the muscular pulmonary arteries had thickened media and in a few the intima was thickened by fibrous tissue. Many hemosiderin laden macrophages were present in alveolar spaces and the alveolar lining cells were cuboidal in shape and increased in number. The interlobular septa were thickened by fluid, fibrous tissue and dilated lymphatic channels.

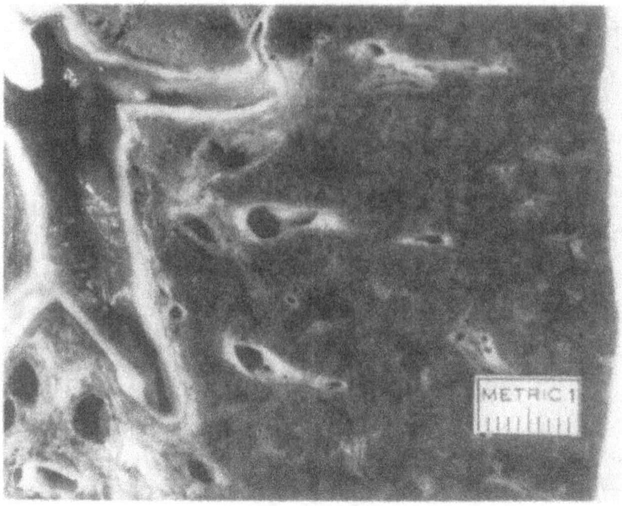

FIGURE 4. Close-up view of a longitudinal section of the lung showing a thickened large pulmonary artery. The aorta was free of atherosclerosis.

During life this patient was believed to have primary pulmonary hypertension, but at necropsy no plexiform lesions were present in the lungs, a finding essential for this diagnosis.[2] The medial thickening of the pulmonary arteries is simply an anatomic manifestation of severe pulmonary hypertension and not an indication of its cause. Study at necropsy of histologic sections of the wall of the pulmonary trunk indicated an adult configuration of the medial elastic fibers, a finding that indicates that the pulmonary hypertension was acquired rather than having persisted from birth.[1] The calcific bar in the ventricular septum and left ventricular free wall, of course, is not observed in patients with primary pulmonary hypertension, but again, its cause was not revealed by anatomic study. Thus, both the cause of the severe pulmonary arterial and venous hypertension and of the cardiac ventricular calcific deposit remain unexplained.

References

1. Heath D, Wood EH, DuShane JW, Edwards JE. *The structure of the pulmonary trunk at different ages and in cases of pulmonary hypetension and pulmonary stenosis. J Path Bact 1959;77:443–456.*

2. Wagenvoort CA, Wagenvoort N. *Primary pulmonary hypertension: a pathologic study of the lung vessels in 156 clinically diagnosed cases. Circulation 1970;42:1163–1184.*

Aneurysm of the Pulmonary Trunk Unassociated with Intracardiac or Great Vessel Left-to-Right Shunting

DEBORAH J. BARBOUR, MD
WILLIAM C. ROBERTS, MD

In contrast to aneurysm of the aorta, which is fairly common, aneurysmal dilation of the pulmonary trunk (PT) or of the right or left main pulmonary arteries is rare except in congenital heart disease with an intracardiac or great artery shunt. During the past 27 years we have studied at necropsy 3 patients with aneurysms (diameter more than 4 cm) of the PT and of 1 or both of its 2 major branches unassociated with congenital heart disease. This report describes findings in these 3 patients and summarizes findings in 3 previously reported necropsy patients with PT aneurysms unassociated with congenital heart disease.[1-3]

Certain findings in our 3 patients are summarized in Table I. All were women aged 40, 58 and 63 years. Patient 1 had hypertrophic cardiomyopathy (Fig. 1) and a pulmonary arterial systolic pressure of 54, 51 and 35 mm Hg on 3 occasions in the last 2 years of life. Patient 2 had systemic sarcoidosis and scleroderma with interstitial pulmonary fibrosis (Fig. 2) and a pulmonary arterial systolic pressure of 85 mm Hg. In patient 3, the cause of the PT aneurysm, which contained a large intraaneurysmal thrombus, could not be determined (Fig. 3). The PT aneurysms were 5, 7 and 7 cm in maximal diameter. Histologic study of the wall of the aneurysm disclosed it to be abnormal in patients 2 and 3 and normal in patient 1. The numbers of elastic fibers in the media in patients 2 and 3 clearly were decreased compared with normal (Fig. 3). Histologic study of 34 sections of lung in these 3 patients disclosed the pulmonary arterial intima and media to be thickened in all, but none had plexiform lesions (indicative of irreversible pulmonary hypertension).

Three previously reported patients with PT aneurysms unassociated with shunts included a 57-year-old man and 45- and 64-year-old women. The man had chronic lung disease and was an opium smoker; 1 woman was presumed to have primary pulmonary hypertension with pulmonary plexiform lesions and a pulmonary arterial mean pressure of 66 mm Hg; the other woman had no apparent explanation for the PT aneurysm which, like our patient 3, had an intraaneurysmal thrombus. All 3 had decreased numbers (compared with normal) of elastic fibers in the media of the PT.

From the Pathology Branch, National Heart, Lung, Blood Institute, National Institutes of Health, Bethesda, Maryland 20892.
Manuscript received and accepted June 18, 1986.

Aneurysms of the PT have been reported by other investigators in patients with primary pulmonary hypertension,[2] mitral stenosis,[4] the Marfan syndrome[5–7] and syphilis.[4–8] Since 1959, approximately 8,000 hearts have been examined in our laboratory and only the 3 patients included herein had aneurysms of the PT unassociated with left-to-right shunts. Of our 435 patients studied at necropsy with mitral stenosis, of 25 with primary pulmonary hypertension, and of 26 with the Marfan syndrome, none had an aneurysm of the PT.

The mechanism of development of PT aneurysm unassociated with left-to-right shunting is unclear. Pulmonary hypertension is usually present but it does not have to be severe as seen in our patient 1. The wall of the aneurysm may be abnormal as demonstrated by loss of elastic fibers in the media, but the wall may not be abnormal as was observed in our patient 1.

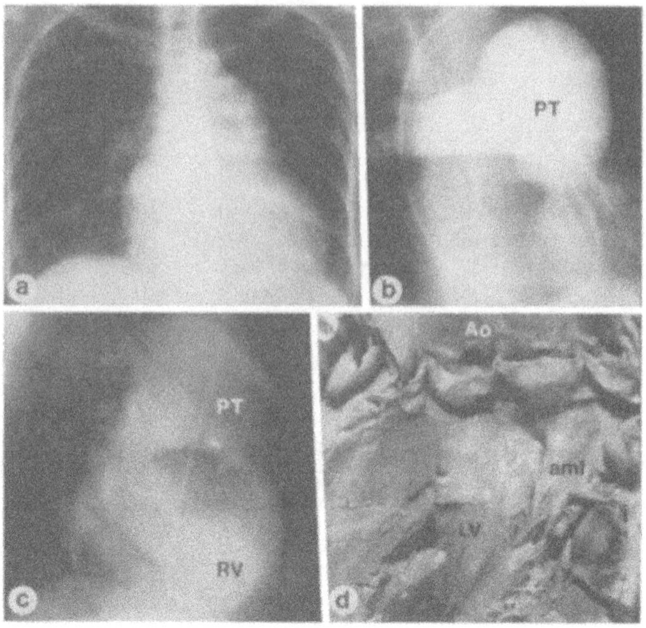

FIGURE 1. Patient 1 (Table I). Heart and radiograph. *a*, posteroanterior chest radiogram showing marked dilatation of the pulmonary trunk. *b*, posteroanterior angiogram with injection of contrast material into the huge pulmonary trunk (PT). *c*, lateral view of the same angiogram demonstrating aneurysm. *d*, opened left ventricular (LV) outflow tract showing a mural endocardial plaque in opposition to the anterior mitral leaflet (AMI) and a normal aortic valve. The mural endocardial plaque is typical of hypertrophic cardiomyopathy. Ao = ascending aorta; RV = right ventricle.

1. Shilkin KB, Low LP, Chen BTM. *Dissecting aneurysm of the pulmonary artery. J Pathol 1969;98:25–29.*

2. Luchtrath H. *Dissecting aneurysm of the pulmonary artery.* Virchows Arch *(Pathol Anat) 1981;391:241–147.*

3. Chiu B, Magil A. *Idiopathic pulmonary arterial trunk aneurysm presenting as cor pulmonale: report of a case. Hum Pathol 1985;16:947–949.*

4. Deterling RA, Clagett OT. *Aneurysm of the pulmonary artery: review of the literature and report of a case. Am Heart J 1947;34:471–499.*

5. Tung HL, Liebow AA. *Marfan's syndrome. Observations at necropsy: with special reference to medionecrosis of the great vessels. Lab Invest 1952;1:382–405.*

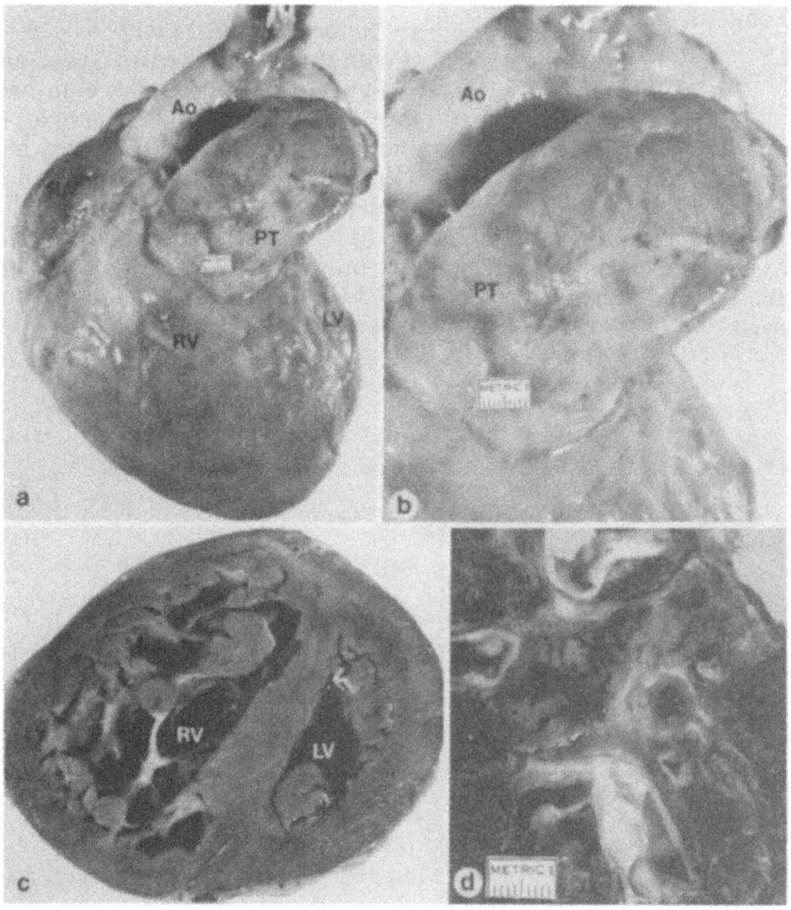

FIGURE 2. Heart and lung. *a* and *b*, exterior view of the anterior surface of the heart at necropsy showing the severely dilated pulmonary trunk (PT). The right ventricular (RV) cavity is much larger than the left ventricular (LV) cavity. *c*, transverse section through the ventricles at the level of the papillary muscles showing severe right ventricular (RV) wall thickening. *d*, longitudinal section through the lung near the hilum showing atherosclerotic plaques in the pulmonary arteries and enlarged perihilar lymph nodes containing noncaseating granulomas typical of sarcoidosis. Ao = aorta; RA = right atrium.

TABLE I Clinical Findings in Three Patients

Case	Necropsy Number	Age (yr)	Pressures (mm Hg) PA (s/d)	RV (s/d)	RA (m)	SA (s/d)	LV (s/d)	Diameter (cm) PT Aneurysm	↓EF in PT
1	A63-77	40	35/17	35/5	4	130/85	125/12	7	0
2	A86-14	58	85/32	85/9	...	140/60	...	7	++
3	A85-29	63	...	...	...	...	...	5	+

EF = elastic fibers; LV = left ventricle; m = mean; PA = pulmonary artery; PT = pulmonary trunk; RA = right atrium; RV = right ventricle; SA = systemic artery; s/d = systolic/diastolic.

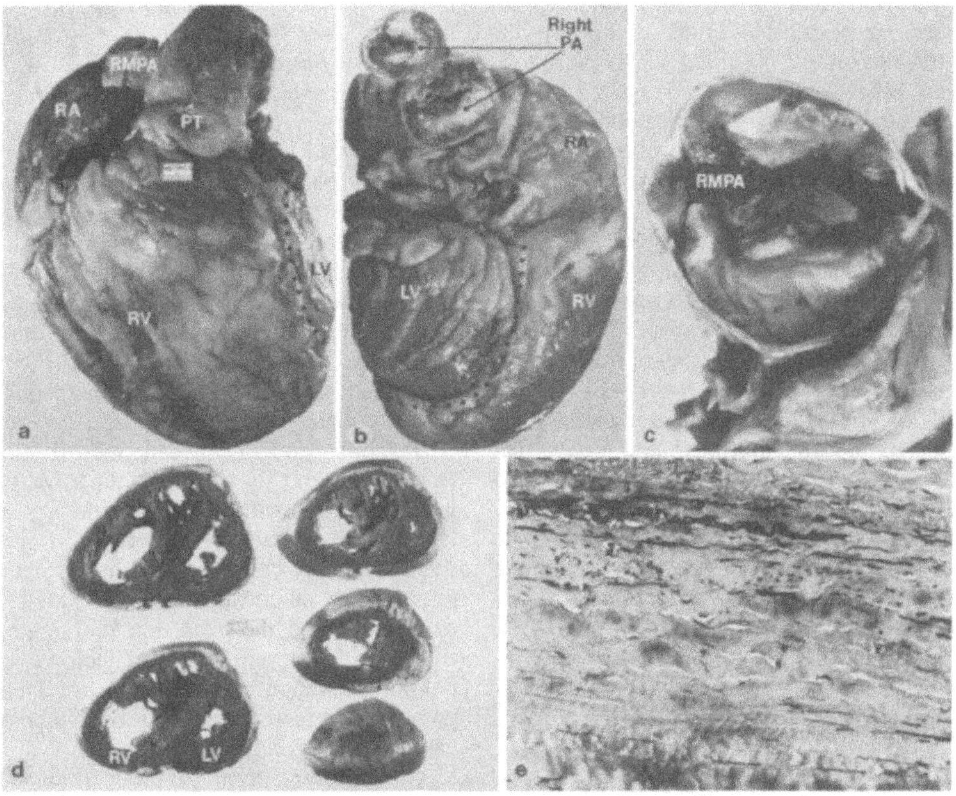

FIGURE 3. Patient 3. Heart (*a, b and d*) and pulmonary trunk (*b, c and e*). *a*, anterior view of the heart at necropsy. The right ventricle (RV) is massively enlarged and forms the cardiac apex. The pulmonary trunk (PT) and right main pulmonary artery (RMPA) are markedly dilated. *b*, posterior view of heart and right pulmonary artery (PA) at the level of its bifurcation showing extension of the PT aneurysm into the right upper and lower lobe main arterial branches, both of which are filled with organized mural thrombus. *c*, cross section through the right main pulmonary artery (RMPA) showing the aneurysmally dilated lumen to be markedly narrowed by organized thrombus. *d*, transverse sections through right (RV) and left ventricular (LV) chambers extending from base (*top left*) to apex (*bottom right*). The right ventricular cavity is markedly dilated while the left ventricular cavity is of normal dimension. No myocardial necrosis or fibrosis was present. *e*, photomicrograph of portion of wall of PT showing severe depletion of elastic fibers.

6. Headley RN, Carpenter HM, Sawyer CG. *Unusual features of Marfan's syndrome including two postmortem studies. Am J Cardiol 1963;11:259–266.*
7. Roberts WC, Honig HS. *The spectrum of cardiovascular disease in the Marfan syndrome: a clinicomorphologic study of 18 necropsy patients and comparison to 151 previously reported necropsy patients. Am Heart J 1982;104:115–135.*
8. Boyd LJ, McGavack TH. *Aneurysm of the pulmonary artery. A review of the literature and report of two new cases. Am Heart J 1939;18:562–578.*

Fatal Cor Pulmonale Caused by Extensive Tumor Emboli in the Small Pulmonary Arteries Without Emboli in the Major Pulmonary Arteries or Metastases in the Pulmonary Parenchyma

Michael J. Domanski, MD, Robert E. Cunnion, MD, Daniel J. Fernicola, MD, and William C. Roberts, MD

Microscopic-sized tumor emboli are an uncommon cause of cor pulmonale.[1–4] We report 2 patients who had precipitous terminal courses of respiratory insufficiency caused by extensive tumor emboli in the small pulmonary arteries.

Both patients were young (aged 38 and 27 years), both had recognized cancers (breast and pancreas) for short periods (12 and 9 months), and both had acute dyspnea for the first time beginning a short time before death (17 days and 1 day) with tachypnea and tachycardia. During the final acute dyspneic period, both had clear lung fields by chest radiographs and no neoplasm in the lung parenchyma at necropsy; both had elevated pulmonary arterial pressures (58/38 and 68/40 mm Hg), normal-sized cardiac silhouettes on chest radiograph and normal-sized hearts at necropsy (270 and 330 g); both had dilated right ventricular cavities (with normal-sized left ventricular cavities) and severe tricuspid regurgitation by echocardiogram; both had hypoxemia and respiratory alkalosis, and both had thrombocytopenia (40,000 and 44,000 cu mm) and anemia (hematocrits 33 and 27%). One patient (case 2) had schistocytes in peripheral blood. Pulmonary arteriogram (recorded only in patient 1) was normal (Figure 1); perfusion lung scan (recorded only in patient 2) was normal; cytology of pulmonary venous blood (analyzed only in patient 2) was positive for cancer cells. At necropsy, both had numerous small pulmonary arteries containing tumor emboli (Figure 2) without emboli in the major pulmonary arteries and without metastases in the pulmonary parenchyma, and both had widespread metastases in liver, lymph node and bone.

The 2 patients described in this study had rapidly progressive pulmonary and cardiovascular compromise resulting from extensive tumor emboli in the small pulmonary arteries. Diagnosis of this mechanism of dyspnea is rarely suspected antemortem.[2,3] Adenocarcinomas and trophoblastic neoplasms are the most frequently reported causes but other malignancies have been implicated.[3,5] Gastric carcinoma is the neoplasm giving rise most frequently to this syndrome.[5]

Patients generally present with dyspnea, tachypnea, tachycardia and hypoxemia with a normal chest radiograph and a nondiagnostic pulmonary arteriogram.[2,3,6] Progressive pulmonary hypertension is typical. Treatment is usually unsuccessful.[6] In our patient 1, a correct presumptive diagnosis was made based upon the clinical picture and the exclusion of large-artery thromboembolism by arteriography. Cytologic examination of pulmonary venous blood withdrawn through a wedged pulmonary artery catheter can be diagnostic,[7] as was the case in the second patient.

Small artery tumor emboli should be considered whenever a patient with a known malignancy presents

From the Clinical Trials and Cardiology and Pathology Branches, National Heart, Lung, and Blood Institute, and the Critical Care Medicine Department, National Institutes of Health, Bethesda, Maryland 20892. Manuscript received December 31, 1992, and accepted February 6, 1993.

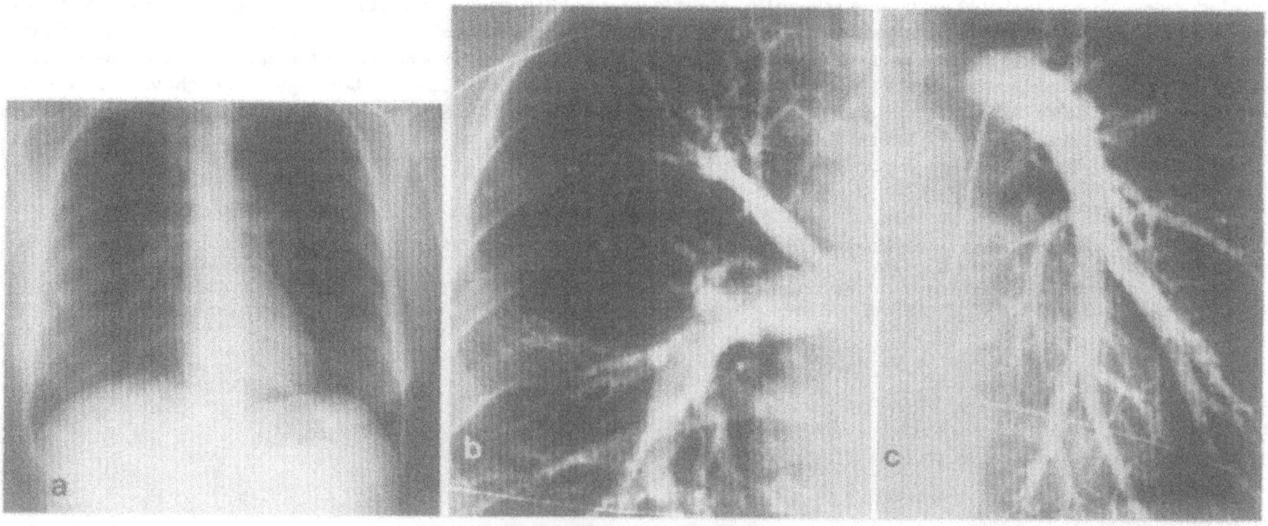

FIGURE 1. Case 1. Posteroanterior chest radiograph and pulmonary arteriograms. The chest radiograph *(a)*, obtained 2 days before death, is normal. No filling defects are seen on right *(b)* or left *(c)* pulmonary arteriograms obtained 1 day before death.

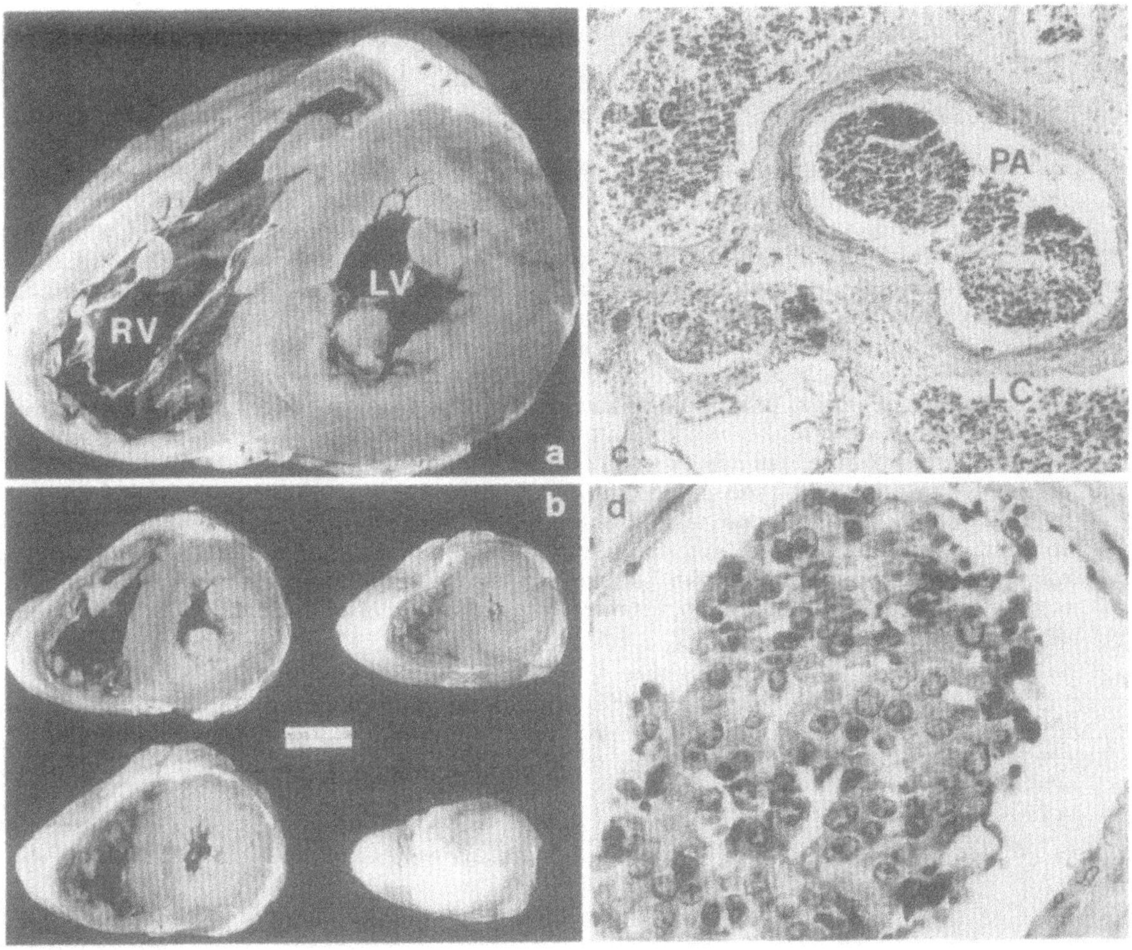

FIGURE 2. Case 1. Transverse cuts of the cardiac ventricles *(a and b)* showing a dilated right ventricle (RV) and a normal-sized left ventricle (LV). Microscopic sections of the lung show tumor emboli in *(c and d)* small pulmonary arteries (PA) and metastatic tumor in *(c)* lymphatic channels (LC). Hematoxylin-eosin stain × 100 *(c)*; Movat stain × 630 *(d)*; both reduced by 29%.

with progressive, unexplained dyspnea or pulmonary hypertension. Cytology of pulmonary venous blood may be diagnostic and antineoplastic therapy may be useful.

1. Kane RD, Hawkins HK, Miller JA, Noce PS. Microscopic pulmonary tumor emboli associated with dyspnea. *Cancer* 1975;36:1473–1482.
2. Marini JJ, Bilnoski W, Huseby JS. Acute cor pulmonale resulting from tumor microembolism. *West J Med* 1980;132:77–80.
3. Schriner RW, Ryu JH, Edwards WD. Microscopic pulmonary tumor embolism causing subacute cor pulmonale: a difficult antemortem diagnosis. *Mayo Clin Proc* 1991;66:143–148.
4. von Herbay A, Illes A, Waldherr R, Otto HF. Pulmonary tumor thrombotic microangiopathy with pulmonary hypertension. *Cancer* 1990;66:587–592.
5. Scully RE, ed. Case records of the Massachusetts General Hospital: case 30-1987. *N Engl J Med* 1987;317:225–235.
6. Altemus L, Lee R. Carcinomatosis of the lung with pulmonary hypertension: pathoradiologic spectrum. *Arch Intern Med* 1967;119:32–38.
7. Masson RG, Krikorian J, Lukl P, Evans GL, McGrath J. Pulmonary microvascular cytology in the diagnosis of lymphangitic carcinomatosis. *N Engl J Med* 1989; 321:71–76.

Clinical and Morphologic Features of Acute, Subacute and Chronic Cor Pulmonale (Pulmonary Heart Disease)

William Clifford Roberts, MD[a,b,c,*], Alexis E. Shafii, MD[d], Paul A. Grayburn, MD[a,b], Jong Mi Ko, BS[a], Matthew R. Weissenborn, MD[e], Randall L. Rosenblatt, MD[b], and Joseph M. Guileyardo, MD[c]

Described are certain clinical and morphologic features of one patient with *acute*, another with *subacute*, and one with *chronic* cor pulmonale. All 3 had evidence of severe pulmonary hypertension. The patient with acute cor pulmonale 4 days after coronary bypass for unstable angina pectoris suddenly developed severe breathlessness with cyanosis and had fatal cardiac arrest and necropsy disclosed massive pulmonary embolism. The patient with subacute cor pulmonale had severe right-sided heart failure for 5 weeks and necropsy disclosed microscopic-sized neoplastic pulmonary emboli from a gastric carcinoma without parenchymal pulmonary metastases. The patient with chronic cor pulmonale had evidence of right-sided heart failure for years, the result of primary or idiopathic pulmonary hypertension almost certainly present from birth because the pattern of elastic fibers in the pulmonary trunk was that seen in newborns where the pressure in the pulmonary trunk and ascending aorta are similar. The patient with chronic cor pulmonale had plexiform pulmonary lesions indicative of irreversible pulmonary hypertension. Neither the acute nor the subacute patient had chronic pulmonary vascular changes. All 3 patients had dilated right ventricular cavities and non-dilated left ventricular cavities and only the patient with chronic cor pulmonale had right ventricular hypertrophy. **(Am J Cardiol 2015;115:697−703)**

In Paul Dudley White's third edition of his *Heart Disease* published in 1951, sixteen pages were devoted to acute and chronic cor pulmonale.[1] In Braunwald's ninth edition of *Heart Disease* published in 2012, cor pulmonale was not mentioned in the index, although many pages were devoted to pulmonary hypertension,[2] the common denominator of acute, subacute, and chronic cor pulmonale. Cor pulmonale may be defined as dilatation of the right ventricular cavity without hypertrophy of its wall (*acute* and *subacute* cor pulmonale) or both dilatation of the right ventricular cavity and hypertrophy of its wall (*chronic* cor pulmonale), secondary to pulmonary hypertension not caused by a condition involving the left side of the heart. Although chronic cor pulmonale appears to have been recognized by Laennec by 1821,[3] acute cor pulmonale was not described until 1935 by McGinn and White[4] and the subacute form was described initially by Brill and Robertson in 1937.[5] Although the echocardiographic or computed tomographic features of acute cor pulmonale have been well described, we were unable to find any published reports describing clinical and morphologic features in patients with all 3 forms of cor pulmonale. Our purpose herein is simply to illustrate these characteristic features in 3 patients, 1 each with the acute, the subacute, and the chronic forms of cor pulmonale.

[a]Baylor Heart and Vascular Institute, Departments of [b]Internal Medicine, [c]Pathology, [d]Cardiothoracic Surgery, and [e]Radiology, Baylor University Medical Center, Dallas, Texas. Manuscript received November 6, 2014; revised manuscript received and accepted December 5, 2014.

Support for this investigation was provided by the Baylor Health Care System Foundation.

See page 703 for disclosure information.

*Corresponding author: Tel: (214) 820-7911; fax: (214) 820-7533.

E-mail address: wc.roberts@baylorhealth.edu (W.C. Roberts).

Table 1
Clinical and Morphologic Findings in the 3 Patients with Cor Pulmonale

Variable	Acute	Subacute	Chronic
Age (Years)	67	52	33
Sex	Man	Woman	Woman
Duration of symptoms of heart failure	< 1 hour	5 weeks	20 years
Cause of pulmonary hypertension	Massive PE	PE (Neoplastic)	PPH
Echocardiogram			
Dilated right ventricular cavity	-*	3+/4+	3+/4+
Dilated right atrial cavity	-*	0/4+	2+/4+
Thickened right ventricular wall	-*	0/4+	4+/4+
Left ventricular ejection fraction (%)	65	55	55
Pressures (mm Hg)			
Pulmonary artery wedge (a/v/mean)	-	6/10/6	16/18/14†
Pulmonary artery (s/d)	-	70/30	94/45†
Right ventricle (s/d)	-	70/14	94/31†
Right atrium (a/v/mean)	-	13/10/8	19/15/15†
Systemic artery (s/d)	-	115/70	90/50
Cardiac index (L/min/m^2)	-	1.7	-
Hematocrit (%)	43	37	41
Body mass index (Kg/m^2)	43	32	21
Children	1	3	0
Heart and lung transplant	0	0	+
Heart weight (g)	570	385	430
Floating heart‡	+	+	+

a = a wave; PE = pulmonary embolism; PPH = primary pulmonary hypertension; s/d = peak systolic/end diastolic; v = v wave.

* Unable to access because of severe obesity.

† At age 27 years.

‡ Indicative of severe cardiac adiposity.

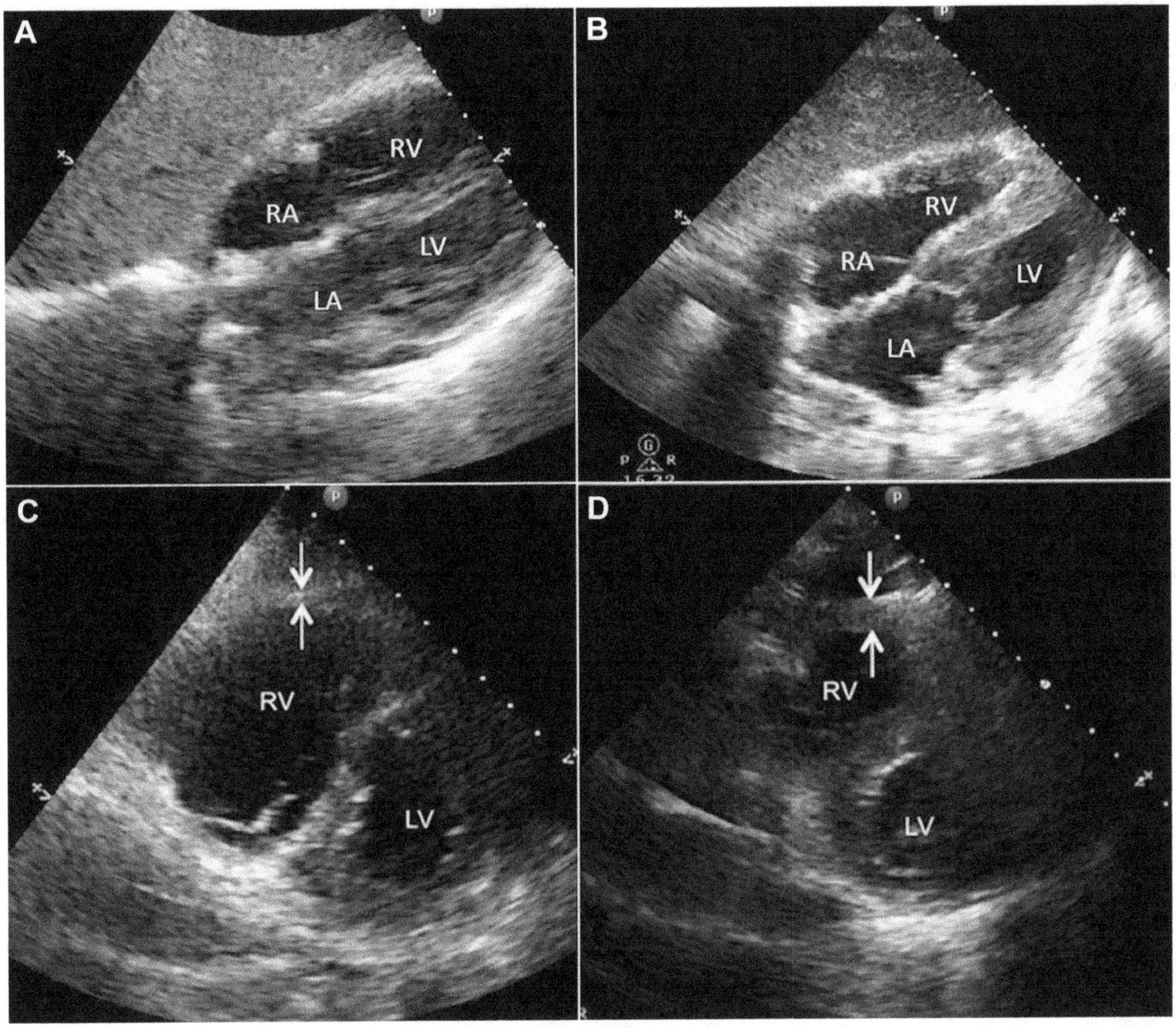

Figure 1. Echocardiograms in the patients with subacute *(A* and *C)* and chronic *(B* and *D)* cor pulmonale. *A* and *B* represent 4-chamber views and *C* and *D* represent cross-sectional views. The right ventricular (RV) cavity is dilated in both patients and the left ventricular (LV) cavity is not dilated in either patient. The RV wall is very thick in the patient with chronic cor pulmonale *(B* and *D)* but not in the patient with subacute cor pulmonale *(A* and *C)*. LA = left atrium; RA = right atrium. The arrows indicate normal RV wall thickness in *C* and abnormally thick RV in *D*.

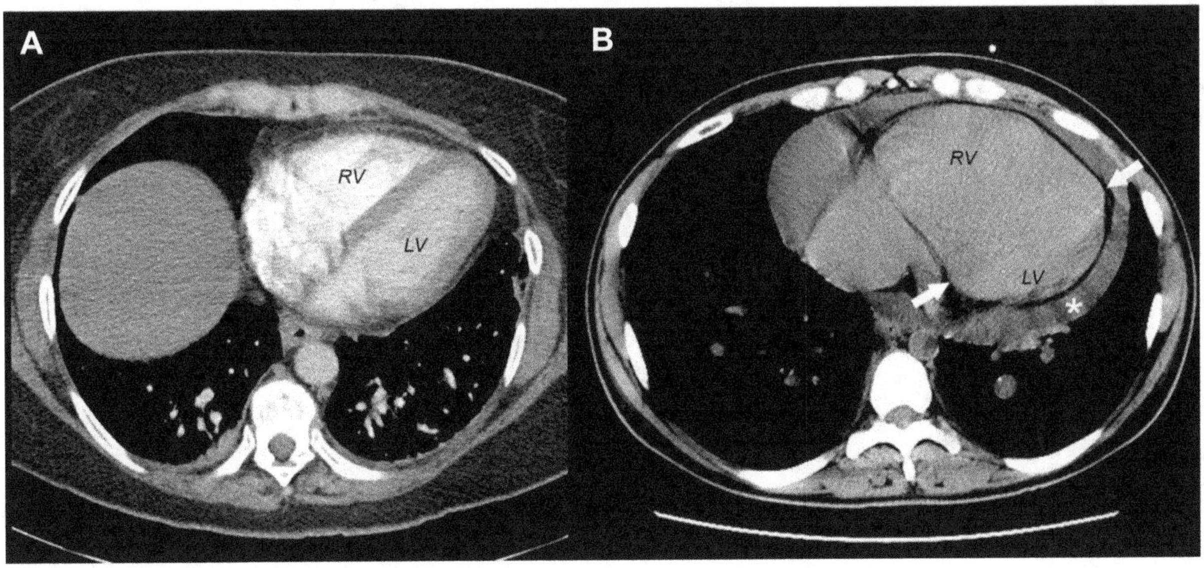

Figure 2. Computed tomographic pictures in the subacute patient *(A)* and in the chronic patient *(B)*. The right ventricular cavity is greatly dilated. A pericardial effusion is present in *B*. The left ventricular cavity in *B* is minute. The arrows point to the ventricular septum. LV = left ventricle; RV = right ventricle; * = pericardial effusion.

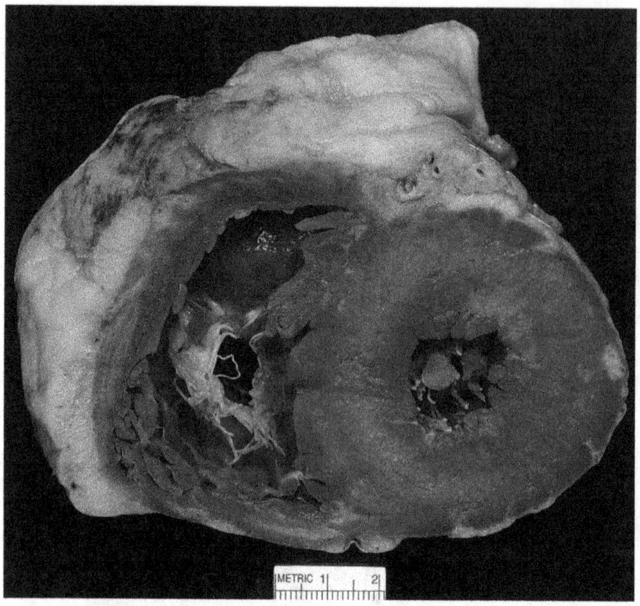

Figure 3. Acute cor pulmonale. Cross sections of the cardiac ventricles showing a dilated right ventricle and a normal size left ventricular cavity. The right ventricular wall is not thickened. The quantity of subepicardial adipose tissue is so extensive that the heart floated in a container of formaldehyde (body mass index 43 Kg/m^2).

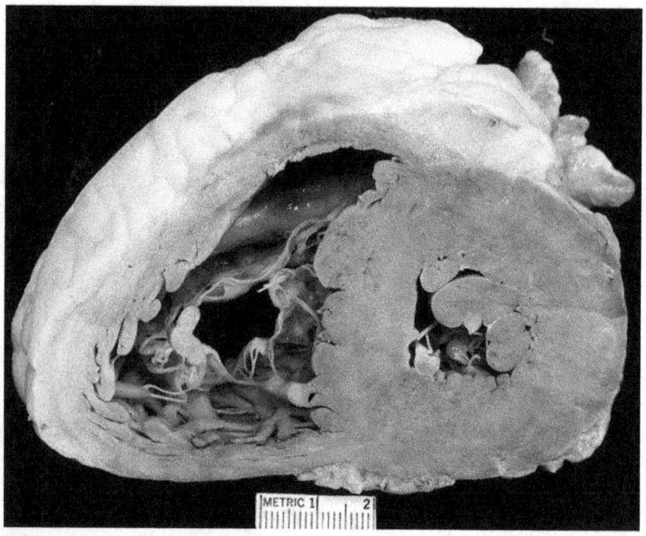

Figure 4. Subacute cor pulmonale. Transverse view of the ventricles showing the tricuspid valve and mitral valve. The right ventricular cavity is greatly dilated but the left ventricular cavity is not. The right ventricular wall is not thickened. The quantity of subepicardial adipose tissue is greatly increased such that the heart floated in a container of formaldehyde.

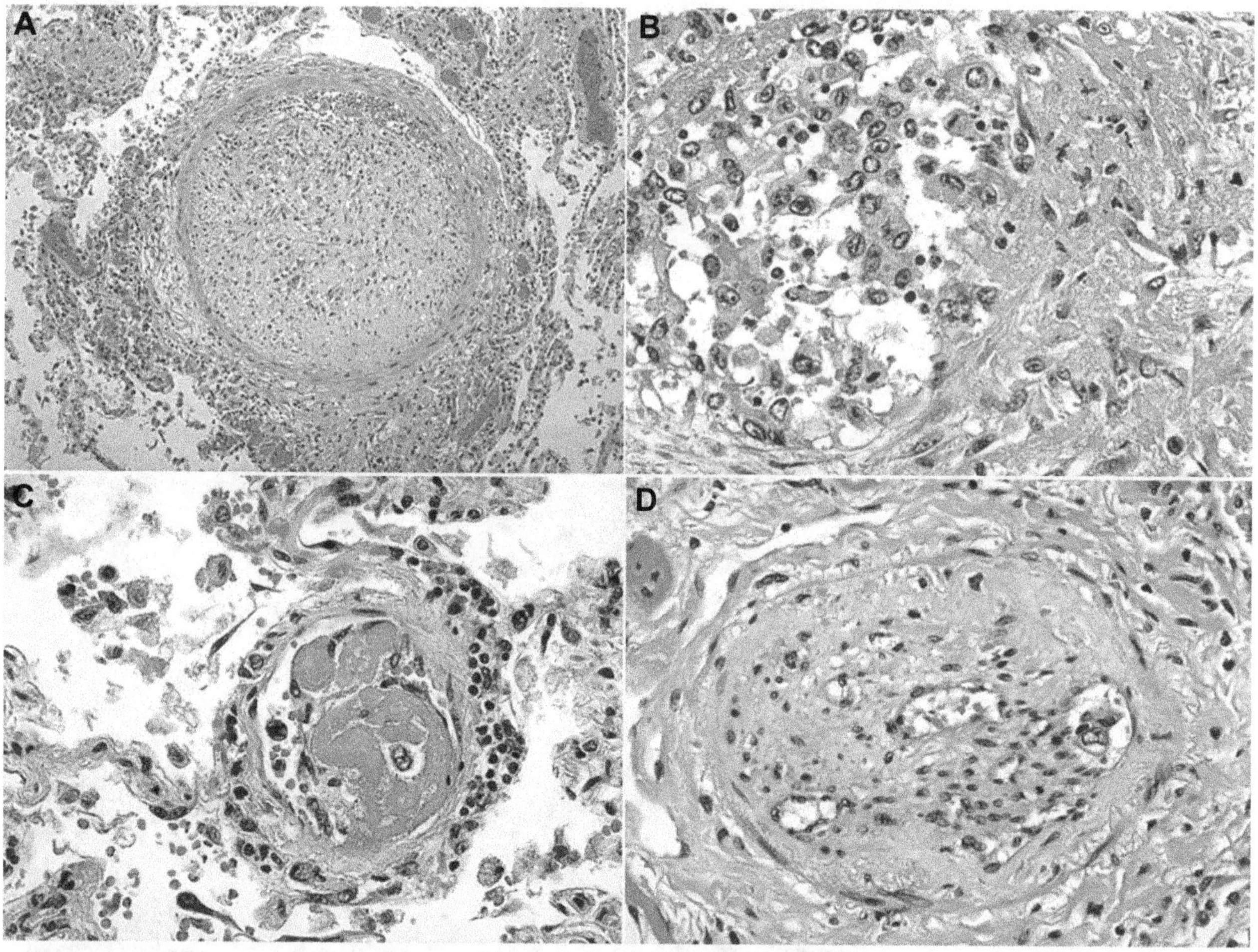

Figure 5. Subacute cor pulmonale. Photomicrographs of intrapulmonary arteries occluded or narrowed by metastatic cells within the lumen and with superimposed thrombus. The artery in *A* is virtually occluded. The gastric cancer cells are easily seen in the pulmonary artery illustrated in *B* and there is also some fibrin deposits within the lumen. *C* This small pulmonary artery is narrowed mainly by fibrin but a few gastric carcinoma cells are present. *D* This pulmonary artery contains organized thrombus and 4 small recanalized channels indicating that the emboli to the lungs probably occurred during the 5 symptomatic last weeks of this patient's life. Hematoxylin-eosin stains: X 100 *(A)*; X 400 *(B, C* and *D)*.

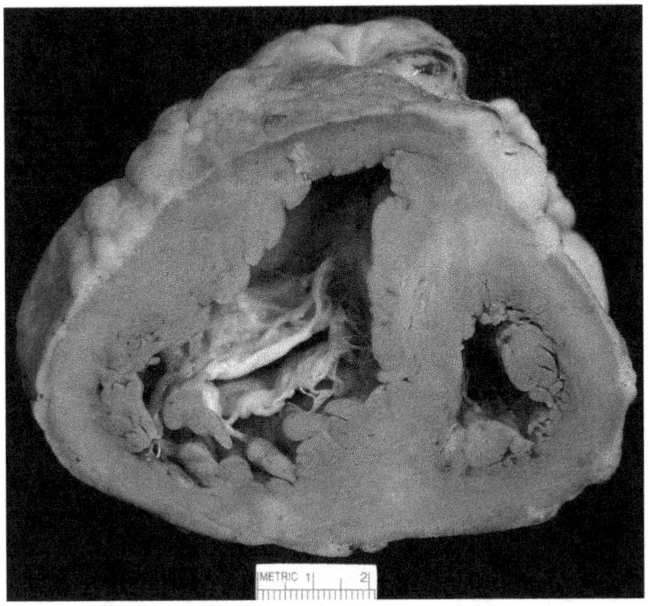

Figure 6. Chronic cor pulmonale. Transverse section of the ventricles in the patient with primary pulmonary hypertension. The right ventricular cavity is considerably dilated and the left ventricular is not. The right ventricular wall is about as thick as the left ventricular wall. The margins of the tricuspid valve leaflets are thickened, presumably the result of the very high closing pressure (peak right ventricular systolic pressure). The ventricular septum is thicker than either the right or left ventricular free walls.

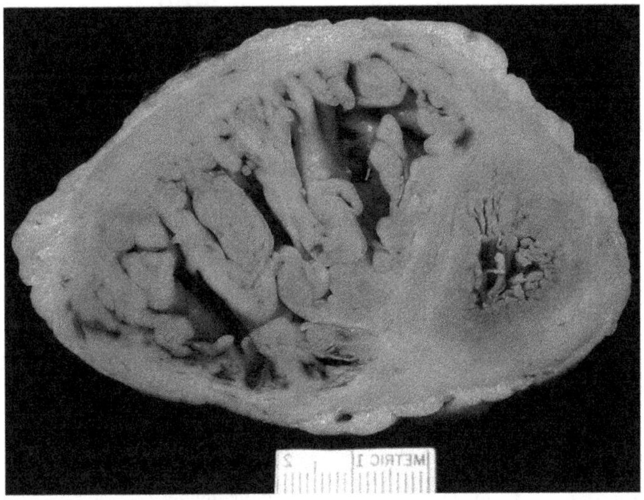

Figure 7. Chronic cor pulmonale. This view is a transverse cut in the apical half of the cardiac ventricles and it is shown to show how thick the pectinate muscles are in the right ventricular cavity. In this view the anterior and posterior right ventricular walls are really not thickened but the pectinate muscles are enormously thickened. Thickening of the pectinate muscles is one of the best signs of right ventricular hypertrophy, better than wall thickness. The left ventricular cavity is minute.

Patient Descriptions

Pertinent features of each of the 3 patients are summarized in Table 1. Echocardiographic and computed tomographic features in the subacute and chronic cases are shown in Figures 1 and 2. The acute patient, aged 67, had symptoms

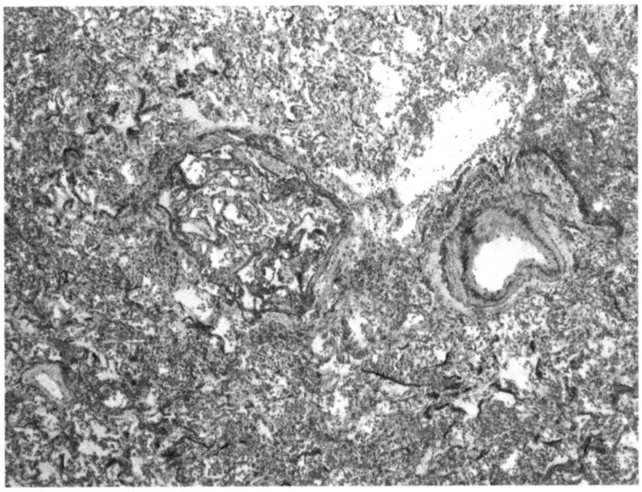

Figure 8. Chronic Cor pulmonale. Photomicrograph of a portion of lung showing a large plexiform lesion and a muscular pulmonary artery with thickening of its media and of its intima. Erythrocytes have entered most of the alveolar spaces. Movat stain, x100.

suggesting a respiratory catastrophe for only several minutes and necropsy disclosed massive pulmonary emboli (Figure 3); the subacute patient, aged 52, had symptoms for 5 weeks, determined at necropsy to be the result of multiple microscopic-sized pulmonary neoplastic emboli without parenchymal lung metastases from carcinoma of the stomach (Figures 4 and 5), and the chronic patient, only 33 years old, had symptoms of right-sided heart failure and periodic substernal chest pain for about 20 years (Figures 6–8). All 3 had very dilated right ventricular cavities, the acute and subacute patients without right ventricular wall thickening, and the chronic patient with both right ventricular dilatation and severe right ventricular wall thickening. The subacute and chronic patients had documented severely elevated right ventricular and pulmonary arterial peak systolic pressures (70 and 94 mm Hg, respectively), and the acute patient almost certainly did as well. Neither the acute nor the subacute patients had thickened walls of the pulmonary arteries and neither had plexiform lesions. The chronic patient, in contrast, had classic findings of primary pulmonary hypertension (medial and intimal thickening of the pulmonary arteries and numerous pulmonary plexiform lesions) (Figure 8). Sections of the pulmonary trunk in the acute and subacute patient disclosed a typical adult pattern of the medial elastic fibers whereas in the chronic patient the pattern was that present at birth and similar to the medial elastic fiber pattern of the aorta (Figures 9 and 10).

Discussion

Each of the 3 patients described herein fulfilled a definition of acute, subacute, and chronic cor pulmonale. The causes of the pulmonary hypertension in them, however, were quite different. The acute patient had a massive pulmonary embolus and died within a few minutes. The patient with the subacute syndrome had extensive neoplastic emboli to the small pulmonary arteries without emboli to the major pulmonary arteries or metastases from her gastric cancer to the pulmonary parenchyma and had symptoms of right-sided heart failure for

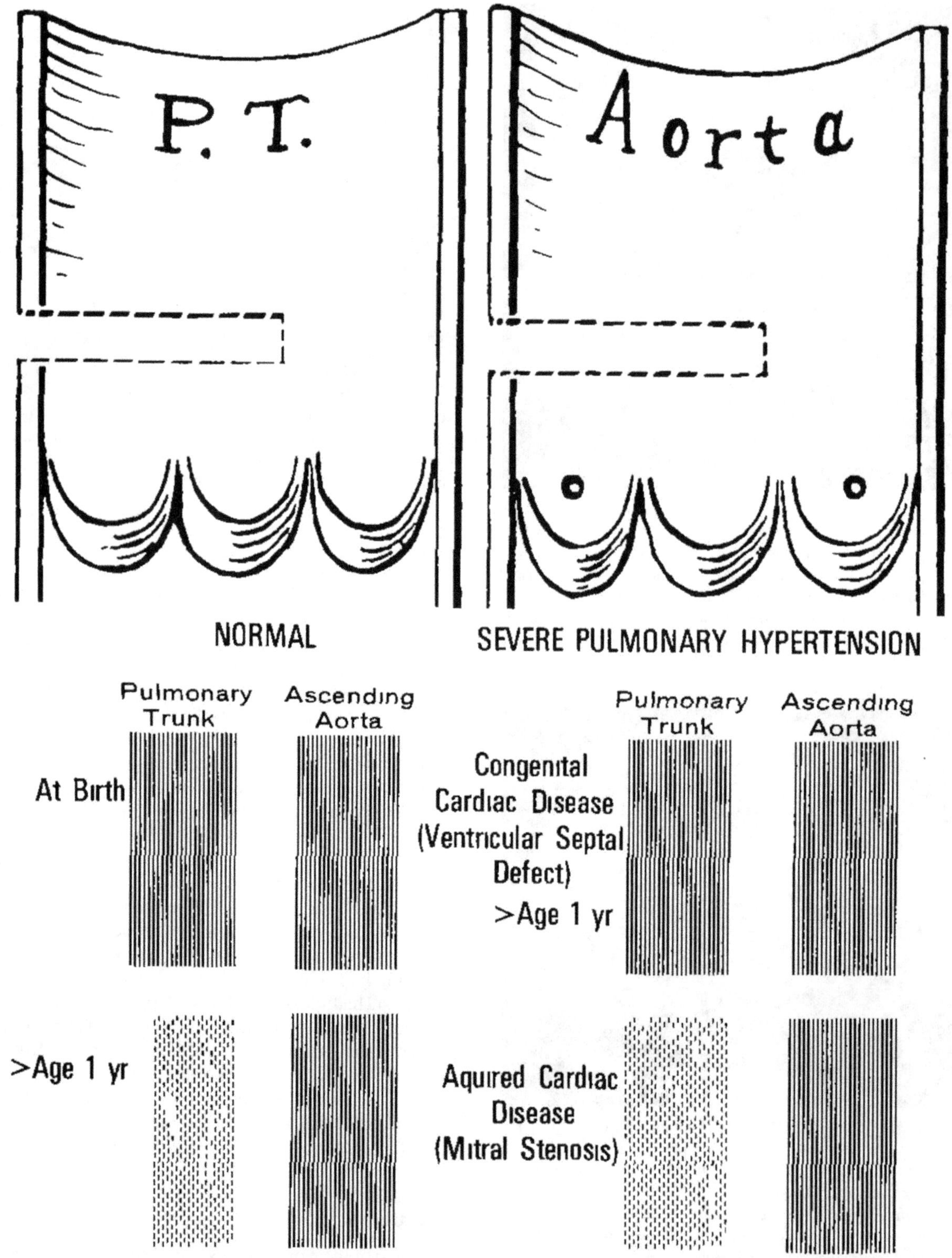

Figure 9. Configuration of elastic fibers in the pulmonary trunk at birth, after 1 year of age, with pulmonary *hypertension from birth* (VSD), and with an acquired condition (*mitral stenosis*). The sketch (*top*) shows the sites in the pulmonary trunk (PT) and aorta at which the sections for histologic examination were taken. At birth the configuration of the elastic fibers in both the pulmonary trunk and ascending aorta are identical and wall thicknesses are similar. Normally, after a year of age the number of elastic fibers in the pulmonary trunk diminishes considerably to reach an "adult configuration," and the thickness of the wall also diminishes. If a large ventricular septal defect or a aorticopulmonary defect is present from birth, both the configuration of the elastic fibers and wall thickness of the pulmonary trunk remains similar to that of the normal aorta. The information on the configuration of elastic fibers in the pulmonary trunk is based on original work by Heath and associates.[9,10]

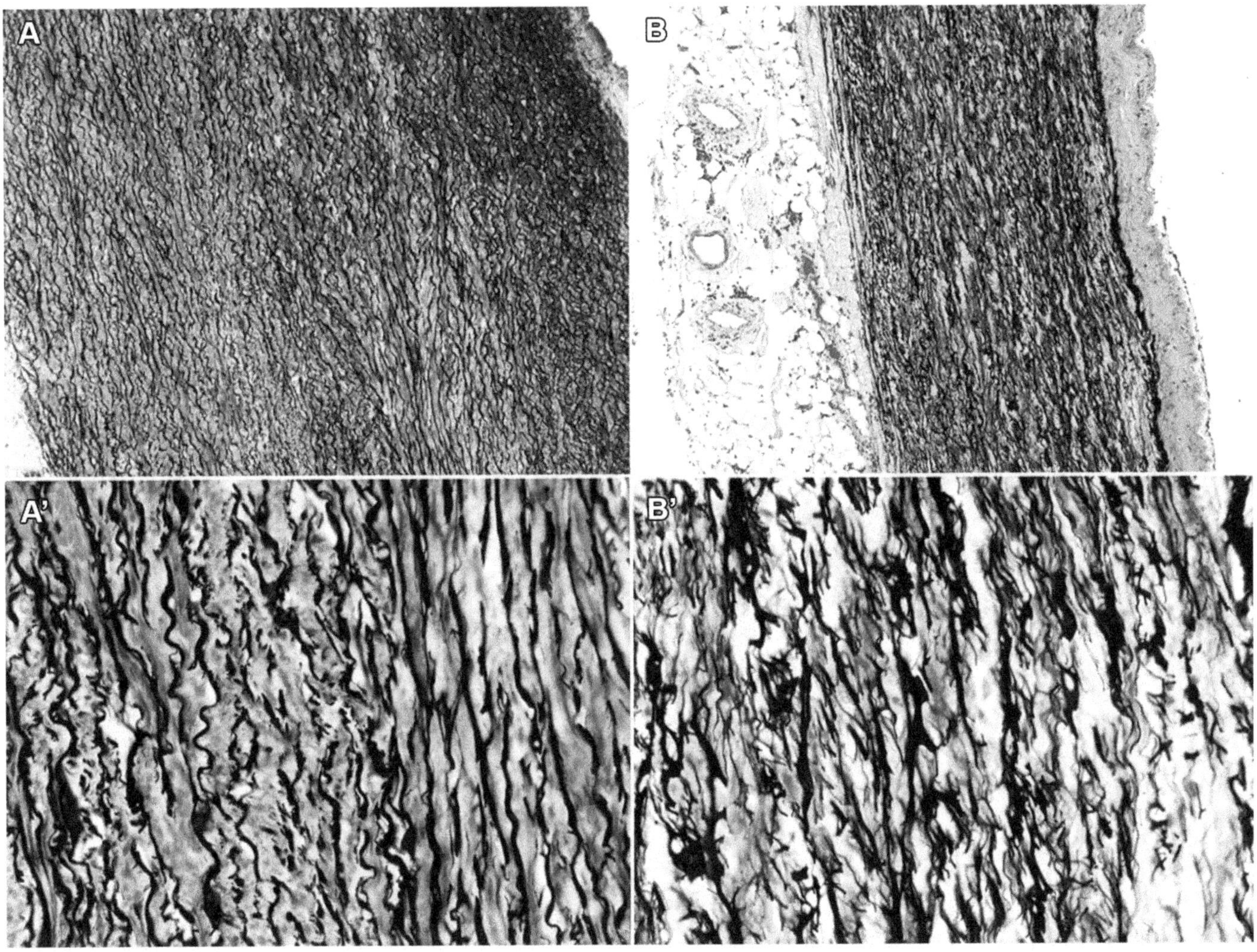

Figure 10. Chronic cor pulmonale. *A* and *A'* are sections of the ascending aorta stained for elastic fibers, and *B* and *B'* are sections of the pulmonary trunk stained for elastic fibers. The aorta is much thicker than is the pulmonary trunk but the configuration of the elastic fibers in the aorta and pulmonary trunk are similar, indicating that the pulmonary hypertension was almost certainly present from the time of birth. Movat stains X 100 *(A* and *B)*; X 400 *(A'* and *B')*.

5 weeks. Microscopic pulmonary neoplastic emboli without pulmonary parenchymal metastases was originally described by Brill and Robertson[5] in 1937 and they termed the condition "subacute cor pulmonale." Subsequently, a number of such cases has been reported.[6–8]

The patient with chronic cor pulmonale had primary or idiopathic pulmonary hypertension.[9] The unusual feature is that pulmonary hypertension appears to have been present from the time of birth. The evidence comes from studies by Heath and colleagues[10] and Heath and Edwards[11] who examined histologic sections of the pulmonary trunk and ascending aorta and found from study of patients with large left-to-right shunts (ventricular septal defect or patent ductus arteriosus) that the configuration of the elastic fibers in each of these arteries was similar when the pulmonary hypertension was present from birth, whereas in the patients who acquired pulmonary hypertension later in life (for example, from mitral stenosis) the pulmonary trunk had few elastic fibers and those present were disrupted (The aorta retains its fetal pattern of medial elastic fibers throughout life.). At birth, peak systolic pressures in the pulmonary trunk and ascending aorta are similar and therefore the configuration of elastic fibers in both pulmonary trunk and ascending aorta are similar. By one year of age, the peak systolic pressure in the pulmonary trunk has fallen to about one fifth of the peak systolic pressure in the ascending aorta and the elastic fibers have also decreased by approximately 80%, proportional to the reduction in peak systolic pressure.

Heath and Edwards[11] also found that some patients with primary pulmonary hypertension retain the fetal elastic pattern in the pulmonary trunk suggesting that the high pressure in the pulmonary circuit persisted from birth. A similar study by Roberts[12] in 1963 found the classic fetal pattern of elastic fibers in the pulmonary trunk in 1 and probably in 2 of 5 adults with primary pulmonary hypertension studied by him, again strongly suggesting that the high pulmonary pressure present at birth was retained into adulthood.

Neither our acute nor subacute cor pulmonale patient had medial or intimal thickening of the intrapulmonary

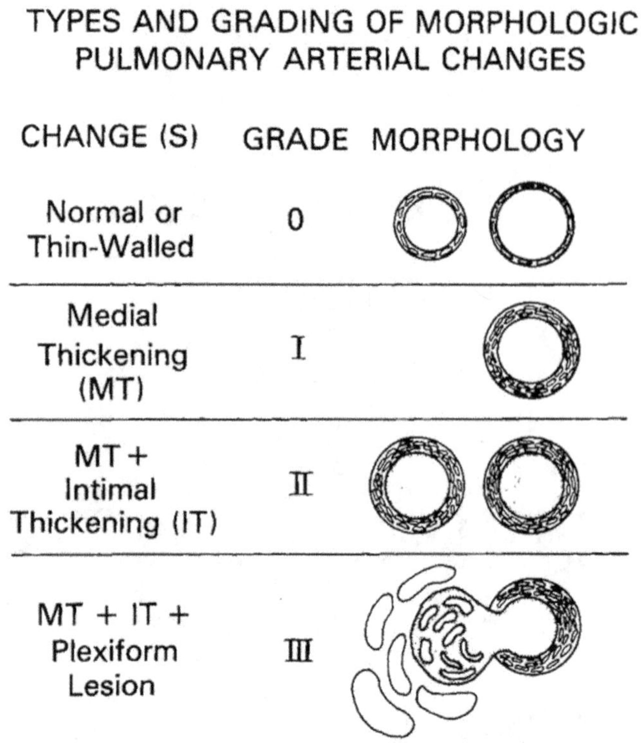

Figure 11. Diagram showing the types and grading of morphologic arterial changes in the lungs. Any elevation of pulmonary arterial pressure can cause medial thickening and if the pressure persists also intimal thickening. Plexiform lesions have occurred only in patients with severe pulmonary hypertension, usually pulmonary artery systolic pressures equivalent to aortic peak systolic pressures and indicate that the pulmonary hypertension is irreversible.

pulmonary arteries or plexiform lesion, whereas our chronic cor pulmonale patient had intrapulmonary arteries with thickened intima and media and numerous plexiform lesions (Figure 11). The plexiform lesions are indicative of irreversible pulmonary hypertension.[13]

Disclosures

The authors have no conflicts of interest to disclose.

1. White PD. Heart Disease. Fourth Edition. New York: The McMillan Company, 1951:1015.
2. Bonow RO, Mann DL, Zipes DP, Libby P, eds. Braunwald's HEART DISEASE. A Textbook of Cardiovascular Medicine. Ninth Edition. Philadelphia: Elsevier Saunders, 2012:1961.
3. Laennec RTH, Forbes J. A Treatise on the Diseases of the Chest and on Mediate Auscultation. London: Thomas & George Underwood, 1829: 736.
4. McGinn S, White PD. Acute cor pulmonale resulting from pulmonary embolism: its clinical recognition. *JAMA* 1935;104:1473–1480.
5. Brill IC, Robertson TD. Subacute cor pulmonale. *Arch Intern Med* 1937;60:1043–1057.
6. Mason DG. Subacute cor pulmonale. *Arch Intern Med* 1940;40: 1221–1229.
7. Schriner RW, Ryu JH, Edwards WD. Microscopic pulmonary tumor embolism causing subacute cor pulmonale: A difficult antemortem diagnosis. *Mayo Clin Proc* 1991;66:143–148.
8. Domanski MJ, Cunnion RE, Fernicola DJ, Roberts WC. Fatal cor pulmonale caused by extensive tumor emboli in the small pulmonary arteries without emboli in the major pulmonary arteries or metastases in the pulmonary parenchyma. *Am J Cardiol* 1993;72:233–234.
9. Simonneau G, Gatzoulis MA, Adatia I, Celermajer D, Denton C, Ghofrani A, Gomez Sanchez MA, Krishna Kumar R, Landzberg M, Machado RF, Olschewski H, Robbins IM, Souza R. Updated clinical classification of pulmonary hypertension. *J Am Coll Cardiol* 2013;62:D34–41.
10. Heath D, DeShane JW, Wood EH, Edwards JE. The structure of the pulmonary trunk at different ages and in case of pulmonary hypertension and pulmonary stenosis. *J Pathol Bacteriol* 1959;77:443.
11. Heath D, Edwards JE. Configuration of elastic tissue of pulmonary trunk in idiopathic pulmonary hypertension. *Circulation* 1960;21:59.
12. Roberts WC. The histologic structure of the pulmonary trunk in patients with "primary" pulmonary hypertension. *Am Heart J* 1963;65:230–236.
13. Roberts WC. A simple histologic classification of pulmonary arterial hypertension. *Am J Cardiol* 1986;58:385–386.

www.ingramcontent.com/pod-product-compliance
Lightning Source LLC
LaVergne TN
LVHW062149200926
848484LV00007B/1885